MANUAL OF
CONSCIOUS
SEDATION

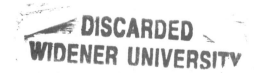

MANUAL OF CONSCIOUS SEDATION

MICHAEL KOST, MSN, CRNA

Program Director
Frank J. Tornetta School of Anesthesia at Montgomery Hospital
Norristown, Pennsylvania

Adjunct Faculty
Saint Joseph's University
Philadelphia, Pennsylvania

President
Specialty Health Consultants
Blue Bell, Pennsylvania

W.B. SAUNDERS COMPANY
A Division of Harcourt Brace & Company

Philadelphia   London   Toronto   Montreal   Sydney   Tokyo

W.B. SAUNDERS COMPANY
A Division of Harcourt Brace & Company

The Curtis Center
Independence Square West
Philadelphia, Pennsylvania 19106

NOTICE

Anesthesia is an ever-changing field. Standard safety precautions must be followed, but as new research and clinical experience broaden our knowledge, changes in treatment and drug therapy become necessary or appropriate. Readers are advised to check the product information currently provided by the manufacturer of each drug to be administered to verify the recommended dose, the method and duration of administration, and contraindications. It is the responsibility of the treating physician relying on experience and knowledge of the patient to determine dosages and the best treatment for the patient. Neither the publisher nor the author assumes any responsibility for any injury and/or damage to persons or property.

THE PUBLISHER

Library of Congress Cataloging-in-Publication Data

Kost, Michael.
  Manual of conscious sedation / Michael Kost.
     p.   cm.
  ISBN 0-7216-7194-2
  1. Conscious sedation.   2. Intravenous anesthesia.   I. Title.
  [DNLM: 1. Conscious Sedation—nurses' instruction.   2. Anesthesia,
  Intravenous—nurses' instruction.   WO 200 K861 1998]
  RD85.C64K67   1998
  617.9'62—dc21
  DNLM/DLC
                                                                98-14401

All continuing education test materials have been developed by the author in cooperation with **Nursing Spectrum. Nursing Spectrum** is solely responsible for the development, administration, billing, processing, and grading of the tests, as well as for issuing the credit hours for continuing education.

MANUAL OF CONSCIOUS SEDATION   ISBN 0-7216-7194-2

Printed in the United States of America

Last digit is the print number: 9   8   7   6   5   4   3

ABOUT THE AUTHOR

Michael Kost, MSN, CRNA, is program director of the Frank J. Tornetta School of Anesthesia at Montgomery Hospital, Norristown, Pennsylvania. He is president of Specialty Health Consultants, a firm that specializes in educational and consulting services to health care facilities and organizations. He received his bachelor of science in nursing from Widener University, Chester, Pennsylvania, CRNA certificate from the Montgomery Hospital School of Anesthesia, and a master of science in anesthesia from Saint Joseph's University, Philadelphia, Pennsylvania. Recently completing the clinical nurse specialist program in gerontology, he received a master of science in nursing from Gwynedd Mercy College, Gwynedd Valley, Pennsylvania. He has presented to national and local chapters of professional organizations and is a frequent lecturer and author on conscious sedation, ambulatory anesthesia, postanesthesia care, and pharmacology topics.

Preface

The administration of intravenous conscious sedation has become common practice in a variety of clinical settings. The increased use of conscious sedation has produced a demand for *qualified* providers to assess, diagnose, and intervene on behalf of the patient. This manual focuses on the preprocedural, procedural, and postprocedural care of the patient presenting for conscious sedation. It is a concise reference guide designed for quick and easy access, as well as an educational resource tool and a means for periodic evaluation. *Manual of Conscious Sedation* is the first comprehensive manual to incorporate the latest information available on the practice of conscious sedation, patient preparation, postprocedure care, and education. Written for clinicians engaged in the administration of conscious sedation, it also functions as a practical guide for clinicians practicing in the ambulatory care setting. For information on obtaining continuing education credits from **Nursing Spectrum,** see the details printed on the last page of the text.

The book is written in three parts. Part I addresses preprocedural patient care issues. Chapter 1 defines the concept of conscious sedation and addresses statutory, regulatory, and recommended practice requirements related to the clinical applications of conscious sedation. Chapter 2 combines comprehensive preprocedure assessment strategies related to organ systems, pathophysiologic disease processes, and recommended treatment modalities. A focus on preparation and reduction of patient anxiety is the hallmark of Chapter 2.

Part II incorporates the procedural care of the patient receiving conscious sedation. The administration of sedative medications requires a thorough understanding of the pharmacokinetic and pharmacodynamic effects of each medication administered. Chapters 3 and 5 feature a concise review of absorption, distribution, metabolism, and systemic effects of each pharmacologic agent administered. Techniques of administration (single dose, bolus administration, continuous infusion) are also highlighted in Chapter 5.

A common complication associated with the administration of sedative medications is respiratory depression. Upper airway anatomy and airway evaluation (Mallampati classification) coupled with emergency airway management are outlined in Chapter 4. This comprehensive review provides the clinician with a systematic assessment tool and intervention protocol. Recommended and required monitoring modalities (continuous electrocardiogram, blood pressure, and pulse oximetry) as prescribed by regulatory, statutory, and recommended practice are reviewed in Chapter 6. Dysrhythmia characteristics and recommended treatment protocols in Chapter 6 provide a valuable reference tool for the clinician.

Chapter 7 recognizes the specific needs from both ends of the patient care spectrum (pediatrics and geriatrics). Preprocedure assessment, physiologic variations, pharmacologic considerations, and sedative techniques specific to each population are reviewed. Intravenous insertion techniques are richly illustrated in Chapter 8 to serve as a step-by-step outline for the experienced clinician as well as the student clinician responsible for establishing intravenous access. Signs and symptoms, etiology, and treatment and prevention of systemic and local complications associated with intravenous cannulation are summarized. Fluid and electrolyte profiles of intravenous solutions are also combined with peripheral catheter care guidelines. Consideration is given to the administration of conscious sedation in a wide variety of practice settings: critical care areas, emergency rooms, operating rooms, ambulatory surgical centers, radiology departments, and physician offices. Specific procedures and patient care considerations are detailed in Chapter 9.

Part III encompasses the monitoring requirements and postprocedure care of the patient. Postprocedure care, documentation, discharge planning, and recovery scoring mechanisms are reviewed and available for easy reference in Chapter 10. A special chapter has been included for educators and managers to assist in the implementation of a conscious sedation educational training program. Numerous tables, illustrations, and figures in Chapter 11 address conscious sedation position description, credentialing, and departmental documentation issues related to the administration of intravenous conscious sedation. Risk reduction strategies and quality improvement methodology complete Part III. Recommendations on risk reduction strategies include use of a conscious sedation data base program approach to provide proof of compliance associated with the regulatory, statutory, and recommended practice requirements of conscious sedation in any practice setting.

The appendixes provided in the manual complement the preprocedural, procedural, and postprocedural patient care aspects outlined in Chapters 1 through 11. Appendix A highlights the Joint Commission on Healthcare Organizations' sample policies and procedures related to the administration of conscious sedation. Appendix B provides recommended standards of care from the Association of Operating Room Nurses' "Recommended Practices for Managing the Patient Receiving Conscious Sedation/Analgesia." Because of the prevalence of latex allergy, The American Association of Nurse Anesthetists' Latex Allergy Protocol is featured in Appendix C. A text on conscious sedation would not be complete without a complete pharmacologic review of sedative, hypnotic, opioid, and reversal medications. Appendix D provides the clinician with a comprehensive pharmacologic profile of each medication used in the conscious sedation practice setting. Dysrhythmia characteristics and recommended treatment protocols featured in Chapter 6 are enhanced when combined with the advanced cardiac life support algorithms featured in Appendix E. The American Academy of Pediatrics Committee on Drug's guidelines for the management of sedated pediatric patients are outlined in Appendix F. The final appendix focuses on clinical competencies for the nurse engaged in the administration of conscious sedation. These clinical competencies may be used by nurse managers for periodic review or as an individual self-assessment tool by the clinician engaged in the administration of intravenous conscious sedation.

MICHAEL KOST, MSN, CRNA

Acknowledgments

Sincere thanks to Maura Connor, nursing editor, W.B. Saunders, for her continued support and guidance throughout this entire project, and to Marge Johnson, administrative assistant, Specialty Health Consultants, for her timely manuscript preparation and friendship. Special thanks to the reviewers, who through their efforts have enhanced the content of this book.

MICHAEL KOST, MSN, CRNA

Contents

PART II PROCEDURAL CARE OF THE PATIENT DURING CONSCIOUS SEDATION, 63

3 Pharmacologic Concepts, 65

4 Airway Management and Management of Respiratory Complications, 75

APPENDIXES, 241

INDEX, 321

PART I

Preprocedure Care of the Patient

Goals, Objectives, and Legal Scope of Practice

CHAPTER 1

AORN RECOMMENDED PRACTICE I

Registered nurses should know the goals and objectives of intravenous conscious sedation/analgesia.

The administration of conscious sedation for brief surgical and diagnostic procedures has gained widespread popularity over the last several years. Not only has the number of procedures requiring the administration of conscious sedation increased but also the variety of procedures in the surgical and diagnostic caseload. Surgical and diagnostic procedures conducted with conscious sedation are listed in Table 1–1. The rationale for the proliferation of the administration of conscious sedation is varied. As healthcare reimbursement continues to evolve, a critical review of practice patterns has ensued. Patients receiving conscious sedation demonstrate shorter recovery time than patients receiving general or regional (spinal, epidural) anesthesia.[1] As healthcare continues to focus on efficiency coupled with an increase in outpatient surgical procedures, conscious sedation offers the clinician a desirable alternative for specific diagnostic and surgical procedures. The use of intravenous conscious sedation has increased the demand for *qualified* providers. Registered nurses have responded to this demand through implementation of educational programs, definition of clinical competencies, and promulgation of recommended practice guidelines by professional practice organizations and state board of nursing position statements.[2–5]

Recent pharmacologic advances have also contributed to the increased use of conscious sedation for specific patient populations. The introduction of intravenous medications with shorter half-lives, no active metabolites, and minimal cumulative effects has increased the margin of safety and efficacy associated with the administration of conscious sedation. Recent monitoring advances have also had a significant impact on the delivery of conscious sedation.[6] The advent of pulse oximetry introduced into clinical practice in the 1980s produced the ability to assist the clinician in the diagnosis of hypoxic states. This ability has greatly enhanced the margin of safety associated with administration of conscious sedation.

DEFINITION OF CONSCIOUS SEDATION

It is important to define the combination of amnestic, anxiolytic, and analgesic medications used to achieve a state of conscious sedation. The term *conscious sedation* was first described by Dr. C. R. Bennett. In a paper entitled

3

TABLE 1-1. *Conscious Sedation Procedures*

SPECIALTY	TYPE OF PROCEDURE
Burns	Dressing changes
Cardiology	Angioplasty
	Cardiac catheterization
	Cardioversion
	Electrophysiologic ablation
	Insertion of invasive lines
	Pacemaker insertion
	Transesophageal echo
	Vascular access
Cosmetic surgery	Blepharoplasty
	Chemical peels
	Dermabrasion
	Liposuction
	Otoplasty
	Rhinoplasty
	Rhytidectomy
	Skin laser enhancement
Gastroenterology	Colonoscopy
	Endoscopy
	Endoscopic retrograde cholangio-pancreatography (ERCP)
	Liver biopsy
General surgery	Hernia repair
	Incision and drainage
	Lipoma excision
	Superficial biopsies
Gynecologic	Dilatation and curettage (D & C)
	Dilatation and evacuation (D & E)
	Cone biopsy
	Hysteroscopy
	Incision and drainage
	In vitro fertilization
	Laparoscopy
	Lesion fulguration
Ophthalmology	Blepharoplasty
	Cataract extraction
	Lens implant
Oral surgery	Dental caries
	Odontectomy
	Periodontal
Orthopedic	Arthroscopy
	Closed fracture reduction
	Hand surgery
	Joint manipulation

TABLE 1–1. *Conscious Sedation Procedures* Continued

SPECIALTY	TYPE OF PROCEDURE
Pulmonology	Biopsy
	Bronchoscopy
	Endotracheal intubation
	Chest tube insertion
Radiology	Arteriography
	Computed tomography scan
	Embolization
	Localization and biopsy
	Magnetic resonance imaging
Urologic	Cystoscopy
	Lithotripsy
	Vasectomy

This is not an all-inclusive list.

"Conscious Sedation in Dental Practice," he presented information related to the administration of intravenous sedative medications in conjunction with local anesthetics.[7] The technique used sedative and analgesic medications combined with local anesthetics in the affected area. In this way, the patients maintained their protective reflexes and were provided a minimally depressed level of consciousness.

"**Intravenous conscious sedation** is produced by the administration of amnestic, analgesic and sedative pharmacologic agents. A patient receiving conscious sedation has a 'depressed level of consciousness.' " However, they "retain the ability to independently and continuously maintain a patent airway and respond appropriately to physical and verbal stimuli."[8] To satisfy the definition of conscious sedation, it is important to adhere to three clearly delineated criteria:

- Ability to retain protective airway reflexes
- Ability to independently and continuously maintain a patent airway
- Ability to respond appropriately to physical and verbal stimuli

The objectives of conscious sedation listed in Table 1–2 were initially presented in 1985 by Scammon, Klein, and Choi. The primary goal of intravenous conscious sedation is to allay patient fear and anxiety associated with the proposed procedure. The goal of conscious sedation techniques is to use the *least* amount of sedation while providing for patient comfort. Additional goals of intravenous conscious sedation include

- Mood alteration
- Enhanced patient cooperation
- Elevation of pain threshold
- Stable vital signs
- Amnesia
- Rapid recovery

TABLE 1–2.   *Objectives of Conscious Sedation*

1. **Maintain adequate sedation with minimal risk.** The patient's ability to communicate is preserved. Physiologic monitoring is employed and emergency resuscitation is on hand.
2. **Relieve anxiety and produce amnesia.** These objectives are accomplished by means of good preoperative communication and instruction and low levels of visual and auditory stimuli.
3. **Provide relief from pain and other noxious stimuli.** Opioids are given to supplement local or topical anesthetics and to block pain sensations remote from the operative site.

From Scammon FL, Klein SL, Choi WW. Conscious sedation for procedures under local or topical anesthesia. *Ann Otol Rhinol Laryngol.* 1985;94:21.

DEEP SEDATION

The administration of conscious sedation depends on individual patient response and the total dose of medication administered. Varied patient response or overuse of a conscious sedation technique may lead the patient into a state of deep sedation. *Deep sedation* is defined as a controlled state of depressed consciousness, accompanied by partial or complete loss of protective reflexes, including the inability to respond purposefully to verbal or physical command.[9] A differentiation of the characteristics of conscious sedation versus deep sedation is presented in Table 1–3. Deep sedation may predispose the patient to an increased incidence of respiratory depression, decreased response to the hypoxic drive, and cardiovascular depression. *Unconsciousness and unresponsiveness are not objectives of conscious sedation.*

TABLE 1–3.   *The Differences Between Conscious Sedation and Deep Sedation*

CONSCIOUS SEDATION	DEEP (UNCONSCIOUS) SEDATION
Mood altered	Patient unconscious
Patient cooperative	Patient unable to cooperate
Protective reflexes intact	Protective reflexes obtunded
Vital signs stable	Vital signs labile
Local anesthesia provides analgesia	Pain eliminated centrally
Amnesia may be present	Amnesia always present
Shorter recovery room stay	Occasional prolonged recovery room stay or overnight admission required
Perioperative complications infrequent	Perioperative complications are reported in 25% to 75% of cases
Uncooperative or mentally handicapped patient cannot always be managed	Useful in managing difficult or mentally handicapped patients

Copyright *Comprehensive Accreditation Manual for Hospitals: The Official Handbook.* Oakbrook Terrace, IL: Joint Commission on Accreditation of Healthcare Organizations, 1997, 77–78. Reprinted with permission.

TABLE 1–4.　*Components of General Anesthesia and Conscious Sedation*

GENERAL ANESTHESIA	CONSCIOUS SEDATION
Amnesia	Amnesia
Unconsciousness	Analgesia
Muscle relaxation	Anxiolysis
Attenuation of stress response	

SYNERGISM

Pharmacologic medications used to achieve a state of conscious sedation include

- Benzodiazepines: amnesia, anxiolysis
- Opioids: analgesia
- Sedative hypnotics: anxiolysis

Combinations of these carefully titrated medications give the clinician the ability to perform surgical and diagnostic procedures while the patient is under altered levels of consciousness. The administration and combination of benzodiazepines, opioids, and sedative hypnotics may produce profound synergistic effects. These synergistic effects may lead to a state of deep sedation or general anesthesia. In 1990 Bailey reported in *Anesthesiology* more than 80 deaths directly attributed to the administration of conscious sedation with benzodiazepines specifically when combined with an opioid.[10] This demonstrated synergism combined with preexisting medical conditions and varied patient response may lead to the development of hypoxemia, apnea, deep sedative states, or general anesthesia. As shown in Table 1–4, many of the components of general anesthesia are also components of conscious sedation. To prevent the development of an unconscious state during diagnostic or surgical procedures, it is important to understand the pharmacokinetic and pharmacodynamic profile of the intravenous agents used to produce conscious sedation. The clinician must also appreciate the potency and synergistic action of combined medications used to produce the sedative state.

LEGAL SCOPE OF PRACTICE

An understanding of the definition of conscious sedation and adherence to the criteria outlined are required for registered nurses to maintain compliance with legal scope-of-practice issues in many jurisdictions. As registered nurses prepare to respond to the increased number of procedures that require conscious sedation, they must be cognizant of legal scope-of-practice issues. Legal scope-of-practice issues related to nursing are delegated and administered through state boards of nursing. Individual state statutes define the practice of nursing. As registered nurses have become more involved in the administration of conscious sedation and patient monitoring, scope-of-practice issues have been raised in many states.

In the late 1980s, the demand for registered nurses to participate in the administration of conscious sedation procedures and the monitoring of patients re-

COMMONWEALTH OF PENNSYLVANIA

Pennsylvania Code

Title 49. Professional and Vocational Standards

DEPARTMENT OF STATE

CHAPTER 21. STATE BOARD OF NURSING

49 § 21.413   Conscious Sedation   **Pt. I**

As used in this subsection, "conscious sedation" is defined as a minimally depressed level of consciousness in which the patient retains the ability to independently and continuously maintain an airway and respond appropriately to physical stimulation and verbal commands. The registered nurse who is not a certified registered nurse anesthetist may administer intravenous conscious sedation medications, under § 21.14, during minor therapeutic and diagnostic procedures, when the following conditions exist:

(1) The specific amount of intravenous conscious sedation medications has been ordered in writing by a licensed physician and a licensed physician is physically present in the room during administration.

(2) Written guidelines specifying the intravenous medications that the registered nurse may administer in a particular setting are available to the registered nurse.

(3) Electrocardiogram, blood pressure and oximetry equipment are used for both monitoring and emergency resuscitation purposes pursuant to written guidelines which are provided for minimum patient monitoring. Additional emergency resuscitation equipment is immediately available.

(4) The patient has a patent intravenous access.

(5) The registered nurse involved in direct patient care has completed a course in advanced cardiac life support (ACLS) or pediatric cardiac life support, which establishes competency in airway management and resuscitation appropriate to the age of the patient.

(6) The registered nurse possesses the knowledge, skills and abilities related to the management of patients receiving intravenous conscious sedation with evaluation of competence on a periodic basis. This includes, but is not limited to, arrhythmia detection, airway management and pharmacologic action of drugs administered. This includes emergency drugs.

(7) The registered nurse managing the care of the patient receiving intravenous conscious sedation medication may not have other responsibilities during the procedure. The registered nurse may not leave the patient unattended or engage in tasks which would compromise continuous monitoring.

(8) The registered nurse monitors the patient until the patient is discharged by a qualified professional authorized to discharge the patient in accordance with established criteria of the facility.

Source: The provisions of this § 21.413 adopted February 20, 1987, effective February 21, 1987, 17 Pa.B. 811; amended June 21, 1991, effective June 22, 1991, 21 Pa.B. 2818; amended January 17, 1992, effective January 18, 1992, 22 Pa.B. 300; amended November 12, 1994, effective November 13, 1994, 24 Pa.B. 5404; amended November 12, 1994, effective November 13, 1994, 24 Pa.B. 5404; amended March 25, 1997, effective March 26, 1997.

ceiving it increased dramatically.[11] In response, registered nurses concerned with legal scope-of-practice issues contacted their individual state boards of nursing to inquire about the conscious sedation practice patterns that were developing in their institutions. Responses from state boards of nursing varied in their position regarding the administration of conscious sedation and the monitoring of patients receiving it. Some state boards have adopted formal position or policy statements that delineate the responsibility of professional registered nurses engaged in the administration of conscious sedation. Many state boards of nursing have enacted formal policy statements that define and identify prescriptive responsibilities and requirements of the registered nurse participating in the conscious sedation process. Some state boards of nursing have not yet taken formal action on the issue. A few select state boards of nursing may not have statutory authority to enact such legislation, whereas some continue to gather information on the issue. An example of a state board of nursing that has enacted a formal policy statement under the Professional Nursing Law is the Pennsylvania State Board of Nursing,[12] which adopted by majority vote its proposed policy statement related to the administration of intravenous sedation by registered nurses (see p 8). Registered nurses must be aware of their state's specific requirements associated with the clinical practice of conscious sedation (Advanced Cardiac Life Support [ACLS], monitoring requirements, intravenous access, etc.).

Physicians also are subject to statutory authority related to the administration of conscious sedation and the monitoring of patients receiving it. In 1991 the state of New Jersey enacted legislation that required "all physicians wishing to perform intravenous conscious sedation in the hospital setting to be credentialed by the Department of Anesthesia within that institution."[13] The purpose of this legislation was to increase physician awareness of the medications used for conscious sedation procedures. It is also a mechanism to enhance the physician's understanding of monitoring modalities used during performance of the diagnostic procedure.

JOINT COMMISSION ON ACCREDITATION OF HEALTHCARE ORGANIZATIONS

In addition to state statutory regulations, standards related to the administration of conscious sedation have also been published by the Joint Commission on Accreditation of Healthcare Organizations (JCAHO) and several professional organizations. The mission of the JCAHO is to improve the quality of care provided to the public. Healthcare organizations may apply for and undergo a full accreditation survey every 3 years. The accreditation process focuses on an assessment of an organization's compliance with standards developed by the JCAHO. Standards and intents developed by the JCAHO to improve quality patient care are listed in Table 1–5. The JCAHO has taken an active role in the development of policies, standards, and intents specific to the administration of conscious sedation. In the "Planning and Providing Care" section it is stated that *staff members provide care according to their scope of practice, standards of practice and hospital policies.*[14] Anesthesia care standards further delineated under the "Care of Pa-

TABLE 1–5. *JCAHO Standards and Intents*

I. PATIENT-FOCUSED FUNCTIONS
- Patient rights and organization ethics
- Assessment of patients
- Care of patients
- Education
- Continuum of care

II. ORGANIZATIONAL FUNCTIONS
- Improving organization performance
- Leadership
- Management of the environment of care
- Management of human resources
- Management of information
- Surveillance, prevention, and control of infection

III. STRUCTURES WITH FUNCTIONS
- Governance
- Management
- Medical staff
- Nursing

---

tients" section are applied to patients receiving not only general, spinal, and other major regional anesthesia but also sedation (with or without analgesia), which in the manner used may be reasonably expected to result in the loss of protective reflexes. Loss of protective reflexes is defined as an inability to handle secretions without aspiration or to maintain a patent airway independently.[14] Sedation is a continuum, and it is not always possible to predict how an individual patient receiving sedation will respond. Therefore it is the obligation of each institution to develop appropriate protocols for patients receiving sedation that may result in a loss of protective reflexes. The Joint Commission further states that these protocols should be consistent with *professional standards* and address at least the following[15]:

- Sufficient qualified individuals* must be present to perform the procedure and monitor the patient (TX.2–TX.2.2, LD.2.7, LD.2.9, HR.1, HR.2).
- Appropriate equipment for care and resuscitation is present (LD.1.3.2, EC.2.13).
- Appropriate monitoring of vital signs—heart rate, respirations, and oxygenation—using pulse oximetry equipment (TX.1, TX.2–TX.2.2, TX.3–TX.3.9, TX.5–TX.5.4).
- Care is properly documented (IM.7.3–IM.7.4).
- Outcome measurement (PI.3.1–PI.3.2.7).

Qualified Individual: An individual who is qualified to participate in one or all of the mechanisms outlined in the standards by virtue of one or more of the following: education, experience, competence, applicable professional licensure, regulation or certification, registration, and privileges.

Position Statement on the Role of the Registered Nurse (RN) in the Management of Patients Receiving Intravenous Conscious Sedation

A. Definition of Intravenous Conscious Sedation

Intravenous conscious sedation is produced by the administration of pharmacologic agents. A patient under conscious sedation has a depressed level of consciousness, but retains the ability to independently and continuously maintain a patent airway and respond appropriately to physical and verbal commands.

B. Management and Monitoring

It is within the scope of practice of a registered nurse to manage the care of patients receiving intravenous conscious sedation during therapeutic, diagnostic or surgical procedures provided the following criteria are met:

- Administration of IV conscious sedation medications by nonanesthetist RNs is allowed by state laws and institutional policy, procedures and protocol.
- A qualified anesthesia provider or attending physician selects and orders the medications to achieve IV conscious sedation.
- Guidelines for patient monitoring, drug administration and protocols for dealing with complications or emergency situations are available and have been developed in accordance with accepted standards of anesthesia practice.
- The registered nurse managing the care of patients receiving IV conscious sedation shall have no other responsibilities that would leave the patient unattended or compromise continuous monitoring.
- The registered nurse managing the care of patients receiving IV conscious sedation and medications:
  - Demonstrates the acquired knowledge of anatomy, physiology, cardiac arrhythmia recognition and complications related to IV conscious sedation and medications.
  - Assesses total patient care requirements during IV conscious sedation and recovery. Physiologic measurements should include, but not be limited to, respiratory rate, oxygen saturation, blood pressure, cardiac rate and rhythm and the patient's level of consciousness.
  - Understands the principles of oxygen delivery, respiratory physiology, transport and uptake, and demonstrates the ability to use oxygen delivery devices.
  - Anticipates and recognizes potential complications of IV conscious sedation in relation to the type of medication being administered.
  - Possesses the requisite knowledge and skills to assess, diagnose and intervene in the event of complications or undesired outcomes and to institute nursing interventions in compliance with orders (including standing orders) or institutional protocols or guidelines.
  - Demonstrates skill in airway management resuscitation.
  - Demonstrates knowledge of the legal ramifications of administering IV conscious sedation, including the RN's responsibility and liability in the event of an untoward reaction or life threatening complications.

The institution or practice setting has in place an educational/competency validation mechanism that includes a process for evaluating and documenting the individuals who are related to the management of patients receiving IV conscious sedation. Evaluation and documentation of competence occurs on a periodic basis according to institutional policy.

Continued on following page

Position Statement on the Role of the Registered Nurse (RN) in the Management of Patients Receiving Intravenous Conscious Sedation *Continued*

C. Additional Guidelines

- Intravenous access must be continuously maintained in the patient receiving IV conscious sedation.
- All patients receiving IV conscious sedation will be continuously monitored throughout the procedure as well as the recovery phase by physiologic measurements, including but not limited to, respiratory rate, oxygen saturation, blood pressure, cardiac rate and rhythm and patient's level of consciousness.
- Supplemental oxygen will be immediately available to all patients receiving IV conscious sedation and administered per order (including standing orders).
- An emergency cart with defibrillator must be immediately accessible to every location where IV conscious sedation is administered. Suction and a positive pressure breathing device, oxygen and appropriate airways must be in each room where IV conscious sedation is administered.

Provisions must be in place for back-up personnel who are experts in airway management, emergency intubation, and advanced cardiopulmonary resuscitation if complications arise.

Endorsed by:

American Association of Critical-Care Nurses
American Association of Neuroscience Nurses
American Association of Nurse Anesthetists
American Association of Occupational Health Nurses
American Association of Spinal Cord Injury Nurses
American Nephrology Nurses Association
American Nurses Association
American Radiological Nurses Association
American Society of Pain Management Nurses
American Society of Plastic and Reconstructive Surgical Nurses
American Society of Post Anesthesia Nurses

American Urological Association, Allied
Association of Operating Room Nurses
Association of Pediatric Oncology Nurses
Association of Rehabilitation Nurses
AWHONN, Association of Women's Health, Obstetric, and Neonatal Nurses (formerly NAACOG)
Dermatology Nurses Association
National Association of Orthopaedic Nurses
National Flight Nurses Association
National Student Nurses Association
Nurse Consultants Association, Inc.
Nurse Organization of Veterans Affairs
Nursing Pain Association

From American Nurses Association, Washington, DC, November 1991.

These standards were revised and accepted by the Joint Commission's Board of Commissioners. They are identified in the *Comprehensive Accreditation Manual for Ambulatory Care (CAMAC), Comprehensive Accreditation Manual for Hospitals (CAMH), Comprehensive Accreditation Manual for Long Term Care (CAMLTC),* and the *Accreditation Manual for Mental Health, Chemical Dependency, and Mental Retardation/Developmental Disabilities Services (MHM)* manuals.

The JCAHO sample policy and procedures for the administration of conscious sedation are listed in Appendix A. Policies and procedures related to the administration of conscious sedation must be individualized for each practice setting. However, in an attempt to improve quality patient care and promote the safe administration of conscious sedation by qualified persons, these policies and procedures must encompass recommended standards published by professional organizations and adhere to state statutory law. Policies delineated in relation to the administration of conscious sedation must address the following:

- Knowledge of anatomy, physiology, cardiac arrhythmia recognition, and complications related to the administration of intravenous sedation.
- Knowledge of the pharmacokinetic and pharmacodynamic principles associated with conscious sedation medications.
- Preprocedure assessment, monitoring of physiologic parameters, including respiratory rate, oxygen saturation, blood pressure, cardiac rate and rhythm, and patient level of consciousness.
- An understanding of the principles of oxygen delivery and the ability to use an oxygen-delivery device.
- The ability to rapidly assess, diagnose, and intervene in the event of an untoward reaction associated with the administration of conscious sedation.
- Proven skill in airway management.
- Accurate documentation of the procedure and medications administered.
- Postprocedure monitoring and discharge planning.
- Competency validation for training and education mechanisms.

PROFESSIONAL ORGANIZATIONS

In July 1991, the Nursing Organizations Liaison Forum in Washington, D.C., adopted a position statement for the management of patients receiving intravenous conscious sedation for short term therapeutic, diagnostic, or surgical procedures (see pp 11–12). This position statement has been adopted by 23 professional nursing organizations. Professional organizations involved in the development of the position statement are listed in Table 1–6. The Association of

TABLE 1-6. *Professional Nursing Organizations Liaison Forum, Washington, DC—July, 1991*

American Association of Critical Care Nurses (AACN)
American Association of Nurse Anesthetists (AANA)
American Nurses Association (ANA)
Association of Operating Room Nurses (AORN)
Association of Pediatric Oncology Nurses (APON)
American Society of Postanesthesia Nurses (ASPAN)
American Society of Pain Management Nurses (ASPMN)
American Society of Plastic and Reconstructive Surgical Nurses (ASPRN)
Emergency Nurses Association (ENA)
Intravenous Nurses Society, Inc. (INS)
National Flight Nurses Association (NFNA)
Nursing Pain Association (NPA)
Oncology Nursing Society (ONS)
Society of Gastroenterology Nurses and Associates, Inc. (SGNA)

Operating Room Nurses published proposed recommended practice guidelines for nurses administering intravenous conscious sedation/analgesia. These guidelines are presented in Appendix B.

SUMMARY

The administration of conscious sedation for diagnostic or surgical procedures is a highly specialized skill. Clinicians engaged in the art of conscious sedation procedures must realize the fine line between a tranquil amnestic patient and an unconscious, unresponsive patient. To satisfactorily achieve the objectives of conscious sedation and provide adequate sedation with minimal risk, educational preparation and competency validation related to preprocedural patient assessment, pharmacology, anatomy, and physiology of the cardiorespiratory systems, mechanisms of oxygen delivery, physiologic monitoring, and resuscitative techniques will be highlighted throughout this manual.

REFERENCES

1. White PF, Negua JB. Sedative infusions during local and regional anesthesia: a comparison of midazolam and propofol. *J Clin Anesth.* 1991;3:32.
2. Mervick P, Ramsby G. Conscious sedation for imaging and interventional studies. *Radiol Management.* 1994;16:2.
3. Smith C. Preparing nurses to monitor patients receiving local anesthesia. *AORN J.* 1994;59:5.
4. Association of Operating Room Nurses. *Standards, Recommended Practices and Guidelines.* Denver: AORN; 1997:149–154.
5. Newman P. Intravenous conscious sedation: nursing issues. *Specialty Nursing Forum.* 1990;2:3.
6. O'Connor K, Jones S. Oxygen desaturation is common and clinically underappreciated during endoscopic procedures. *Gastrointest Endosc.* 1990;36(suppl 3):S2–S4.
7. Bennett C. *Conscious Sedation in Dental Practice.* 2nd ed. St. Louis: CV Mosby; 1978.
8. American Nurses Association. *Policy Statement on Conscious Sedation.* Washington, DC: The Association; 1991.
9. Stevens M, White P. Monitored anesthesia care. *Anesthesia.* 4th ed. New York: Churchill Livingstone; 1994:1469.
10. Bailey P, Pace N, Ashburn M, et al. Frequent hypoxemia and apnea after sedation with midazolam and fentanyl. *Anesthesiology.* 1990;73:826.
11. Gunn I. The many issues regarding intravenous conscious sedation. *Specialty Nursing Forum.* 1990;2:3.
12. Commonwealth of Pennsylvania, Pennsylvania Code Title 49. *Professional and Vocational Standards.* Department of State, Chapter 21.413. State Board of Nursing, 1995.
13. Nemiroff M. IV conscious sedation: essential techniques of monitoring. *Trends in Health Care Law Ethics.* 1993;8:1.
14. JCAHO. *1996 Accreditation Manual for Hospitals.* vol 1. Standards. Oakbrook Terrace, Ill: JCAHO; 1997.
15. JCAHO. 1996 Joint Commission Videoconference Series: *Anesthesia and Conscious Sedation: Issues and Answers.* JCAHO Satellite Network, Sept. 11, 1996.

Preprocedure Assessment and Patient Selection

CHAPTER 2

AORN RECOMMENDED PRACTICE IV

Each patient who will receive intravenous conscious sedation/analgesia should be assessed physiologically and psychologically before the procedure. The assessment should be documented in the patient's record. [Components of this assessment are listed in Table 2–1.]

JCAHO STANDARD TX.2, TX.2.1, TX.2.2

A preanesthesia assessment is performed for each patient before anesthesia induction. Each patient's anesthesia care is planned. Anesthesia options and risks are discussed with the patient and family prior to administration.

PREPROCEDURE ASSESSMENT

The goals of a thorough preprocedure assessment include the following:

1. Assessment of preprocedure risk factors
2. Assuring that the patient is in the best physical condition before the procedure
3. Reduction of patient anxiety through education and communication
4. Preprocedure planning and patient education
5. Obtain informed consent

Preprocedure assessment must be conducted in an unhurried, reassuring atmosphere. Adequate time must be allotted to alleviate the patient's anxiety while allowing sufficient time to gather data and answer the patient's questions. When feasible, preprocedure assessment should be conducted several days before the proposed procedure. This assessment is best conducted in conjunction *with the registered nurse* who will participate in the administration of conscious sedation. Emergent cases may preclude the clinician's ability to obtain a thorough preprocedure assessment. Nonetheless, a complete assessment is still required before the administration of conscious sedation.

Thorough preprocedure assessment allows the clinician time to gather additional data, order indicated laboratory and diagnostic tests, and implement a conscious sedation plan. The preprocedure assessment period should attempt to identify patient risk factors that may lead to complications, while affording the clinician the opportunity to assure that the patient is in the best physical condition for the planned procedure. A comprehensive preprocedure assessment begins with a review of the medical record. Pertinent information recorded in the pa-

TABLE 2–1.   *Components of Preprocedure Assessment*

- Patient age, height, weight
- Proposed procedure
- Attending physician or service

MEDICAL HISTORY

Cardiac
- Angina
- Coronary artery disease
- Cardiovascular
- Cardiac dysrhythmias
- Exercise tolerance
- Hypertension
- Myocardial infarction

Pulmonary
- Asthma
- Bronchitis
- Dyspnea
- Exercise tolerance
- Cigarette smoking
- Recent cold or flu

Hepatic
- Ascites
- Cirrhosis
- Hepatitis

Renal
- Dialysis
- Renal failure
- Renal insufficiency

Neurologic
- Convulsive disorders
- Headaches
- Level of consciousness
- Stroke
- Syncope
- Vascular insufficiency

Endocrine
- Adrenal disease
- Diabetes
- Hyper/hypothyroidism

Gastrointestinal
- Hiatal hernia
- Nausea
- Recent weight loss
- Vomiting

Hematology
- Anemia
- Aspirin, NSAID use
- Excessive bleeding

Musculoskeletal
- Arthritis
- Back pain
- Joint pain

SURGICAL HISTORY
- Anesthesia complications (nausea, vomiting, delayed emergence)
- Diagnostic procedures
- Family anesthesia history
- Operations

MEDICATIONS
- Name
- Dosage
- Patient compliance

ALLERGIES
- Anaphylactic
- Anaphylactoid
- Side effects

LABORATORY DATA
- Additional laboratory profiles
- Chest x-ray
- ECG
- Electrolytes

DENTITION
- Capped teeth
- Loose/chipped teeth

SOCIAL HISTORY
- Cigarette smoking
- Alcohol use
- Illicit drug use
- Possibility of pregnancy

NPO STATUS
- Instructions
- Liquids
- Solids

INFORMED CONSENT
- Patient questions answered
- Written consent obtained
- Patient instructions given

ASA RISK CLASSIFICATION (OPTIONAL)
- ASA Risk 1–3

NAME AND DATE OF PREPROCEDURE EVALUATOR

tient's chart or record offers insight into the patient's overall health status as well as an opportunity to review the patient's past medical history. In some surgicenters, clinics, or physician offices, previous hospital records are not readily available. Therefore the patient as the medical historian is relied upon to give an accurate past medical history.

In the presence of a well-documented past medical history recorded in the patient's record, the provider may use the preprocedure assessment period to confirm information with the patient. Patients with a significant medical history may require additional laboratory tests and screening before the procedure. By performing preprocedure assessment several days before the scheduled procedure or diagnostic examination, the provider may order indicated tests, obtain specialty consultation, and request previous hospital records for review. To assure that all preprocedure assessments are performed in a consistent manner and avoid the omission of key information, many clinicians use an assessment tool featured on pages 18 to 20.

Initial preprocedure assessment is initiated with a review of the planned procedure. By asking the patient to confirm the planned procedure, the clinician is assured that the patient is aware of the scheduled procedure. Some patients may not be able to specifically repeat the name of the procedure or diagnostic examination. However, a basic understanding of the procedure and the anatomic area should be confirmed to assure that the patient has been advised by the physician as to the nature of the planned procedure.

PATIENT SELECTION

AGE

Next the patient's age should be noted. Although chronologic age does not necessarily correlate with physiologic age, it should be noted on the patient's record. It is equally important to ascertain the psychologic state of the patient at the time of the preprocedure assessment. Psychologic characteristics and the anxiety state of the patient are assessed throughout the entire preprocedure process. During the initial phase of the preprocedure assessment some patients may interject and ask, "What are you going to do to me?" or "What are you going to give me?" It is imperative to reiterate to the patient that once you *conclude* your assessment you will answer questions and explain the conscious sedation procedure. It is premature to comment or recommend an intravenous conscious sedation plan before a complete and thorough preprocedure assessment has been conducted.

HEIGHT AND WEIGHT

It is important to record accurate height and weight before the planned procedure. Broca's index offers a useful way to calculate a patient's ideal body weight.

Broca's Index
1 cm = 2.5 inches; 1 kg = 2.2 pounds
Height (cm) – 100 = IBW (kg): males
Height (cm) – 105 = IBW (kg): females

Intravenous Conscious Sedation
Preprocedure Patient Assessment Tool

Patient Name:_____ Age:_____ Height: _____ Weight: _____

Proposed Procedure:_____ Physician: _____

Scheduled Date: _____/_____/_____   Time: _____ AM PM

MEDICAL HISTORY
Check all that apply

Cardiovascular: **Comments:**

- ☐ Angina
- ☐ CAD
- ☐ Exercise Tolerance
- ☐ Hypertension
- ☐ MI

Pulmonary: **Comments:**

- ☐ Asthma
- ☐ Bronchitis
- ☐ Dyspnea
- ☐ Cold or Flu
- ☐ Cigarette Smoking:

_____ Packs/year

Hepatic: **Comments:**

- ☐ Hepatitis
- ☐ Cirrhosis
- ☐ Ascites

Renal: **Comments:**

- ☐ Insufficiency
- ☐ Dialysis
- ☐ Failure

© 1996, Specialty Health Consultants

Assessment of ideal body weight is important because obesity has a significant impact on the cardiovascular, pulmonary, gastrointestinal, endocrine, and hepatic systems. Obesity is defined as body weight greater than ideal weight. The multisystemic effects of obesity are listed in Table 2–2.

At times, management of the obese patient's airway during a conscious sedation procedure may be tenuous. Because of an increase in body mass and redundant oropharyngeal airway tissue, the patient must not be allowed to progress into a state of deep sedation. A plan of light sedation is indicated when clinicians are requested to provide administration of conscious sedation to obese patients. *Vigilance* in titration of medications is required for this patient population. Obese pa-

Intravenous Conscious Sedation
Preprocedure Patient Assessment Tool *Continued*

Neurologic: Comments:

☐   Insufficiency
☐   Stroke
☐   TIA
☐   Convulsive Disorder
☐   Syncope
☐   LOC:_____

Gastrointestinal: Comments:

☐   Nausea
☐   Vomiting
☐   Hiatal Hernia

PAST SURGICAL HISTORY

Date:_____   Procedure: _____

Anesthesia:_____   Complications:_____

Date:_____   Procedure: _____

Anesthesia:_____   Complications:_____

Date:_____   Procedure: _____

Anesthesia:_____   Complications:_____

MEDICATIONS

Medication: _____

Dose: _____   Last Dose: _____

Medication: _____

Dose: _____   Last Dose: _____

Medication: _____

Dose: _____   Last Dose: _____

                        Continued on following page

tients are also subject to pulmonary aspiration secondary to increased gastric volume and gastric reflux. Obese patients requiring conscious sedation may benefit from preprocedure administration of H_2 blockers (ranitidine) and gastric stimulants (metoclopramide). These medications are discussed in the preprocedure gastrointestinal assessment section of this chapter. Because of significant challenges

Intravenous Conscious Sedation
Preprocedure Patient Assessment Tool *Continued*

Allergies

(a) _____ (d) _____

(b) _____ (e) _____

(c) _____ (f) _____

Laboratory Data

EKG: _____

Hgb. _____ Hct. _____

Electrolytes: Na _____ CL _____ K+ _____

Additional Laboratory Tests: _____

_____

DENTITION
Check all that apply and identify site

☐   Caps: _____

☐   Chipped: _____

☐   Loose: _____

☐   Missing: _____

SOCIAL HISTORY

☐   Alcohol Use _____

☐   Cigarette Smoker _____ _____ Pack/year

☐   Illicit Drug Use _____

☐   Pregnancy _____

     Last Menstrual Period: _____/_____/_____

ASA STATUS
Optional

☐ ASA I   ☐ ASA II   ☐ ASA III

Evaluated by: _____ Date: _____

TABLE 2–2. *Multisystemic Effects of Obesity*

PULMONARY	CARDIOVASCULAR	GASTROINTESTINAL
Chest wall mass ↑	Cardiac output ↑	Intra-abdominal pressure ↑
CO_2 Production ↑	Hypertension	Intragastric pressure ↑
Functional residual capacity ↓↓	Pulmonary hypertension	Risk of aspiration ↑
Pulmonary compliance ↓	Stroke volume ↑	
Total oxygen consumption ↑		
Work of breathing ↑		

associated with management of obese patients, preprocedure concerns may require consultation with a member of the anesthesia care team. Diagnostic tests indicated for the obese patient include a complete blood count, a radiograph of the chest, and a baseline electrocardiogram to rule out ventricular hypertrophy. It is prudent to administer supplemental oxygen to all patients for conscious sedation procedures. Postoperative administration of oxygen should continue until the patient has fully recovered and demonstrates satisfactory return to preprocedure Sao_2 on room air with no signs of hypoxia.

MEDICAL HISTORY: ORGAN SYSTEM ASSESSMENT

CARDIOVASCULAR SYSTEM

The purpose of the cardiac assessment includes the following:

- Estimation of procedural cardiovascular complications
- Comparison of procedural risk versus the effect of not performing the procedure
- Identification of interventions that will decrease the incidence of complications
- Comprehensive cardiovascular assessment

Hypertension

Hypertension is defined as a systolic blood pressure greater than 160 mm Hg or a diastolic blood pressure greater than 95 mm Hg.[1] End organs affected by hypertension include the heart, brain, and kidneys. The heart is predisposed to hypertrophic changes secondary to increased resistance associated with hypertension. Hypertensive damage to the intracerebral vasculature may result in hemorrhage or stroke. End organ renal damage secondary to hypertension reduces glomerular filtration rate and renal blood flow. The incidence of coronary artery disease, myocardial infarction, and stroke is increased in the presence of hypertension.[2] When one is presented with the preprocedure assessment of a hypertensive patient, it is important to ascertain

- When the patient's hypertension was initially diagnosed
- Effectiveness of prescribed treatment plan (diet, salt restriction, medications)

- Identification of medication and dosage used to treat hypertension
- Identification of the patient's preprocedure anxiety level

Preprocedure assessment of the hypertensive patient should initially include recording of the patient's baseline blood pressure. It is equally important to assess the patient's level of compliance with the prescribed treatment plan. During this portion of the cardiovascular assessment, dietary and medication assessment should be ascertained. This includes an accurate assessment and identification of medications used to treat hypertension as well as dietary compliance. Fortunately, many hypertensive patients are well controlled on antihypertensive medication therapy and dietary restriction. To maintain a consistent plasma level of antihypertensive therapy, current recommendations include administration of antihypertensive medications up to and including the day of the scheduled procedure. It is not uncommon for patients presenting for their diagnostic or minor surgical procedure to be hypertensive on the initial preprocedure blood pressure screening. Preprocedure anxiety increases catecholamine release. At times this patient population is normotensive when preprocedure assessment is performed several days before the procedure and hypertensive on the day of the procedure. Management of patients in this group includes thorough patient preparation for the procedure, reassurance, and administration of the patient's morning antihypertensive medication. Once an intravenous line is established, the administration of small doses of benzodiazepines may reduce the patient's anxiety with a resultant decrease in blood pressure. If the blood pressure does not return to the patient's baseline or if the diastolic blood pressure remains elevated (>20%), it may be prudent to cancel the procedure. In this situation, referral of the patient to a specialist (cardiologist, internist) for further evaluation and improved blood pressure control prior to the procedure is recommended. Additional complications of poorly controlled hypertension include altered baroreceptor response, wide fluctuations of blood pressure during the procedure, and volume depletion.

Coronary Artery Disease

When evaluating patients for coronary artery disease, it is important to ascertain a history of chest pain. Questions used by the practitioner to elicit a history of coronary artery disease are listed in Table 2–3. In addition to the questions outlined, patients must describe their chest pain. Factors to be considered include

- Character
- Frequency

TABLE 2–3. *Assessment of Coronary Artery Disease*

- Do you have a history of angina, chest tightness, or heaviness?
- Do you ever have indigestion not associated with eating?
- Have you ever had coronary artery bypass or heart surgery?
- Do you ever get short of breath?
- Have you ever been told you have an abnormal ECG?
- Have you ever felt skipped beats?
- Describe your daily activities and exercise

- Location
- Duration
- Radiation
- Methods of relief

Physical assessment of the patient with coronary artery disease includes assessment of skin color, presence of jugular venous distention, peripheral edema, assessment of baseline blood pressure, and auscultation of heart sounds. An electrocardiogram may reveal normal sinus rhythm, the presence of arrhythmias, or signs of previous infarction. Previous ECGs should be available for comparison. Patients with coronary artery disease must receive their prescribed nitrates, calcium channel blockers, beta blockers, and antihypertensive medications before the scheduled procedure. Postoperative monitoring must also be continued until the patient is fully recovered and demonstrates no signs of cardiovascular instability.

Myocardial Infarction

Preprocedure assessment of patients with previous myocardial infarction must identify the length of time elapsed since the myocardial infarction. Questioning to elicit a history of angina, cardiovascular stability, or shortness of breath is required. If the patient admits to a history of angina, mechanisms of relief must be ascertained. In patients with a history of myocardial infarction, a 30% incidence of reinfarction has been reported to occur if surgery is performed within the first 3 months after infarction. This incidence decreases to 15% when surgery is performed within a 3- to 6-month period. The incidence of reinfarction decreases to approximately 5% after 6 months.[3,4] Many authors have extrapolated these findings and recommend that *elective* procedures be delayed for 6 months after infarction to decrease the incidence of reinfarction. These recommendations have been promulgated regardless of whether the procedure is scheduled for general, regional, or local anesthesia.[5] However, more recent studies indicate no periprocedure myocardial infarctions in noncardiac surgical patients with a history of myocardial infarction within the previous 6 months who received monitored anesthesia care.[6]

Cardiac Arrhythmias

Cardiac arrhythmia may be caused by

- Effects of medications administered
- Hypoxemia
- Hypercarbia
- Electrolyte abnormalities
- Alterations of the autonomic nervous system
- Procedural manipulations
- Preoperative patient anxiety
- Hypovolemia
- Hypotension

In most patients with normal cardiac reserve, arrhythmias are generally well tolerated. Patients with limited cardiac reserve, however, cannot tolerate even the most benign arrhythmias. Newly diagnosed dysrhythmias or dysrhythmias that impair myocardial performance require further evaluation and consultation. Cardiac arrhythmias and treatment protocols are covered in Chapter 6.

Pacemakers

Preprocedure assessment of the patient with a pacemaker must initially evaluate the rationale for the device (sick sinus syndrome, syncope, etc.). Pacemakers are frequently inserted because of bradyarrhythmias. The clinician must recognize not only the indication for placement but also the pacemaker's default rhythm. Electrocautery is sensed by demand pacemakers and may result in asystole or inhibition of firing. Before using electrocautery, the clinician should have the pacemaker programming device available for conversion to a fixed pacemaker rate. Many of the currently used pacemakers are capable of conversion to a fixed rate in the presence of electrocautery. However, for pacemakers without this capability, the technique of converting to a fixed rate should be demonstrated to the attending physician and registered nurse before the planned procedure. The grounding plate should be placed the greatest possible distance from the pacemaker and lead. During the use of bipolar electrocautery, it is important to monitor pulsatile flow with a pulse oximeter. Because electrocautery interferes with ECG monitoring, adequacy of pulsatile flow is assured with pulse oximetry pulsatile display.

Defibrillators (Automatic Internal Defibrillators)

Patients with ventricular tachycardia or fibrillation unresponsive to pharmacologic therapy may be treated with automatic implantable cardioverter defibrillators (AICD). These defibrillators deliver a 25-joule discharge to convert the patient from a life-threatening arrhythmia.[7] Preprocedure consultation with the cardiologist should address postinsertion follow-up, battery strength, status of the pulse generator, and the cardiologist's suggestions for intraprocedural care. If electrocautery use is planned, the generator should be disabled with a magnet. The AICD may be reactivated at the conclusion of the procedure. While the AICD is disabled, an external defibrillator must be immediately available in the clinical setting.

Valvular Heart Disease

Prophylactic antibiotics are indicated for patients with valvular heart disease, ventricular/atrial septal defects, intravascular shunts, and previous endocarditis. Antibiotics are given to protect against the development of endocarditis after bacteremic events. Blood-borne bacteria may lodge on damaged valve leaflets, resulting in bacterial endocarditis. Bacteremic events include instrumentation of the gallbladder, gastrointestinal/genitourinary tract, and oropharynx. The American Heart Association recommendations for prevention of bacterial endocarditis are listed in Table 2–4.

Completion of the preprocedure cardiac evaluation should incorporate the findings of the patient's history, physical examination, and a review of laboratory

TABLE 2–4. *Endocarditis Antibiotic Prophylaxis*

ADULTS	CHILDREN
DENTAL, ORAL, NASAL, PHARYNGEAL, OR UPPER AIRWAY PROCEDURES	
Standard	
Amoxicillin, 3 g PO, 1 h before and 1.5 g 6 h after the procedure	Amoxicillin, 50 mg/kg PO 1 h before and 25 mg/kg, 6 h after the procedure
Penicillin Allergy	
Erythromycin, 1 g PO 2 h before and 500 mg 6 h afterward	Erythromycin, 20 mg/kg PO 2 h before and 10 mg/kg 6 h afterward
or	*or*
Clindamycin, 300 mg PO 2 h before and 150 mg 6 h afterward	Clindamycin, 10 mg/kg PO 2 h before and 5 mg/kg 6 h afterward
High Risk (Prosthetic Valve or Prior Endocarditis)	
Ampicillin, 2 g IV or IM, and gentamicin, 1.5 mg/kg (up to 80 mg) IV or IM 30 min before, and amoxicillin, 1.5 g PO 6 h afterward or repeat IV regimen 8 h later	Ampicillin, 50 mg/kg IV or IM, and gentamicin, 2 mg/kg IV or IM 30 min before, and amoxicillin, 50 mg/kg PO 6 h afterward or repeat IV regimen 8 h later
High Risk with Penicillin Allergy	
Vancomycin, 1 g IV 1 h before (infuse over 1 h)	Vancomycin, 20 mg/kg IV 1 h before (infuse over 1 h)
GENITOURINARY AND GASTROINTESTINAL PROCEDURES	
Standard	
Ampicillin, 2 g IV or IM, and gentamicin, 1.5 mg/kg (up to 80 mg) IV or IM 30 min before, and amoxicillin, 1.5 g PO 6 h afterward	Ampillin, 50 mg/kg IV or IM, and gentamicin, 2 mg/kg IV or IM 30 min before, and amoxicillin, 50 mg/kg PO 6 h afterward
Penicillin Allergy	
Vancomycin, 1 g IV 1 h before (infuse over 1 h), and gentamicin, 1.5 mg/kg (up to 80 mg) IV	Vancomycin, 20 mg/kg IV 1 h before (infuse over 1 h), and gentamicin, 2 mg/kg IV
Low Risk	
Amoxicillin, 3 g PO 1 h before and 1.5 g 6 h after the procedure	Amoxicillin, 50 mg/kg PO, 1 h before and 25 mg/kg 6 h after the procedure

data. Patients with a recent myocardial infarction, unstable angina, poor exercise tolerance, cardiac arrhythmias, dyspnea, fatigue, coronary artery disease, or hypertension may require cardiac consultation. When indicated, additional cardiac testing (stress test, echocardiogram, or cardiac catheterization) may reveal valuable information that will alter preprocedure and intraprocedure management of the conscious sedation procedure. The American College of Cardiology/American Heart Association Task Force recently published *Guidelines for Perioperative Cardiovascular Evaluation for Noncardiac Surgery* featured in Figure 2–1. Adequate time must be allotted to assure that the patient is hemodynamically stable and in optimum cardiovascular condition before the planned procedure.

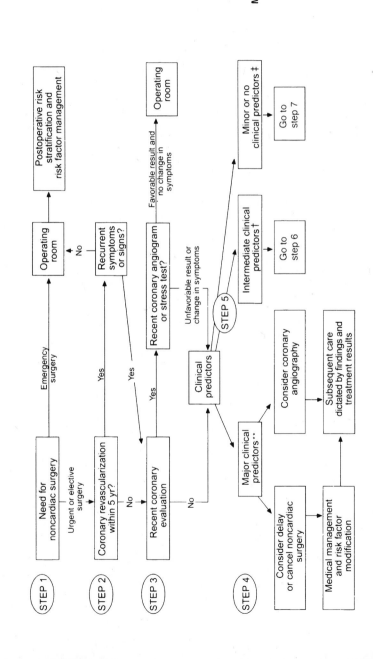

STEP 1

Need for noncardiac surgery → Emergency surgery → Operating room → Postoperative risk stratification and risk factor management

↓ Urgent or elective surgery

STEP 2

Coronary revascularization within 5 yr? → Yes → Recurrent symptoms or signs? → No → Operating room

↓ No ↓ Yes

STEP 3

Recent coronary evaluation → Yes → Recent coronary angiogram or stress test? → Favorable result and no change in symptoms → Operating room

↓ No ↓ Unfavorable result or change in symptoms

Clinical predictors

→ Major clinical predictors**

→ Intermediate clinical predictors† → Go to step 6

→ Minor or no clinical predictors‡ → Go to step 7

STEP 4

Major clinical predictors**

→ Consider delay or cancel noncardiac surgery

→ Consider coronary angiography → Subsequent care dictated by findings and treatment results

Medical management and risk factor modification

STEP 5

**Major Clinical Predictors **

· Unstable coronary syndromes
· Decompensated CHF
· Significant arrhythmias
· Severe valvular disease

26

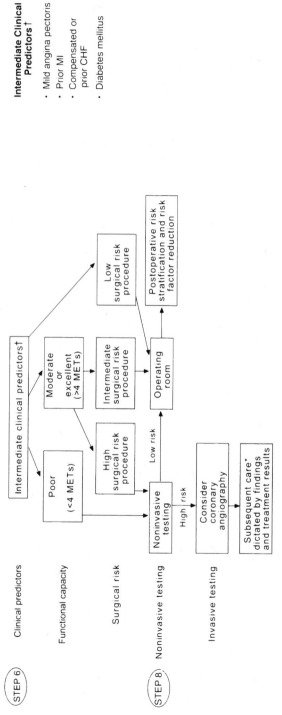

FIGURE 2–1. Stepwise approach to preoperative cardiac assessment. Subsequent care may include cancellation or delay of surgery, coronary revascularization followed by noncardiac surgery, or intensified care. (From American College of Cardiology/American Heart Association Cardiovascular Evaluation Guidelines. *J Am Coll Cardiol.* 1996;27(4):910–948.)

Figure continued on following page

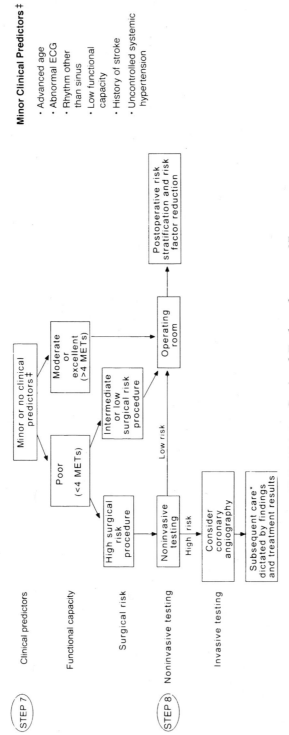

FIGURE 2–1. *Continued.* For legend see page 27.

PULMONARY ASSESSMENT

Sedative and analgesic medications interfere with the regulation of spontaneous pulmonary ventilation. Therefore, prevention of respiratory complications, including respiratory failure, atelectasis, and hypoxia, require careful preoperative assessment and planning. Preprocedure pulmonary assessment must address the type, severity, and reversibility of preexisting pulmonary disease. Symptoms of pulmonary disease must be ascertained by the clinician before the anticipated procedure. Pulmonary symptoms that predispose the patient to increased risk include the following:

- Chronic cough
- Sputum production
- Rhinitis
- Sore throat
- Dyspnea
- Cigarette smoking
- Previous pulmonary complications
- Hemoptysis

The presence of dyspnea on preprocedure evaluation may be an ominous sign. Dypsnea occurs when the requirement for ventilation is greater than the patient's ability to physiologically respond to the increased oxygen demand. Causes of dyspnea are listed in Table 2–5. Patients with a history of dyspnea require further preprocedure pulmonary evaluation. Assessment of dyspnea at rest or at specific levels of exertion is an important indicator of the severity of preexisting pulmonary disease. A general rule of thumb used by many clinicians is the absence of dyspnea after the ascent of two flights of stairs. Use of this criteria suggests satisfactory cardiorespiratory function.[8] This absence of dypsnea on moderate exertion generally signifies that preexisting lung disease is nonexistent or so minor that it will not present any problems.

Preprocedure radiographs of the chest are indicated in patients based on the severity of pulmonary disease and the magnitude of the planned procedure. Indications for preprocedure chest x-ray examination are identified in Table 2–6. The

TABLE 2–5. *Causes of Dyspnea*

A. Obstructive Pulmonary Disease
- Asthma
- Bronchitis
- Emphysema
- Upper airway obstruction

B. Restrictive pulmonary disease

C. Cardiomyopathy

D. Left ventricular failure

E. Obesity

F. Anemia

G. Neuromuscular disease

TABLE 2-6.   *Indications for Preprocedure Chest X-Ray*

- Blood-tinged or colored sputum
- Cigarette smoking greater than 20 pack years
- Exposure to tuberculosis
- History of congestive heart failure
- Malignancy
- Presence of cardiovascular disease
- Productive cough
- Pulmonary infection
- Sudden change in pulmonary/cardiovascular symptoms

---

clinician ordering the chest film must assess the benefits of the film versus the diagnostic benefit associated with use of the examination. Regardless of the preexisting pulmonary disease, the purpose of the preprocedure pulmonary assessment should focus on identification and treatment of acute infections with appropriate antibiotic therapy. Relief of bronchospastic disease through use of bronchodilators, implementation of mechanisms to improve sputum clearance (postural damage and incentive spirometry), and cessation of cigarette smoking attempt to optimize the patient's preprocedure pulmonary condition.

Chronic Obstructive Pulmonary Disease

Patients with chronic obstructive pulmonary disease frequently have a history of cigarette smoking. Dyspnea, cough, and wheezing may be present. As the disease progresses, barrel chest develops, use of accessory muscles for respiratory excursion, and pursed-lip breathing may ensue.

Asthma

Asthma affects approximately 5% of the adult population and 7% to 10% of children in the United States. Asthma is a chronic condition characterized by airway inflammation and the potential for bronchospasm. Asthma is accompanied by a combination of clinical features, which include the following:

- Wheezing
- Airway obstruction with reversibility
- Increased airway responsiveness
- Decreased mucociliary clearance
- Increased mucus production

Preoperatively, the asthmatic patient should exhibit no signs of respiratory infection (fever, productive cough). Eradication of acute and chronic infection with antibiotics is essential. The absence of wheezing, dyspnea, or recent attacks most likely indicates the patient is in a stable phase of the disease. Preprocedure assessment must include pharmacologic evaluation of the asthmatic patient. Beta agonists (albuterol) are used to produce bronchial dilation. Corticosteroids decrease airway inflammation, and anticholinergic agents (ipratropium bromide) inhibit muscarinic receptors in the autonomic nervous system with resultant bronchodilation. Additional preprocedure assessment includes identification of the last asthma attack, severity, mechanisms used to relieve the attack, and conditions that aggravate the condition. The patient treated with beta agonists should use his or her metered-dose inhaler before the planned procedure. Metered-dose inhalers (MDIs), oxygen, and breathing treatment equipment should also be available in the procedure room. *Morphine sulfate* is contraindicated in the asthmatic patient population because of its histamine-releasing properties. Fortunately, through identification of the last attack, its severity, the mechanism of relief, and continuation of the patient's prescribed pharmacologic protocol, many asthmatic patients tolerate the administration of intravenous conscious sedation without incident.

Bronchitis

Bronchitis is a common cause of chronic obstructive pulmonary disease. Permanent or minimally reversible obstruction to airflow occurs during exhalation. The presence of cough, dyspnea, and sputum production may require supplemental oxygenation to avoid hypoxemia and allow the patient the ability to carry out the activities of daily living. Preprocedure assessment of the patient with chronic obstructive pulmonary disease requires a determination of the severity of dyspnea, hypoxia, and infection. Supplemental oxygen (no more than 2 L) is recommended during the procedure and should remain in place until all residual respiratory depressant effects have dissipated.

HEPATIC ASSESSMENT

The liver is responsible for the synthesis of proteins and clotting factors and for detoxification of pharmacologic agents and metabolic byproducts. The liver also excretes bodily waste products, stores iron and vitamins, and supplements the body's energy stores. It is the largest organ in the body and receives approximately 29% of cardiac output.[9] Treatment of patients with impaired hepatic function should attempt to prevent further hepatic deterioration. Patients presenting for conscious sedation may have acute or chronic liver disease. These patients are predisposed to symptoms associated with hepatic disease, which include the following:

- Ascites
- Portal hypertension
- Arteriolar vasodilitation
- Arterial desaturation
- Decreased hematocrit
- Encephalopathy
- Electrolyte disturbances

Enzyme Induction

An important pharmacologic function of the liver is the breakdown of lipid-soluble medications into water-soluble compounds via the cytochrome P-450 microsomal enzyme system. The degree of metabolism of pharmacologic compounds is dependent on hepatic blood flow and enzyme activity in the endoplasmic reticulum. In some cases, patients with significant liver impairment may exhibit resistance to conscious sedation medications because of the accentuated drug metabolism attributed to enzyme induction. Conversely, patients with liver disease may be extremely sensitive to pharmacologic medications because of a decrease in hepatic blood flow and destruction of the hepatocytes, which contain the microsomal enzyme system. Therefore, with acute or chronic liver failure, careful titration and vigilance are required to assess patient response to medications administered.

Hepatitis

Hepatitis is characterized by inflammation of the hepatocytes. Characteristics of hepatitis are listed in Table 2–7. The diagnosis of hepatitis is often confirmed only after presentation with fatigue, anorexia, dark urine, fever, hepatomegaly, ascites, esophageal varices, and peripheral edema. A combination of these symp-

TABLE 2–7. *Characteristic Features of Viral Hepatitis*

TYPE A	TYPE B	TYPE C	TYPE D
TRANSMISSION			
Fecal-oral, contaminated shellfish	Percutaneous, venereal	Percutaneous	Percutaneous
INCUBATION PERIOD (d)			
20–37	60–110	35–70	60–110
RESULTS OF SERUM ANTIGEN AND ANTIBODY TESTS			
IgM early and IgG during convalescence	HBsAg and anti-HBc early and persist in carriers	Anti-HVC in 6 months	Anti-HVD late and may be short-lived
IMMUNITY			
45% have antibodies	5–15% have anti-HBs	Unknown	Protected if immune to type B
COURSE			
Does not progress to chronic liver disease	Chronic liver disease develops in 1–10%	Chronic liver disease develops in >50%	Coexists with type B
PREVENTION			
Pooled gamma globulin	Hepatitis B vaccine, hepatitis B immunoglobulin	Unknown	Unknown
MORTALITY			
≤0.2%	0.3–1.5%	Unknown	2–20%

HBcAg, hepatitis B core antigen; HBsAg, hepatitis B surface antigen; HVC, HVD, herpes virus types C and D; IgG, IgM, immunoglobulins G and M.
From Stoelting R, Dierdorf S. *Anesthesia and Coexisting Disease.* 3rd ed. New York: Churchill Livingstone; 1993:257.

toms may signify severe hepatic disease. The treatment of hepatitis often focuses on the presenting symptoms. Attention to the nutritional support and hydration status of the patient is imperative. Preprocedure preparation of the patient with hepatitis should discourage the use of alcohol. Assessment of the coagulation profile, nutritional status, and optimization of presenting symptoms is required before the planned procedure.

Cirrhosis

Cirrhosis is a liver disease that results in scarring and destruction of liver cells. Decreased hepatic blood flow occurs with increased resistance of flow through the portal system. Cirrhosis and portal hypertension also affect the cardiopulmonary system in the cirrhotic patient. The cardiovascular effects associated with cirrhosis include a hyperdynamic circulation, cardiomyopathy, and portal vein hypertension. Pulmonary considerations associated with cirrhosis include decreased oxygen affinity for the hemoglobin molecule accompanied by varying degrees of oxygen desaturation. This predisposition to desaturation and hypoxemia requires careful titration and dosage reduction of conscious sedation medications. In cases of advanced liver disease, ascites secondary to portal hypertension, hypoalbuminemia, and edema also predispose cirrhotic patients to hypoxemia. Patients presenting with hepatic disease require careful assessment to ascertain the magnitude of the disease. Predisposition to hypoxemia and decreased drug metabolism require attentive monitoring and careful titration and dosage reduction of all medications.

RENAL ASSESSMENT

Preprocedure assessment of the renal system is required to assess impairment prior to the scheduled conscious sedation procedure. Functions of the kidney include the following:

- Regulation and maintenance of fluid status
- Acid-base maintenance system
- Excretion of waste products and electrolyte balance
- Detoxification of pharmacologic agents

The kidneys perform these tasks via filtration, reabsorption, and secretion. Preprocedure evaluation of renal function consists of assessment of the patient for a history of renal surgery or any degree of renal impairment. A history of minor urologic or renal impairment may include cystitis, incontinence, and benign prostatic disease. There are distinct groups of patients with renal impairment who require preprocedure evaluation.

Renal Insufficiency

For patients with renal insufficiency presenting for conscious sedation procedures, optimization of hydration status is a priority. The goal of the provider is to preserve normal renal function throughout the procedure and in the immediate postprocedure period. Depending on the state of hypovolemia or hypervolemia, many authors advocate titration of saline solution, mannitol, furosemide, or low-dose dopamine.[10-16] Although it is not practical to measure urine output during short diagnostic procedures, urine output should be measured and documented both before and after the procedure. Attention to volume status is assured through adequate preprocedure assessment of skin turgor, weight, blood pressure, and heart rate. Patients who appear hypervolemic may also require diuretic therapy before the procedure.

Dialysis

For patients with little or no existing renal function, preprocedure assessment and planning should focus on preservation of the remaining organ systems in the body. The vascular cannulation site used for dialysis must be carefully guarded against insult. Blood pressure measurement must not be done on the side of the vascular access site. Infection is a leading cause of morbidity and death in patients with compromised renal function. Strict adherence to aseptic or sterile technique must be used for all invasive procedures and intravenous cannula insertion. Anephric patients may be anemic as a result of decreased erythropoeitin secretion. Erythropoeitin secreted by the kidney is required for the synthesis of hemoglobin molecules. This anemia predisposes the patient to the development of hypoxia. Preprocedure laboratory work may reveal hyperkalemia, increased blood urea nitrogen, calcium, and creatinine levels, and acidosis requiring dialysis. Dialysis before the procedure is beneficial to many patients. However, hypovolemia associated with dialysis may predispose the patient to hypotension during the procedure. Careful titration of intravenous medications is required to avoid hypotension and hypoxemia in this specific patient population.

Characteristics associated with chronic renal failure include anemia, metabolic acidosis, pruritus, hypertension, altered fluid and electrolyte status, and susceptibility to infection. During preprocedure assessment, the clinician must ascertain the following:

- Degree of renal insufficiency
- Whether the insufficiency is chronic or acute
- The last dialysis treatment noted on the chart

Once assessment is completed, preprocedure treatment of renal disease must address presenting symptoms and focus on the following:

- Fluid volume
- Homeostasis
- Electrolyte balance
- Renal clearance
- Hormonal secretion

Hypertension associated with renal disease is a common finding. Hypertension secondary to renal disease is a result of hypervolemia or alterations in the renin-angiotensin mechanism. Hypertension associated with renal disease is often treated as essential hypertension until end-stage renal failure ensues. Patients with preexisting electrolyte disturbances (serum potassium > 5.5 mmol/L) may benefit from dialysis prior to the scheduled procedure. A focus on euvolemia, normotension, correction of electrolyte disturbances, normokalemia, and correction of clinically significant anemia should precede any conscious sedation procedure.

Pharmacologic Effects of Renal Disease

The presence of preexisting renal disease decreases protein binding, which results in accentuation of pharmacologic effects for highly protein bound intravenous conscious sedation medications. Midazolam is 98% protein bound. In the presence of renal failure and a decrease in protein binding, there is an increase in the active pharmacologic component of midazolam. Therefore accentuation of benzodiazepine effect may be greatly enhanced in patients with renal disease. Patients with renal impairment also have a greater risk of adverse drug reaction.[17-19] As outlined earlier, pharmacologic effects are accentuated secondary to increased plasma levels of the drug, decreased protein binding, and drug accumulation. Careful titration and reduction of dose must be combined with careful assessment of the cardiopulmonary response to sedative medications in all settings, particularly in those patients with preexisting renal dysfunction.

NEUROLOGIC ASSESSMENT

Preprocedure assessment of the patient with neurologic disease attempts to elicit a history of mental deficiency, cerebral vascular insufficiency, or intrinsic metabolic neurologic disease. The goal of a complete neurologic assessment is to ascertain and document preprocedure levels of consciousness and to evaluate the presence of preexisting neurologic disease.

Cerebrovascular Insufficiency

Cerebrovascular disease may present as:

1. Transient ischemic attacks (TIAs) with reversible temporary cerebral dysfunction.
2. Minor cerebrovascular accident with return to a near-normal physiologic state.
3. Major stroke with resultant severe cerebral dysfunction or death.

Transient ischemic attacks are temporary, reversible, ischemic attacks with full recovery in periods ranging from minutes to 24 hours. Temporary interruption of cerebral blood flow may result from plaque or debris, with recovery occurring after dissolution of the debris. The finding of TIAs on preprocedure assessment may indicate impending severe neurologic dysfunction or stroke.

Carotid Artery and Vertebral Basilar Disease

Cerebral ischemia may also result from insufficient blood flow to the circle of Willis. The circle of Willis receives blood flow for cerebral circulation from the internal carotid artery and the vertebral arteries, which converge to form the posterior basilar artery. Collection of arterial plaque in the carotid artery results in decreased cerebral circulation with resultant neurologic symptoms, which include the following:

- Visual loss
- Paresis
- Numbness and tingling of the contralateral extremities

Patients with TIAs or carotid disease may be treated medically or surgically. Medical management consists of antiplatelet medications and anticoagulant therapy. Surgical treatment is indicated when plaque buildup results in lesions that obstruct 80% of blood flow with repeated TIAs. Surgical excision of the obstructive lesion generally results in improvement of the patient's neurologic status. It is important to assess coagulation status during preprocedure assessment if the planned procedure may predispose the patient to blood loss. Documentation of the incidence and severity of TIAs coupled with a history of the length and resolution of the TIA must be documented. Specific documentation must address focal neurologic deficits and any functional neurologic limitations *prior to the procedure.* This documentation is important if a new postprocedure deficit is reported to the clinician.

Stroke

Preprocedure neurologic assessment may reveal a history of hemorrhagic or ischemic stroke. Hemorrhagic insult associated with stroke results from subarachnoid or intracerebral bleeding. Preprocedure neurologic symptoms that warrant additional investigation include the following:

- Headache
- Vomiting
- Loss of consciousness
- Seizures
- Slurred speech
- Unsteady gait
- Hemiparesis

These preprocedure neurologic symptoms require documentation and consultation before the administration of conscious sedation.

Convulsive Disorders

Patients with a history of epilepsy or convulsive disorder require a thorough assessment of their disease state. Epileptic seizures result from a discharge of abnormally excitable neurons. This excitation may be triggered by discontinuation of medications, infection, neoplasm, drug or alcohol use, electrolyte disturbance, and hypoxia. Preprocedure assessment must focus on the underlying cause of the seizure. Recommendations for antiseizure medications include maintenance of therapeutic plasma levels with administration of the morning dose of antiseizure medication on the morning of the planned procedure.[20-22] Initial assessment of patients with seizures requires differentiation of the specific type of seizure. Grand mal seizures are characterized by

- Tonic-clonic convulsions
- Unconsciousness
- Severe muscle clonus
- Incontinence
- Postictal state

Petit mal seizures are characterized by

- Brief periods of staring
- Unresponsiveness

Petit mal or focal seizures are generally associated with pediatric patients. Assessment of epileptic patients with a seizure history must ascertain compliance with prescribed medications and treatment protocol. Postponement of the procedure should be considered for noncompliant patients or patients who have not received appropriate evaluation and therapy.

Peripheral Nervous System Assessment

Evaluation of the peripheral nervous system includes assessment of extremity strength, color, pallor, temperature, capillary refill, and peripheral pulses. Sensory deficits and decreased reflexes may also signify peripheral sensory impairment. When neurologic assessment reveals a peripheral neuropathy, the degree, change over time, and the exact nature of the specific neuropathy must be documented before the procedure.

ENDOCRINE SYSTEM

Preprocedure assessment of the endocrine system may reveal primary diseases associated with overproduction or decreased production of hormones or by alterations in the stress response.

Diabetes

Diabetes is a chronic disease that is characterized by disruption of glucose metabolism. This altered glucose metabolism results in excessive plasma glucose levels. Hyperglycemia is a result of impaired synthesis, secretion, or use of endogenous insulin. The diagnosis of diabetes is indicated when fasting blood sugar levels are higher than 140 mg/dl or a 2-hour postprandial blood glucose level is greater than 140 mg/dl.[23] Diabetes affects more than 12 million people in the United States. Ninety percent of diabetic patients do not require insulin and maintain adequate blood sugar levels through dietary restriction, exercise, and weight control. Some patients may require oral hypoglycemic agents. Oral hypoglycemic agents work in one of two ways; they increase insulin release from the pancreas or increase the peripheral response to insulin.[24] This patient population is classified as having type II or non-insulin-dependent diabetes (NIDDM). Specific characteristics of type II diabetes include a gradual decline in pancreatic

TABLE 2–8. *Clinical Types of Diabetes Mellitus*

EVENT	TYPE I INSULIN-DEPENDENT	TYPE II NON-INSULIN-DEPENDENT
Age at onset	Childhood	Middle age or elderly
Timing of onset	Abrupt	Gradual
Predisposing factors	Genetic	Obesity, pregnancy, drugs
Islet beta cell mass	90% loss	Mild to moderate decrease
Plasma insulin level	Absent or minimal	Normal, increased, or decreased
Control of diabetes	Insulin required	Diet, exercise may be enough
Acidosis, ketosis	Common	Rare

From Barash P, Cullen B, Stoelting R. *Clinical Anesthesia.* 2nd ed. Philadelphia: JB Lippincott; 1992: 553.

function. There is evidence of a genetic link related to non-insulin-dependent diabetes mellitus.

Type I diabetes is called insulin-dependent diabetes mellitus (IDDM) and occurs in the remaining 10% of diabetic patients. Type I patients tend to be younger and not predisposed to obesity; their disease is referred to as juvenile-onset diabetes. Clinical characteristics of type I and II diabetes are listed in Table 2–8. Type I patients are predisposed to hyperglycemia, acidosis, and ketosis. Diabetes may result in end-organ impairment, which includes the following:

- Hypertension
- Coronary artery disease
- Nephropathy
- Retinopathy
- Neuropathy
- Peripheral vascular disease

Hypertension and coronary disease associated with diabetes mellitus may increase the incidence of cardiovascular complications (labile blood pressure, ST segment depression, chest pain) during the administration of conscious sedation medications for diagnostic or brief surgical procedures. Autonomic neuropathy may present as silent myocardial ischemia and postural hypotension. Gastroparesis secondary to autonomic neuropathy increases the risk of aspiration and regurgitation.

KETOACIDOSIS. Ketoacidosis may be triggered by infection, stress, trauma, poor insulin regimen compliance, or the proposed procedure itself. Ketoacidosis leads to an increased resistance to insulin. Characteristics of ketoacidosis include hyperglycemia, hyperosmolarity, hyperkalemia, hyponatremia, and intracellular dehydration with osmotic diuresis. These characteristics predispose the patient to hypotension and hypovolemia. Symptoms of ketoacidosis include nausea, vomiting, lethargy, and hypovolemia. Correction of ketoacidosis includes administration of regular insulin, volume replacement with intravascular fluids, and correction of electrolyte disturbances.

TABLE 2–9.   *Classification of Insulin Preparations*

| | HOURS AFTER SUBCUTANEOUS ADMINISTRATION (ESTIMATED) | | |
	ONSET	PEAK	DURATION
Fast-acting			
Regular*	0.5–1	2–4	6–8
Semilente	1–3	5–10	16
Intermediate-acting			
Isophane (NPH)†	2–4	6–12	18–26
Lente*	2–4	6–12	18–26
Long-acting			
Protamine zinc	4–8	14–24	28–36
Ultralente	4–8	14–24	28–36

*Available as human insulin (Humulin).
†NPH, neutral (N) solution, protamine (P), with origin in Hagedorn's laboratory (H).
From Stoelting R, Dierdorf S. *Anesthesia and Coexisting Disease.* 3rd ed. New York: Churchill Livingstone; 1993.

INSULIN.   A variety of insulin is marketed for supplementation to the diabetic patient. Pork, beef, and human insulin are currently available for the treatment of diabetes mellitus. The pharmacologic profile of insulin types is presented in Table 2–9.

ORAL HYPOGLYCEMIC AGENTS.   Oral hypoglycemic agents are used when diet and exercise regimens can no longer control blood glucose levels. Oral hypoglycemic agents are listed in Table 2–10. The prolonged duration of action of oral hypoglycemic agents predisposes the patient to hypoglycemia during the procedure and in the immediate postprocedure period. Oral hypoglycemic agents should be withheld on the morning of the planned procedure to prevent hypoglycemia in the presence of the morning fast. Signs of hypoglycemia include changes in level of consciousness and documentation of preprocedure blood sugar levels.

Preprocedure assessment of the diabetic patient includes identification of the type of diabetes. Compliance with diet, exercise, and medication must also be documented. A thorough assessment for coronary artery disease, hypertension, autonomic neuropathy, and gastroparesis is required prior to the administration of

TABLE 2–10.   *Oral Hypoglycemic Agents*

AGENT	DURATION OF ACTION (HOURS)
Tolbutamide	6–10
Tolazamide	16–24
Chlorpropamide	24–72
Glyburide	18–24
Glipizide	16–24

conscious sedation. For type I diabetic patients treated with insulin, an attempt should be made to maintain blood sugar levels between 120 and 200 mg/dl. A variety of techniques have been advocated to control blood sugar during surgery.[25-32] No matter which diabetic management protocol is selected, it is important to set clear guidelines (blood sugar ranges) and to monitor and document glucose levels frequently. Carefully planned procedures of short duration should be scheduled as early in the morning as possible. Early scheduling allows time to obtain a preprocedure blood sugar reading and complete the procedure. When fully recovered, the patient may receive the morning dose of insulin or oral hypoglycemic agent along with supplemental nutrition.

Disorders of the Thyroid Gland

The thyroid gland is responsible for regulation of the thyroid hormone. The thyroid gland responds to the pituitary gland's production of thyroid-stimulating hormone (TSH). Increased TSH results in an increase in thyroxine (T_4), which operates through a negative feedback loop. This negative feedback process decreases the release of TSH from the anterior pituitary gland. It is important to ascertain the status of thyroid function secondary to the thyroid hormone's function of regulating metabolic activity.

HYPERTHYROIDISM. Hyperthyroidism produces an increased basal metabolic rate (BMR) secondary to increased secretion of the thyroid hormone. Symptoms of hyperthyroidism include weight loss, heat intolerance, tachycardia, nervousness, tremors, and warm moist skin. This increase in thyroid hormone production may result from thyroiditis, adenoma, or dysfunction of the pituitary gland. Preprocedure management must focus on return of the patient to a euthyroid state. Procedures on a hyperthyroid patient should be postponed until the patient becomes euthyroid. It may take 2 to 6 weeks on propylthiouracil to decrease the synthesis and conversion of T_4 sufficiently to create a euthyroid state.[25]

Beta adrenergic antagonists may be prescribed to control tachycardia and hypertension. Additional treatment modalities for hyperthyroidism include gland removal or radioactive iodine. Preprocedure examination must assess the prescribed hyperthyroid treatment protocol, cardiovascular status, and the state of patient anxiety. During preprocedure assessment it is important to assess the size of the thyroid gland. Visual assessment of gland size is recommended because frequent manual palpation of the gland releases thyroxine into the bloodstream. The T_4 produces an increase in basal metabolic rate, heart rate, and blood pressure. Additional considerations related to the enlarged thyroid gland include difficult airway management because of increased tissue mass. Because of the increased basal metabolic rate, the pharmacologic effects of intravenous sedatives and analgesics may be reduced in the presence of hyperthyroidism.

HYPOTHYROIDISM. Hypothyroidism results from insufficient circulating thyroid hormone. Symptoms of hypothyroidism include intolerance to cold, bradycardia, cardiomegaly, dry skin, hair loss, fatigue, congestive heart failure, decreased mentation, and periorbital edema. Causes of hypothyroidism include surgical ablation, pituitary or hyperthalamic dysfunction, or decreased hormonal biosynthesis. Diagnosis of hypothyroidism includes decreased T_4 and increased TSH on a preprocedure thyroid serum panel. Treatment of hypothyroidism consists of supplemental thyroid medication. Exogenous T_4 requires 10 days for physiologic effect, whereas triiodothyronine (T_3) exerts physiologic effects in 6 hours.[23] Levothyroxine is often used as an exogenous replacement because of its long half-life and its ability to produce consistent plasma T_4 levels.

Hypothyroid patients generally have a marked sensitivity to intravenous sedatives, analgesics, and hypnotics. Hypothyroidism also reduces the ventilatory response to $Paco_2$ and Pao_2. This marked sensitivity requires a critical reduction in the dose of intravenous conscious sedation medications. Careful titration of sedatives, analgesics, or hypnotics is required, as even markedly reduced doses have resulted in profound central nervous system and respiratory depression. Patients with hypothyroidism may also have large tongues. This increase in tissue mass coupled with the marked sensitivity to pharmacologic medications requires careful attention to airway management. Upper airway obstruction is not tolerated in this patient population and airway obstruction requires immediate intervention.

DISEASES OF THE ADRENAL CORTEX

The adrenal cortex produces glucocorticosteroids, mineralocorticosteroids, and androgens. These hormones are under the control of the anterior pituitary gland through the secretion of adrenocorticotropic hormone (ACTH). Adrenal cortical disease may occur from decreased or increased production of these hormones. The following conditions may be encountered on preprocedure assessment of the patient presenting for intravenous conscious sedation.

Glucocorticoid Overproduction: Cushing's Disease

Glucocorticoid steroids regulate protein, carbohydrate, and nucleic acid metabolism. Under normal conditions, approximately 20 to 30 mg of cortisol is produced each day. Cortisol production is significantly increased in the presence of stress, infection, and anxiety. In the face of surgery or diagnostic procedures, the adrenal gland may produce 75 to 150 mg/d.[34] During periods of extreme stress, the adrenal gland secretes 200 to 500 mg/d. Cushing's disease may be caused by increased production of ACTH, malignant tumors, or iatrogenic overtreatment with exogenous steroids. Glucocorticoid steroids also antagonize the effects of antidiuretic hormone (ADH). As result of excess cortisol production, the symptoms of Cushing's disease include the following:

- Hypertension
- Hyperglycemia
- Polyuria
- Osteoporosis
- Hypokalemia
- Truncal obesity
- Moon face
- Skin striations
- Hypovolemia

Preprocedure preparation of the patient with Cushing's disease must focus on correction of fluid and electrolyte abnormalities, treatment of hypertension, and regulation of blood sugar prior to the anticipated procedure.

Decreased Cortisol Production: Addison's Disease

Decreased cortisol production may result from hemorrhagic destruction of the adrenal cortical cells, carcinoma, or adrenal cortical suppression secondary to use of exogenous steroids. Use of exogenous steroids to treat asthma, allergy, or associated inflammatory conditions leads to adrenal cortisol suppression. The administration of exogenous steroids on a short-term basis of a 7- to 10-day treatment protocol decreases cortisol-releasing hormone and ACTH release. This decreased hormone release generally returns to normal within several days after cessation of exogenous steroid therapy. However, long-term exogenous steroid supplementation in the presence of inflammatory bowel disease, asthma, and associated inflammatory conditions of more than 10 days' duration may result in adrenocorticol insufficiency. The presenting symptoms may mimic hypovolemic shock. Additional symptoms associated with adrenal insufficiency include hypovolemia, hypoglycemia, nausea, vomiting, hypotension, and hemoconcentration. The use of supplemental exogenous steroids has been advocated to prevent intraoperative adrenal crisis. There are limited numbers of documented cases of acute adrenal crisis in the anesthesia literature. However, because of the significant morbidity and mortality associated with adrenal crisis and the minimal side effects associated with exogenous steroid supplementation, many authors advocate the use of exogenous steroid supplementation to prevent the development of adrenal insufficiency. Preprocedure steroid replacement is based on the *degree of stress and the magnitude of the procedure.* Preprocedure steroid coverage may range from no additional exogenous steroids for minor surgical procedures to 200 to 300 mg/70 kg for major surgical or diagnostic procedures.

Mineralocorticosteroid Production

CONN'S SYNDROME. Conn's syndrome results from excess production of mineralocorticosteroids. Mineralocorticosteroids regulate extracellular fluid volume and potassium balance. Increased mineralocorticosteroid production may result from adenomas or adrenal hyperplasia. Symptoms associated with hyperaldosteronism include hypokalemia, hyponatremia, muscle weakness, hypertension, tetany, and polyuria. Hypokalemia is responsible for the kidney's inability to concentrate urine, polyuria, and muscle weakness associated with Conn's syndrome. Preprocedure preparation of the patient with Conn's disease includes replacement of potassium, administration of antihypertensive agents, and correction of fluid volume status. Preprocedure serum electrolytes are also warranted.

HYPOALDOSTERONISM. Hypoaldosteronism results in hyperkalemia, with resultant heart block, cardiac conduction defects, hyponatremia, and hypotension. Causes of decreased aldosterone secretion include diabetes, renal failure, and adrenalectomy. Preprocedure treatment of decreased aldosterone secretion includes return of the patient to a eukalemic state, liberal fluid and sodium intake, and administration of exogenous mineralocorticosteroids (fludrocortisone).

Pheochromocytoma

Catecholamine-secreting tumors located in the adrenal medulla or chromaffin tissue are termed *pheochromocytomas*. Additional sites of catecholamine-secreting tumors include the spleen, ovary, bladder, and right atria. Symptoms associated with pheochromocytoma are related to an increase in catecholamine release. Classic symptoms include palpitations, headache, weight loss, diaphoresis, hypertension, flushing, and hyperglycemia. Confirmative diagnosis of pheochromocytoma is made after a 24-hour urine collection reveals excess free norepinephrine levels. The combination of diaphoresis, tachycardia, and headache, particularly in young to middle-aged patients, is highly suggestive of the presence of pheochromocytoma. The presence of pheochromocytoma requires additional consultation concerning surgical excision of the catecholamine-producing tumor prior to additional diagnostic or minor surgical procedures. Before the procedure, antihypertensive treatment with alpha blockers is required to promote vasodilatation and restore blood volume. Phenoxybenzamine (Dibenzyline) or phentolamine (Regitine) may be given to counteract the alpha effects (peripheral vasoconstriction) associated with the increased release of catecholamines. Cardiac arrhythmias may be controlled with beta blockers. Correction of hypertension with a return of controlled heart rate facilitates a return of volume status. Seventy-five percent of patients who undergo surgical removal of the tumor return to baseline blood pressure within 10 days.[35] Patients presenting for intravenous conscious sedation procedures should be past this window period for stabilization of hemodynamic parameters before additional diagnostic procedures commence.

GASTROINTESTINAL ASSESSMENT

Gastrointestinal assessment includes not only evaluation for obesity but also the following conditions:

- Nausea
- Vomiting
- Diarrhea
- Gastrointestinal (GI) bleeding
- Gastric reflux

The presence of persistent nausea, vomiting, or diarrhea predisposes the patient to electrolyte abnormalities. Correction of electrolyte status and fluid volume is required before the administration of intravenous conscious sedation is initiated. Dryness of mucous membranes, decreased skin turgor, and a large, swollen tongue may indicate significant hypovolemia. Hematocrit, serum osmolality, blood urea nitrogen level, electrolyte profile, and urine output are indicators to quantify volume deficit. Anemia secondary to diarrhea, nausea, vomiting, or GI bleeding requires careful assessment of hemoglobin and hematocrit. Risks and benefits of transfusion must be examined before the procedure. Severe diarrhea

TABLE 2–11.   *H₂ Antagonist and Gastrokinetic Agent Dosage Schedule*

MEDICATION	DOSAGE	HALF-LIFE (h)	ONSET OF ACTION (min)	DURATION OF ACTION (h)
H₂ ANTAGONIST				
Cimetidine	300 mg hs and 75 min before the procedure	2	45–60	3–4
Ranitidine	150 mg PO hs and 1–1½ h before the procedure	2½–3	60–90	8–9
Famotidine	20 mg PO 1–1½ h before the procedure	2½–3½	60	10–12
GASTROKINETIC AGENT				
Metoclopramide*	10 mg PO	2–4	30–60	
	0.15 mg/kg IV over 3–5 min	2–4	1–3	1–2

*Action: dopamine antagonist that stimulates upper gastrointestinal motility and gastric emptying and increases gastroesophageal sphincter tone.

results in the excretion of large amounts of water, sodium, and potassium through the colon. In severe cases, shock and cardiovascular compromise may occur. Emergent colonoscopy or endoscopic examination raises several concerns. Bleeding into the stomach or upper GI tract increases gastric volume and the incidence of regurgitation. Anemia and decreased oxygen-carrying capacity of the hemoglobin molecule also increase the risk of hypoxemia. Preprocedure assessment of GI bleeding must focus on restoration of blood volume, supplemental oxygenation, and light sedation.

H₂ ANTAGONISTS

Patients with a history of pregnancy, recent opioid ingestion, diabetes, pain, abdominal distention, gastric acid reflux, hiatal hernia, or obesity may benefit from the administration of an H₂ (histamine) blocker such as cimetidine, ranitidine, or famotidine to increase gastric pH.[36] An H₂ dosage schedule is presented in Table 2–11.

ANESTHESIA AND SURGICAL HISTORY

Preprocedure assessment of the patient's anesthesia and surgical history must ascertain patient recollection of past anesthetics, surgical procedures, and complications related to these procedures. Since medical records and charts may not be readily available from other institutions or physician offices, it is important to obtain an accurate surgical and anesthesia history. Questions related to anesthetic and surgical history may be stated: "What operations have you had in the past?" "Do you recall what type of anesthesia you had?" This question is generally answered with "I went to sleep" or "They knocked me out." It is important to consider the amnestic effects of the benzodiazepines and sedatives used in the operating room. Many patients are under the impression that they received a general anesthetic when in essence they received a local anesthetic with sedation or a regional anesthetic with sedation and monitoring. On solicitation of information concerning past anesthesia and surgical procedures, a sufficient amount of time must be allotted for the patient to answer the question: "Do you recall any anesthesia complications associated with these procedures?" Additional questioning related to past surgery and anesthesia include: "Has anyone in your family ever had any anesthesia complications?" An initial response to this question may be an immediate, "No." However, with some prompting, patients may recall a negative past anesthetic experience. This prompting includes: "Have you ever had nausea or vomiting after any past surgical or diagnostic procedures or been admitted to the intensive care unit unexpectedly?" Positive responses must be followed up with contact with physician offices, hospitals, or surgicenters to ascertain specific complications associated with prior surgical or diagnostic procedures. If previous anesthesia records are secured for review, the following items should be documented:

- Response to preoperative sedative medications
- Verification of ease of airway management
- Vascular access
- Intraoperative complications
- Drug reactions
- Hemodynamic parameters
- Documented postoperative complications

MEDICATION EVALUATION

The purpose of the preprocedure evaluation is to decrease morbidity and optimize the patient's condition before the proposed procedure. After organ system assessment, it is important to identify currently prescribed medications and therapeutic rationale. A medication review during preprocedure assessment includes asking the patient, "What medications are you currently taking?" This question allows the patient to answer with prescription and over-the-counter medications they may be using.

When one is questioning the patient about medications, it is important to evaluate and ascertain drug dosage and last dose administered. Once the medication history is complete, it is important to give the patient accurate preprocedure instructions related to medication. An example of this includes the continuation of antihypertensive medications up to and including the morning of the procedure to promote cardiovascular stability. When indicated, aspirin and nonsteroidal anti-inflammatory drugs should be discontinued secondary to bleeding potential associated with platelet dysfunction. Rarely, a patient may indicate uncertainty regarding which medication he or she is taking or report taking "two little white pills and a red pill." It is important to ascertain the name, dosage, and last ingestion of these medications. This may be accomplished after questioning a family member or a significant other. If the patient or family member cannot identify a medication, it may be necessary to contact the prescribing physician or the physician's office staff for confirmation of the prescribed treatment protocol. During the preprocedure assessment, it is important for the clinician to ascertain not only which medications the patient is taking but also the patient's compliance with the prescribed treatment protocol and the efficacy of treatment.

ALLERGIES

A continuation of preprocedure medication assessment includes the patient's allergy history. Questions related to an allergy history include "Are you allergic to any medication?" At this point, many patients respond with "No" or with a list of several allergies. Allergies reported may include nausea associated with the use of analgesics or gastrointestinal upset with the use of antibiotics. The side effects associated with the use of pharmacologic agents are separate and distinct from an allergic reaction. Side effects may be classified as unpleasant reactions or adverse reactions to prescribed drugs. True allergies to pharmacologic agents occur with less frequency and are manifested by the following conditions:

- Bronchospasm
- Circulatory collapse
- Edema
- Hives
- Hypotension
- Pruritus
- Skin wheals
- Wheezing

Fortunately, true allergic reactions are rare and the patient's recollection may be insufficient. Many patients may recall rashes and hives, and yet few may recall the development of cardiovascular collapse. This information must be elicited from patient recollection, review of a previous chart, or observation of the patient after a medication has been administered.

ANAPHYLACTIC VS. ANAPHYLACTOID

Anaphylaxis refers to a life-threatening drug reaction of a severe magnitude. Anaphylactic drug reactions are mediated via the IgE immunoglobulin within the immune system. Therefore anaphylactic reactions are life-threatening drug reactions mediated by antibodies. The term *anaphylactoid* is used when there is no antibody involvement in the reaction.[37] Differentiation of anaphylactic vs. anaphylactoid reaction during the administration of medications or during the procedure is not important. What is important is the *identification* of an allergic response. Presenting symptoms of allergic reaction include urticaria, hypotension, oropharyngeal edema, hives, wheezing, bronchoconstriction, and cardiovascular compromise requiring immediate diagnosis and treatment. The treatment protocol of allergic reaction is listed in Table 2–12.

TABLE 2–12. *Treatment of Allergic Reactions*

• Preparation	• Epinephrine (In the presence of CV col-
• Discontinue suspected allergen	lapse)
• Airway maintenance	• Diphenhydramine
• Intravenous volume (Several liters	• Terbutaline
[20 ml/kg] may be required if there is	• Aminophylline
massive vasodilatation)	• Corticosteroids

Preprocedure assessment of the patient with multiple allergies or documentation of a true anaphylactic or anaphylactoid reaction requires careful preparation and planning before the administration of intravenous conscious sedation. The initial step in the prevention of an allergic reaction includes identification of the allergen. It may be difficult to identify an allergen in the patient's history or previous anesthetic records. When antibiotics, local anesthetics, sedatives, hypnotics, and analgesics have been combined and administered, it may be extremely difficult to specify which medication precipitated the allergic response. Allergy testing may not be conclusive or may not have been conducted. Preprocedure assessment of the patient with a suspected allergy to benzodiazepines may require the administration of a hypnotic (propofol) or a barbiturate substitute (thiopental [Pentothal] or methohexital) to achieve the desired sedative effects. A true IgE-mediated allergy to narcotics is rare. In the case of this rare phenomenon, the new nonsteroidal analgesic ketorolac may offer the clinician an analgesic alternative without the need for narcotic adjuncts. Allergic reactions secondary to contrast media are discussed in Chapter 10. A complete latex allergy protocol is featured in Appendix C.

REVIEW OF LABORATORY DATA

The current state of healthcare reimbursement dictates conscientious, efficient preprocedure laboratory testing and screening. In the past, laboratory or diagnostic testing was reimbursed on a fee-for-service basis. As reimbursement continues to evolve into a capitated system, the clinician must focus on specific laboratory or diagnostic tests that yield beneficial information about the patient.[38] Achievement of these goals in a cost-effective way is a challenge in a capitated healthcare system. Random laboratory testing in the absence of suspicious clinical features or symptoms is not only expensive, it is time consuming and inconvenient for the patient. It is important to use these preprocedure assessment tools in an efficacious manner to avoid expensive office, surgicenter, or hospital delays on the day of the procedure. To have diagnostic testing yield beneficial information, it is important to conduct a thorough patient history and physical examination before considering which laboratory tests to order. After completion of a thorough chart review, history, and physical examination, determining factors for laboratory testing include the following:

- Patient age
- Specific disease state

- Magnitude of planned procedure
- Medication history
- Degree of pathophysiologic state

Although there are no clear-cut guidelines for required laboratory testing, an additional benefit of preprocedure testing is that it yields baseline comparison in addition to revealing important quantitative data. Therefore the goals of preprocedure laboratory testing are to identify underlying pathophysiologic disease conditions, confirm the presence and degree of specific disease states, and complement the preprocedure process in its goal to decrease morbidity and mortality. Preprocedure testing indications listed in Table 2–13 are dependent on the severity of the disease state, symptoms, and magnitude of the planned procedure.

As the practice of quality patient care continues to be the provider's goal, the judicious ordering of laboratory and diagnostic testing yields additional clinical data. These data should be used to prevent intraprocedure complications, decrease morbidity and mortality, and reduce preprocedural delays. On the basis of the broad variety of surgical and diagnostic procedures that may be performed

TABLE 2–13. *Preprocedure Testing Indications*

ECG
- Angina
- Age: males greater than 40 years; females greater than 50 years
- CHF
- Cigarette smoking greater than 20 pack years
- Coronary artery disease
- Diabetes
- Electrolyte abnormality
- Heart murmur
- History of myocardial infarction
- History of rheumatic heart disease
- History of palpitations or arrthymia
- Hypertension
- Malignancy
- Obesity
- Pulmonary disease
- Shortness of breath with minimal exertion

CHEST X-RAY
- Blood-tinged or colored sputum
- Cigarette smoking greater than 20 pack years
- Exposure to tuberculosis
- History of CHF
- Malignancy
- Presence of cardiovascular disease

- Productive cough
- Pulmonary infection
- Sudden change in pulmonary/cardiovascular symptoms

HEMOGLOBIN AND HEMATOCRIT
- Age greater than 40
- History of blood dyscrasia
- History of malignancy
- Menstruating females
- Recent blood donor (within 1 month)
- Recent surgery or trauma
- Renal disease

ELECTROLYTES
- Diabetes
- Renal disease
- Utilization of medications:
  – Digoxin
  – Diuretics
  – Steroids

LIVER FUNCTION TESTS
- Alcohol abuse
- Black stools or change in bowel habits
- Bleeding disorder
- Coffee ground emesis
- Drug abuse
- Jaundice
- Recent weight loss

TABLE 2-14. *Summary of Preprocedure Test Recommendations*

Age	Asymptomatic Individuals		Individuals Not Receiving General or Major Conduction Anesthesia	
	Men	Women	Sedative Hypnotics for Monitored Anesthesia	Peripheral or IV Nerve Block
6 mo–40 yr	None	Hematocrit ? Pregnancy test	None	None
40–50 yr	Electrocardiogram	Hematocrit ? Pregnancy test	None	None
50–64 yr	Electrocardiogram	? Hematocrit ? Pregnancy test Electrocardiogram	Hematocrit (within 6 mo)	None
65–74 yr	Hemoglobin or hematocrit Electrocardiogram BUN Glucose	Hemoglobin or hematocrit Electrocardiogram BUN Glucose	Hematocrit (within 6 mo) Electrocardiogram (within 1 yr)	Hematocrit (within 6 mo)
>74 yr	Hemoglobin/hematocrit Electrocardiogram BUN Glucose ? Chest x-ray	Hemoglobin/hematocrit Electrocardiogram BUN Glucose ? Chest x-ray	Hematocrit (within 6 mo) Electrocardiogram (within 1 yr) BUN (within 6 mo) Glucose (within 6 mo)	Hematocrit (within 6 mo) Electrocardiogram (within 1 yr)

From Roizen M. *What Is Necessary for Preoperative Patient Assessment?* Philadelphia: Lippincott Raven Publishers: American Society of Anesthesiologists; 1995: Chap. 15, vol. 23, p. 92.

with intravenous conscious sedation, the clinician must decide which laboratory testing is required for the specific patient population. Roizen recently published guidelines for non-blood-loss peripheral diagnostic procedures for symptom-free, healthy patients (Table 2–14). These recommendations may prove beneficial for the attending physician ordering preprocedure laboratory and diagnostic testing.

DENTITION

Preprocedure assessment of dentition includes inquiry and visual examination of the oral cavity. The status of the dentition should be documented for loose, chipped, cracked, or missing teeth. Thorough documentation is beneficial if postprocedure patient claims of loose or missing teeth arise after specific procedures. Medial or lateral chipping should be documented before the procedure. Additional anomalies should be noted, as well as identification of specific dental sites. See Figure 2–2 for an oral cavity evaluation table.

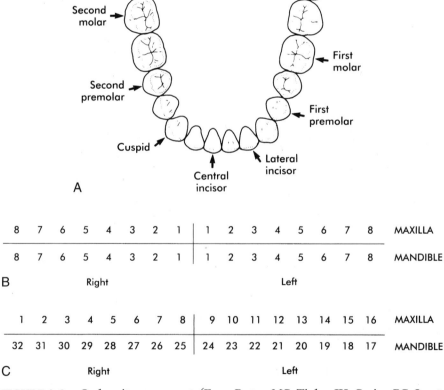

FIGURE 2–2. Oral cavity assessment. (From Rogers MC, Tinker JH, Covino BG, Longnecker DE. *Principles and Practice of Anesthesiology.* St. Louis: Mosby–Year Book; 1993: 2522.)

SOCIAL HISTORY

During preprocedure assessment it is important to obtain a social history from the patient. Components of the social history include cigarette smoking, alcohol intake, illicit drug use, and the possibility of pregnancy. When inquiring into a patient's alcohol, drug, or sexual history, it is best to approach this material via a matter-of-fact approach. Any attempts to belittle or pressure the patient will result in patient withdrawal and, most likely, an inaccurate social history. A variety of mechanisms may be used to solicit this information in a diplomatic and tactful manner.

CIGARETTE SMOKING

A cigarette smoking history must be quantified in pack years and documented on the preprocedure assessment form.

Pack years = Number of packs smoked per day × Number of years smoked

Cigarette smoking increases airway irritability, decreases mucociliary transport, and increases secretions. Patients scheduled for conscious sedation procedures should be counseled to consider cessation of smoking before the procedure. Patients who stop smoking demonstrate a decrease in their level of carboxyhemoglobin and an increase in tissue oxygenation. Several reports in the literature document the length of time required for smoking cessation to yield beneficial cardiopulmonary benefits.[39-40]

DRUG ABUSE—ALCOHOL INTAKE

Textbook questions to solicit alcohol intake include: "Have you ever had a drinking problem?" or "Have you had any alcohol in the last 24 hours?" Aside from appearing abrupt, these questions are also close-ended. When posing these particular questions during preprocedure assessment, many clinicians use a broad lead-in approach. When asked, "How much alcohol do you consume in 1 week?" the patient can respond in a variety of ways: "I have wine with dinner every night," "None," "A couple of beers on the weekend," or "Two or three scotches every evening." These comments generally lead to further discussion of alcohol history and intake. Patients with rare social alcohol use afford minimal concern for multisystemic disease states. However, patients with a history of two or three drinks with lunch or dinner may require additional sedative medication during conscious sedation procedures secondary to increased cytochrome P-450 system activity. Chronic use of alcohol leads to stimulation of the cytochrome P-450 system located in the endoplasmic reticulum of the liver. This stimulation requires increased amounts or doses of sedative and analgesic medications. Chronic ingestion of alcohol is associated with multisystem symptoms. Patients with a history of chronic alcohol use require preprocedure preparation aimed at the presenting symptoms. Chronic alcoholism may lead to cirrhosis, elevated liver enzyme levels, esophageal varices, nutritional disorders, gastritis, psychiatric disorders, cardiac myopathy, electrolyte disturbances, and cerebral atrophy. These symptoms predispose patients to increased risks during the administration of intravenous conscious sedation. As opposed to chronic alcohol ingestion, a general rule of thumb when dealing with acute alcoholism is a decrease in anesthetic requirements. A full stomach and a lack of patient cooperation are also additional risk factors associated with acute alcohol intoxication. If morning preprocedure assessment reveals the odor of alcohol on the patient's breath, blood for determination of serum alcohol levels should be drawn immediately with the patient's permission. If the patient refuses or if the level is indicative of recent alcohol ingestion, the procedure should be canceled. Cancellation is warranted because of probable noncompliance with NPO instructions and the risks associated with increased gastric volume.

STIMULANT MEDICATIONS

Use of stimulants and weight-reduction medications may predispose the patient to cardiac arrythymias, including palpitations and tachycardia. Amphetamine abuse increases the release of catecholamines. Amphetamines may be used for patients with weight disorders, narcolepsy, and attention deficit disorder. Amphetamine abuse is generally via the oral route, but intravenous use is another route of administration. Chronic abuse of amphetamines leads to tolerance and psychotic states secondary to depleted body catecholamine stores. Dieting fads that result in significant weight reduction in short periods of time require additional laboratory data review. ECG, SMA chemistry, and complete blood cell count are required to assess electrolyte status and rule out the presence of cardiac conduction abnormalities before the administration of conscious sedation.

COCAINE ABUSE

It has been estimated that 30 million Americans have used cocaine and 5 million use it on a regular basis. Cocaine is a local anesthetic with vasoconstrictive properties. Its illicit use results in a euphoric sensation. Through its vasoconstricting properties, it leads to hypertension, myocardial ischemia, infarction, cerebral hemorrhage, and seizures. The effects of cocaine use are secondary to the decreased reuptake of norepinephrine into nerve endings for action on dopaminergic receptors. Cocaine is an addictive drug with serious life-threatening consequences. Preprocedure recommendations for the patient with acute cocaine ingestion include postponement of the procedure for 24 to 48 hours.[41] Complications associated with the procedure secondary to cocaine abuse include cardiac dysrhythmias, tachycardia, and increased myocardial oxygen consumption.

OPIOID ABUSE

Opioids are abused via the oral, subcutaneous, or intravenous routes of administration. Opioid ingestion produces a euphoric state with resultant analgesia. Tolerance of the effects of opioids occurs with chronic ingestion. Patients with a history of chronic opioid abuse generally require increased doses of sedative medications during intravenous conscious sedation.

BENZODIAZEPINES

Chronic use of benzodiazepines for skeletal muscle relaxation or as antianxiety medication leads to tolerance and addiction. The benzodiazepine-addicted patient will develop a cross-tolerance not only to benzodiazepine medications but to other sedative and analgesic medications as well.

MARIJUANA

The most common means of ingestion of marijuana is smoking. Smoking marijuana increases tetrahydrocannabinol. A postinhalation euphoric state in conjunction with sympathetic stimulation occurs. This increased sympathetic stimulation increases heart rate, myocardial oxygen consumption, and orthostatic hypotension in some persons. Patients with a history of chronic marijuana use characteristically present with the following symptoms:

- Chronic sinusitis
- Tar deposit in the lung
- Pulmonary impairment
- Conjunctival irritation

The effects of inhaled marijuana last only for several hours. Therefore it is rare to encounter patients who are acutely intoxicated secondary to marijuana ingestion. Patients who admit to marijuana ingestion should have resting heart rate and blood pressure documented before initiation of the procedure. To decrease the incidence of pulmonary complications, symptoms of pulmonary impairment should be resolved before the administration of intravenous conscious sedation.

It is important to approach patients with a history of substance abuse on the basis of the drug abused, the time of last ingestion, and presenting symptoms. Symptoms associated with drug abuse may be life threatening and include the following:

- Cellulitis
- Abscess of the skin
- Cardiomyopathy
- Psychotic behavior
- Aspiration with overdose
- Hepatitis
- Acquired immunodeficiency disease
- Sepsis
- Endocarditis

Counseling and social service support are important for this patient population. It is important to approach these patients individually and to realize that they have a disease of addiction, which requires specific treatment and therapy.

PREGNANCY

Female patients of childbearing age must be questioned regarding the possibility of pregnancy. This question may also be asked in a variety of ways. Some clinicians simply ask, "Is there any possibility that you are pregnant?" A simple "yes" or "no" answer seems to appease some practitioners. However, many providers are becoming more investigative and document the patient's last menstrual period and her denial of pregnancy. Some facilities go one step further and require all women of childbearing age to have a serum pregnancy test the morning of the diagnostic or surgical procedure. If a patient has a positive serum pregnancy test result, the planned procedure *should be canceled*. When diagnostic or minor surgical procedures must be conducted on the confirmed parturient, consultation with a member of the department of anesthesia is warranted.

Cardiovascular Effects of Pregnancy

The pregnant patient population presents the clinician with a variety of physiologic changes that may have an impact on the delivery of intravenous conscious sedation. These physiologic changes affect multiple organ systems, including cardiovascular, pulmonary, gastrointestinal, and hematologic systems. These effects are mediated through hormonal release associated with the pregnant state. Increased oxygen consumption, decreased vascular resistance, increased cardiac output, and increased blood volume are required to meet the metabolic demands of the mother and the fetus. In the second trimester, compression of the vena cava and aorta by the weight of the gravid uterus is a common finding. Decreased venous return of blood to the heart predisposes the mother to tachycardia, faintness, and ultimately fetal distress. Positioning of the pregnant patient during the second trimester and thereafter requires careful attention to avoid aortocaval compression. Methods to prevent compression of the aorta or vena cava include left uterine displacement. Placing the patient in the left lateral position or providing left uterine displacement with a towel pack or blanket placed under the right ischial spine takes the weight of the gravid uterus off of the great vessels and prevents obstruction of venous return and compression of the aorta.

Pulmonary Changes Associated With Pregnancy

Edema of the upper airway and mucous membranes occurs as a result of increased extracellular fluid volume and vascular engorgement. Great care must be taken to maintain a patent airway in this patient population. Epistaxis is a common complication associated with the insertion of nasal airways secondary to the friability of the mucous membrane. As the fetus develops and the uterus enlarges, functional residual capacity decreases, which predisposes the patient to hypoxemia.

Maternal Gastrointestinal Changes

Gastrointestinal changes associated with pregnancy include decreased gastrointestinal motility, decreased food absorption, increased gastric acidity, and decreased lower esophageal sphincter tone. These changes increase the incidence of gastric acid aspiration. If intravenous conscious sedation is required in the pregnant patient, great vigilance and care are required to avoid oversedation and the resultant risk of gastric acid aspiration, hypoxemia, or epistaxis when one attempts to secure an airway.

Anesthesic Management of the Parturient Patient

Objectives for the parturient patient who must receive sedation or anesthesia include the following:

- Avoidance of teratogenic medications
- Avoidance of fetal hypoxia
- Avoidance of premature labor
- Avoidance of fetal acidosis

In general, anomalies may result from the administration of anesthetic medications during organogenesis. The administration of diazepam during the first trimester has been associated with an increased incidence of cleft lip and palate.[42,43] With the numerous physiologic changes associated with pregnancy, pharmacologic implications, and potential airway compromise, it is advised that a member of the anesthesia staff be consulted to care for this specific patient population.

NPO STATUS

Aspiration of gastric contents may result in the development of Mendelson's syndrome, which was first described by Mendelson in 1946. This syndrome occurs in the presence of aspiration of gastric contents greater than 25 ml (0.4 ml/kg) with a pH less than 2.5. Sequelae associated with aspiration of gastric contents depend on the character and volume of the aspirate. Aspiration of solid particulate matter results in an anatomic, mechanical obstruction to gas flow. Aspiration of acidic gastric fluid results in chemical burning of the alveoli with severe ventilatory perfusion mismatch. Aspiration may occur during the administration of intravenous conscious sedation in patients who enter into a state of deep sedation with resultant loss of protective reflexes. Mechanisms to avoid aspiration include administration of H_2 blockers and the avoidance of deep sedation to maintain airway reflexes.

NPO INSTRUCTIONS

Nil per os (NPO) is the Latin term for "nothing by mouth." The NPO principle has been used by anesthesia clinicians and surgeons for years to decrease the risk of gastric acid aspiration. Historically, patients have been instructed to have nothing to eat or drink after midnight. The purpose of the cessation of solid and fluid intake was to assure an "empty" stomach with minimal gastric contents. The NPO phenomenon has been challenged over recent years. Several recent studies are forcing clinicians to revise and reconsider their NPO policy guidelines. Various studies that have led practitioners to reevaluate NPO guidelines lend support to the idea that clear liquids administered 2 to 3 hours before the scheduled procedures do not alter residual gastric volume when compared with the standard

NPO overnight fast.[44-48] Distinct advantages of the NPO policy revision cited by these authors include patient comfort and decreased incidence of hypoglycemia and hypovolemia. Additional studies demonstrate decreased gastric volume and increased pH when compared with standard overnight fasting regimens.[46,49] It should be noted that the majority of these studies used healthy patient control groups who were not identified as being at high risk of aspiration. Patients at risk of aspiration or patients with decreased gastric emptying were not included in many of these studies. However, the formal precedence of strict NPO policy is currently under revision in many institutions. Many practitioners currently allow ingestion of clear liquids up to 3 hours before the planned procedure. Some authors have claimed that the volume of gastric contents and pH did not differ between patients who had coffee with milk or tea and one slice of buttered toast on the morning of surgery and the fasting control group.[50] Simonson recently reported no fasting limitations on the day of surgery. Patients in an outpatient ophthalmic surgicenter were scheduled for conscious sedation with retrobulbar block. General anesthesia was not an option in this study if conscious sedation or the retrobulbar block failed.[51] The significance and importance of NPO guidelines associated with the administration of intravenous conscious sedation are based on varied patient response, total dose of drug administered, and the possibility of patients entering a state of deep sedation. Additional factors that decrease gastric emptying or increase the risk of pulmonary aspiration include the following:

- Delayed gastric emptying
- Diabetes
- Esophageal motility disorders
- Fear
- Obesity
- Opioids
- Pain
- Trauma

TABLE 2-15. *NPO Guidelines*

ADULT PATIENTS
1. NPO after midnight for all solid food
2. **Clear** liquids permitted up to 3 h before the scheduled procedure
3. Oral medications 1–2 h before scheduled surgery, with up to 150 ml of water*
4. An H_2 receptor antagonist should be considered for patients who may be at increased risk

PEDIATRIC PATIENTS
1. No solid foods for 8 h before surgery
2. Clear fluids ad lib up to 3 h before scheduled surgery
3. Clear fluids include glucose water, pulp-free fruit juices, water, or clear broth
4. No milk or breast milk is permitted

---

*Assumes absence of known risk factors.

Methods to reduce gastric volume include fasting, gastric suction, and administration of medications that increase gastrointestinal motility. Gastric suction is an impractical means of decreasing volume in patients presenting for conscious sedation. Use of the gastrokinetic drug metoclopramide combined with an H_2 antagonist effectively decreases gastric volume while increasing pH. When indicated, H_2 antagonists should be administered 1 to 2 hours before the planned procedure. To summarize, the adaptation and incorporation of specific NPO guidelines must be based on a sound rationale. As listed in Table 2–15, recommendations for NPO guidelines have been promulgated by experts in the field of anesthesiology.[51-53]

INFORMED CONSENT

An important risk-management strategy and legal requirement is to obtain informed consent before the administration of conscious sedation. Informed consent requires that the plan, alternatives, and potential complications be explained to the patient in layman's terms. The basis for informed consent stems from the fundamental principle that the patient has the right to exercise control over his or her body and over the treatment plan. Lack of properly obtained informed consent may result in charges of assault and battery. *Assault* is defined as the apprehension or anticipation of the application of unauthorized physical force. *Battery* is defined as the unconsented, unprivileged touching of another person.[54] A separate area on the consent form, which addresses the procedural risks, reasonable alternatives, and expected benefits associated with intravenous conscious sedation, is advised. An example of an appropriate informed consent form for conscious sedation is shown on page 58.

The legal concept of reasonable person is used in obtaining informed consent. The reasonable person doctrine centers on material risk. Material risk is one that the provider knows or ought to know would be significant to a reasonable person in the patient's position of deciding whether or not to submit to a particular medication or treatment procedure.[55] However, all conceivable risks do not require disclosure. Physician responsibility must assess disclosure of remote but devastating complications. In summary, informed consent is an understanding between two persons that incorporates an explanation of the proposed conscious sedation plan and an explanation of risks and alternatives in reasonable layman terms.

ASA RISK-CLASSIFICATION SYSTEM

Incorporation of a risk-classification system is a beneficial addition to the preprocedure assessment form. This physical classification system was developed in 1940 by a committee of the American Society of Anesthetists, currently the American Society of Anesthesiologists.[56] This system was developed to standardize physical status and assign a potential-risk classification. This physical classification system also offers the clinician a numerical summary assessment tool. The ASA Risk Classification is listed in Table 2–16.

Consent for the Administration of Conscious Sedation

I, _____, acknowledge that my doctor has explained that I will have an operation, diagnostic, or treatment procedure. Procedural risks and potential complications have been explained to me. I understand that intravenous conscious sedation is requested so that my doctor can perform the operation or diagnostic procedure. It has been explained to me that all forms of sedation and anesthesia involve some risks. I understand that no guarantees or promises can be made concerning the results of my procedure or sedation technique administered. Complications with intravenous conscious sedation can occur and include the possibility of infection, bleeding, drug reactions, injury to blood vessels, loss of sensation, paralysis, stroke, brain damage, heart attack, or death. I hereby consent to the administration of intravenous conscious sedation either by or under the direction of Doctor _____. Procedural risks, alternatives, and expected benefits have been explained to me in layman's terms, and I have had all questions answered.

_____   _____
Patient Signature   Witness

TABLE 2–16. *American Society of Anesthesiologists (ASA) Classification of Physical Status**

I. Normal, healthy patient with no systemic disease.
II. Mild to moderate systemic disease.
III. Severe systemic disease with functional limitation that is not incapacitating.
IV. Severe systemic disease that is incapacitating and life threatening.
V. A moribund patient not expected to survive 24 hours without surgical intervention.

*Based on the ASA Classification of Physical Status in the American Society of Anesthesiologists Risk Classification System. Reprinted with permission of the American Society of Anesthesiologists, 520 N. Northwest Highway, Park Ridge, Illinois 60068-2573.

PREPROCEDURE PATIENT INSTRUCTION

Preprocedure patient instruction must provide detailed patient-specific instruction pertinent to the planned procedure. Examples of specific instruction include the following:

- NPO
- Time of arrival
- Estimated procedure time
- Presence of a responsible adult for discharge
- Procedure-specific guidelines
  - Bowel preparation
  - Prophylactic antibiotics
  - Dye preparations
  - Loose-fitting clothing

NPO

When instructing patients concerning NPO guidelines, it is important to tell them that they are to have nothing to eat or *drink* after a specific time. A study in *Anaesthesia* reported that only 28% of patients receiving NPO instructions believed that these instructions pertained only to food and not to water.[57] Therefore, when instructing patients regarding NPO status, the clinician must also specify no food, water, juice, coffee, etc. Preoperative oral medications ordered for the morning of the procedure may be taken with 2 to 3 ounces of water. It may be necessary to quantify this amount with the patient to avoid ingestion of large amounts of water.

TIME OF ARRIVAL

Patients should be instructed to arrive at the office or procedure unit at a mutually agreed-upon time. Sufficient time must be allotted to properly register the patient, obtain baseline vital signs, and prepare the patient for the planned diagnostic examination or procedure. When these preprocedure duties are performed in an unhurried atmosphere, the patient's anxiety is decreased through reassurance and proper preparation.

RESPONSIBLE ADULT

Patients must be instructed to arrange for a competent adult to accompany them home. Early notification of this requirement allows the patient time to make arrangements for transportation and recovery at home. *It is not acceptable to discharge a conscious sedation patient to home by taxi.* A responsible adult who will assume postprocedure care and instructions on behalf of the patient must be present.

PROCEDURE-SPECIFIC GUIDELINES

Procedure-specific guidelines (i.e., bowel preparations, prophylactic antibiotics, or dye preparations) must be clearly outlined before the procedure. Written instructions are extremely helpful for many patients and eliminate numerous telephone calls requesting reiteration of preprocedure instructions.

SUMMARY

Patients presenting for diagnostic and minor surgical procedures may have an inherent fear associated with the planned procedure or medications that will be used during the procedure. Preprocedure fears may include the diagnosis of carcinoma, confusion, nausea, vomiting, management of postoperative pain, and in some cases death. During preprocedure assessment the clinician must

- Conduct the interview in an unhurried manner
- Use an organized interview format
- Reassure the patient

Through the mechanisms outlined, the clinician will reassure the patient and achieve the goals of preprocedure assessment. A sincere interest in the patient's procedure and treatment plan decreases patient anxiety.[58,59] When conducted appropriately, preprocedure assessment is a useful mechanism to build a trusting patient-clinician relationship.

REFERENCES

1. Larson P. Evaluation of the patient and preoperative preparation. In: Barash P, Cullen B, Stoelting R. *Clinical Anesthesia.* 2nd ed. Philadelphia: JB Lippincott; 1992:550.
2. Report of the Joint National Committee on Detection, Evaluation and Treatment of High Blood Pressure. *Arch Intern Med.* 1984;144:1045.
3. Tarhan S, Moffitt EA, Taylor WF, Guilani ER. Myocardial infarction after general anesthesia. *JAMA.* 1972;220:1451.
4. Steen PA, Tinker JH, Tarhan S. Myocardial reinfarction after anesthesia and surgery. *JAMA.* 1978;239:2566.
5. Larson P. Evaluation of the patient and preoperative preparation. In: Barash P, Cullen B, Stoelting R. *Clinical Anesthesia.* 2nd ed. Philadelphia: JB Lippincott; 1992:551.
6. Shah KB. Re-evaluation of perioperative myocardial infarction in patients with prior myocardial infarction undergoing noncardiac operations. *Anesth Analg.* 1990;71:231–235.
7. Goldsmith MF. Implanted defibrillators slash sudden death rate in study, thousands more may get them in the future. *JAMA.* 1991;266:3400.
8. Vandam L. *To Make the Patient Ready for Anesthesia.* Addison-Wesley Publishing; 1984:29.
9. Guyton A. *Textbook of Medical Physiology.* 9th ed. Philadelphia: WB Saunders; 1996.
10. Kleinknecht D, Ganeval D, Gonzalez-Duque LA, et al. Furosemide in acute oliguric renal failure: a controlled trial. *Nephron.* 1976;17:51.
11. Siegel DC, Cochin A, Geocaris T, et al. Effects of saline and colloid resuscitation on renal function. *Ann Surg.* 1971;177:51.
12. Hanley MJ, Davidson K. Prior mannitol and furosemide infusion in a mode of ischemic acute renal failure. *Am J Physiol.* 1981;241:556.
13. Davis RF, Lappas DG, Kirklin JK, et al. Acute oliguria after cardiopulmonary bypass: renal functional improvement with low-dose dopamine infusion. *Crit Care Med.* 1982; 10:852.

14. Polson RJ, Park GR, Lindop MJ, et al. The prevention of renal impairment in patients undergoing orthotopic liver grafting by infusion of low dose dopamine. *Anaesthesia.* 1987;42:15.
15. Paul MD, Mazer CD, Byrick RJ, et al. Influence of mannitol and dopamine on renal function during elective infrarenal aortic clamping in man. *Am J Nephrol.* 1986;6:427.
16. Crowley K, Clarkson K, Hannon V, et al. Diuretics after transurethral prostatectomy: a double-blind controlled trial comparing furosemide and mannitol. *Br J Anaesth.* 1990;65:337.
17. Bennett WM, Aronoff GR, Golper TA, et al. Drug prescribing in renal failure. In: *Dosing Guidelines for Adults.* 2nd ed. Philadelphia: American College of Physicians; 1991.
18. *The Medical Letter on Drugs and Therapeutics Handbook on Antimicrobial Therapy.* New Rochelle, NY: The Medical Letter; 1992.
19. Miller R. *Anesthesia.* 4th ed. New York: Churchill Livingstone; 1994.
20. Drugs for epilepsy. *Med Letter Drugs Ther.* 1989;31:1.
21. Montouris GD, Fenichel GM, McLain LW Jr. The pregnant epileptic: a review and recommendations. *Arch Neurol.* 1979;36:601.
22. Shaner DM, McCurdy SA, Herring MO, et al. Treatment of status epilepticus: a prospective comparison of diazepam and phenytoin vs phenobarbital and optional phenytoin. *Neurology.* 1988;38:202.
23. Morgan E, Mikhail M. *Clinical Anesthesiology.* 2nd ed. Stamford, Conn: Appleton & Lange; 1996:565.
24. Davidson J, Eckhardt W, Perese D. *Clinical Anesthesia Procedures of the Massachusetts General Hospital.* 4th ed. Boston: The Hospital; 1993:71.
25. Walts LF, Miller, Davidson MB, et al. Perioperative management of diabetes mellitus. *Anesthesiology.* 1981;55:104.
26. Peterson L, Caldwell J, Hoffman J. Insulin absorbance to poly-vinyl chloride surfaces with implications for constant infusion therapy. *Diabetes.* 1976;25:72.
27. Meyer EJ, Lorenzi M, Bohannon NV, et al. Diabetic management by insulin infusion during major surgery. *Am J Surg.* 1979;137:323.
28. Walsh DB, Eckhauser FE, Ramsburgh SR, et al. Risk associated with diabetes mellitus in patients undergoing gallbladder surgery. *Surgery.* 1982;91:254.
29. Fowkes FGR, Lunn JN, Farrow SC, et al. Epidemiology in anesthesia. III. Mortality risk in patients with coexisting physical disease. *Br J Anaesth.* 1982;54:819.
30. Douglas JS, King SB, Craver JM, et al. Factors influencing risk and benefit of coronary bypass surgery in patients with diabetes mellitus. *Chest.* 1981;80:369.
31. Hjortrup A, Rasmussen BF, Kehlet H. Morbidity in diabetic and nondiabetic patients after major vascular surgery. *Br Med J.* 1983;287:1107.
32. Ransohoff DF, Miller GL, Forsythe SB, Hermann RE. Outcome of acute cholecystitis in patients with diabetes mellitus. *Ann Intern Med.* 1987;106:829.
33. Barash P, Cullen B, Stoelting R. *Clinical Anesthesia.* 2nd ed. Philadelphia: JB Lippincott; 1992:553.
34. Duke J, Rosenberg S. *Anesthesia Secrets.* Philadelphia: Mosby; 1996:337.
35. Jovenich JJ. Anesthesia in adrenal surgery. *Urol Clin North Am.* 1989;16:583.
36. Dubin SA, Silverstein PI, Wakefield ML, et al. Famotidine, a new H2 receptor antagonist. *Anesth Analg.* 1989;68:321.
37. Watkins J. Anaphylactoid reactions to IV substances. *Br J Anaesth.* 1979;51:51.
38. Roizen, MF. Cost effective laboratory testing. *JAMA.* 1994;271:319.
39. Robinson K, Conroy RM, Mulcahy R. When does the risk of acute coronary heart disease in ex-smokers fall to that in non-smokers? *Br Heart J.* 1989;62:16.

40. Rosenberg L, Kaufman D, Helmrich S, Shapiro S. The risk of myocardial infarction after quitting smoking in men under 55 years of age. *N Engl J Med.* 1985;313:1511.

41. Bernard C. Personal Communication (Letter), December, 1996.

42. Saxen I, Saxen L. Association between intake of diazepam and oral clefts. *Lancet.* 1975;2:498.

43. Safra MJ, Oakley GP. Association between cleft lip with or without cleft palate and prenatal exposure to diazepam. *Lancet.* 1975;2:478.

44. Sandhar BK, Goresky GV, Maltby JR, Shaffer EA. Effect of oral liquids and ranitidine on gastric fluid volume and pH in children undergoing outpatient surgery. *Anesthesiology.* 1989;71:327.

45. Splinter WM, Schaefer JD, Zunder IH. Clear fluids three hours before surgery do not affect the gastric fluid contents of children. *Can J Anaesth.* 1990;37:498.

46. Meakin G, Dingwall AE, Addison GM. Effects of fasting and oral premedication on the pH and volume of gastric aspirate in children. *Br J Anaesth.* 1987;59:678.

47. Splinter WM, Schaefer JD. Ingestion of clear fluids is safe for adolescents up to 3 h before anaesthesia. *Br J Anaesth.* 1991;66:48.

48. Splinter WM, Steward JA, Muir JG. The effect of preoperative apple juice on gastric contents, thirst and hunger in children. *Can J Anaesth.* 1989;36:55.

49. Gray J, Santerrel L, Gaudreau HP, et al. Effects of oral cimetidine and ranitidine on gastric pH and residual volume in children. *Anesthesiology.* 1989;71:547.

50. Miller M, Wishart HY, Nimmo WS. Gastric contents at induction of anesthesia: is a 4 hour fast necessary? *Br J Anaesth.* 1983;55:1185.

51. Maziarski FT, Simonson D. NPO status prior to surgery: two different approaches. *CRNA: The Clinical Forum for Nurse Anesthetists.* 1994;5:59.

52. Maltby JR. New guidelines for preoperative fasting. *Can J Anaesth.* 1993;40:R113.

53. Stoelting RK. "NPO" and aspiration pneumonitis: changing perspectives. 40th Annual Refresher Course Lectures and Clinical Update Program. 1995. Lecture No. 432.

54. Scott R. *Legal Aspects of Documenting Patient Care.* Gainesville, Md: Aspen Publications; 1994.

55. Dornette W. *Legal Issues in Anesthesia Practice.* Philadelphia: FA Davis; 1991.

56. Barash P, Cullen B, Stoelting R. *Clinical Anesthesia.* 2nd ed. Philadelphia: JB Lippincott; 1992.

57. Hume MA, Kennedy B, Asbury AJ. Patient knowledge of anaesthesia and perioperative care. *Anaesthesia.* 1994;49:715.

58. Egbert LD, Battit GE, Turndorf H, Beecher HK. The value of the preoperative visit by an anesthetist. *JAMA.* 1963;185:553.

59. Leigh JM, Walker J, Janaganathan P. Effect of preoperative anaesthetic visit on anxiety. *Br Med J.* 1977;2:987.

Procedural Care of the Patient During Conscious Sedation

PART II

Pharmacologic Concepts

CHAPTER
3

As registered nurses prepare patients for the administration of conscious sedation, a working knowledge of the pharmacologic adjuncts used to accomplish
amnesia, analgesia, and hypnosis is required. Basic pharmacologic principles are
presented in this chapter, with an overview of pharmacodynamics and pharmacokinetics. Specific properties of pharmacologic agents used for conscious sedation is presented in Chapter 5. It is important for clinicians engaged in the administration of intravenous conscious sedation to understand the pharmacologic
profile of sedative medications in order to reliably predict side effects associated
with their administration. Pertinent pharmacologic definitions associated with
the administration of intravenous medications are listed in Table 3–1.

PHARMACOKINETICS

Pharmacokinetics is the quantitative study of the absorption, distribution, metabolism, and excretion of injected drugs and their metabolites.[1] In essence, *pharmacokinetics is the study of what the body does to a drug.* The pharmacokinetic profile of a medication considers the following parameters:

- Dose of drug administered
- Drug concentration at the receptor site
- Drug effect
- Patient variability

Before the absorption, distribution, metabolism, and excretion of injected
medications, transfer of the pharmacologic agent across cell membranes must
occur. This transfer is a result of passive diffusion, active transport, or facilitated
diffusion.

1. *Passive diffusion.* Passive diffusion requires the presence of a concentration
   difference on each side of the cell membrane. The degree of pharmacologic

TABLE 3–1. *Pharmacologic Definitions*

Efficacy	The maximum effect that can be produced by a drug.
Hyperreactive	Refers to the patient population that requires **decreased** doses of pharmacologic agents to produce the desired effect.
Hyporeactive	Refers to the patient population that requires **large** doses of pharmacologic agents to produce the expected pharmacologic effect.
Potency	Required pharmacologic dosage required to produce an effect similar to another drug.
Synergism	Synergism occurs when use of one medication in conjunction with another results in a pharmacologic effect greater than the algebraic summation associated with each of the two individual drugs. (1 + 1 = 3).
Tachyphylaxis	Development of an acute tolerance to a drug.
Tolerance	The development of an increased drug requirement to produce a given effect. Results from chronic exposure to medications or toxins, which results in increased dosages of medications required to achieve the desired pharmacologic effect.

transfer is dependent on the magnitude of the concentration gradient across the cell membrane.

2. *Active transport.* Active transport requires energy to move molecules across cell membranes. Energy is required to facilitate movement of pharmacologic compounds and molecules across cell membranes against a concentration gradient.

3. *Facilitated diffusion.* Facilitated diffusion is a process by which a specific carrier transport mechanism is used. Therefore facilitated diffusion cannot move compounds and molecules against an electrochemical or concentration gradient.

PHARMACOLOGIC ABSORPTION

The absorption of a medication is dependent on the rate at which the pharmacologic compound leaves the site of administration. An important consideration associated with absorption is bioavailability. *Bioavailability* is a pharmacologic term used to indicate the extent to which a drug reaches a site of action or the biologic fluid from which the drug gains access to the site.[2] The mode of absorption is also an important characteristic to determine the duration and intensity of pharmacologic effect. Several factors may alter absorption. These factors include solubility of the medication, drug form, circulation at the site of absorption, and protein binding. Generally, highly lipid soluble drugs are capable of crossing cell membranes with ease. The suspension or drug form also affects absorption. To reach the site of action and exert a pharmacologic effect, all drugs must dissolve in water. Therefore pharmacologic adjuncts delivered in an aqueous medium are absorbed faster than those delivered in pill form or suspension. Circulation at the site of absorption also affects bioavailability. An increase in blood flow at the site of absorption increases the rate of absorption. Decreased blood flow at the site of absorption decreases absorption. Factors that decrease blood flow at the site of absorption include hypotension, shock, or utilization of vasoconstrictors.

Protein Binding

Pharmacologic agents bind to plasma proteins to a varying degree. This bound portion of the drug is inactive. The free or unbound portion of a drug is required for pharmacologic effect. Plasma protein binding also contributes to clearance of the drug. The unbound fraction of the drug undergoes metabolism by the hepatic cytochrome P-450 system, glomerular filtration and renal filtration, or both. During preprocedure assessment, patients with nutritional disorders, carcinoma, recent weight loss, renal disease, or decreased plasma protein levels may demonstrate enhanced or exaggerated effects from pharmacologic adjuncts used to achieve conscious sedation. As always, titration of pharmacologic agents is advised in all situations. Careful assessment of patient response is warranted, particularly in patients with altered hepatic or renal function.

Routes of Administration

ORAL. Absorption after ingestion of pharmacologic compounds is dependent on the small intestine and the stomach. Absorption from the gastrointestinal tract generally occurs in the small intestine, where the epithelial lining is thin and has a large surface area.

First-Pass Effect. Medications absorbed through the stomach and intestine require passage (first pass) through the liver before they gain entrance to the systemic circulation. During this process, some of the active pharmacologic compound is inactivated by liver metabolism or biliary excretion, resulting in decreased bioavailability. As a result of this hepatic metabolism or biliary excretion, some oral medications require larger doses than parenteral medications to exert a pharmacologic effect.

SUBLINGUAL. Because of the decreased surface area associated with sublingual administration, the sublingual mode of administration is reserved for highly lipid-soluble medications. Common medications given by the sublingual route include nitroglycerin and nifedipine. Because of venous drainage of the sublingual area directly into the superior vena cava, there is no first-pass effect associated with sublingual administration. Limitations associated with the sublingual route of administration include decreased surface area and the requirement for highly lipid-soluble drugs.

RECTAL. Pharmacologic agents instilled into the rectum are absorbed via the superior hemorrhoidal veins and transported to the liver.[3] Approximately 50% of rectally administered medications undergo first-pass effect. Depending on the site of rectal absorption (proximal or distal), bioavailability varies greatly. Rectal administration is generally reserved for unconscious, uncooperative, or pediatric patients who cannot take oral medications. Rectal administration is not popular because of a wide variation in patient response, rectal mucosal irritation, and diarrhea.

TABLE 3-2. *Techniques of Medication Administration*

METHOD	PATTERN OF ABSORPTION	ADVANTAGES	DISADVANTAGES
Oral ingestion	Lower gastrointestinal tract absorption is dependent on local conditions: • Blood flow • Surface area • Physical state of the drug	Safe Convenient Economical	Emesis secondary to GI upset Drug destruction secondary to digestive enzyme Ineffective in patients with propulsion disorders Requires patient cooperation Requires intact reflexes First-pass effect
Sublingual	Absorption of highly lipid-soluble, nonionized pharmacologic preparations; sublingual venous return empties into the superior vena cava.	Convenient Elimination of first-pass effect	Decreased surface area Need for highly soluble and potent agents Requires patient cooperation
Rectal	Proximal absorption via the superior hemorrhoidal veins; distal absorption bypasses hepatic first-pass effect.	Useful in the presence of emesis and nausea	Mucosal irritation Diarrhea First-pass effect Varied absorption
Subcutaneous	Absorption is dependent on the surface area and the absorbing capillary membrane.	May be used for unconscious, uncooperative patients Vasoconstictors reduce systemic absorption (local anesthetics) Sustained release	Pain, necrosis, tissue sloughing Erratic absorption Suitable for only small volumes of injectate Decreased uptake in the presence of decreased blood pressure

Route		Disadvantages
Intramuscular	Rapid absorption of pharmacologic effect is dependent on blood flow to the muscular bed.	Local irritation
	May be used in the unconscious, uncooperative patient	Erratic absorption
	Sustained release	May result in increased laboratory results (creatine phosphokinase)
	Rapid absorption	
Intravenous	Bypasses absorption processes with resultant immediate blood plasma level of the pharmacologic agent.	Requires vascular access
	Rapid blood plasma level	Side effects and complications are immediate
	Bypasses limiting factors associated with the absorptive process	Requires careful titration
	Utilization of large volumes	
Inhalational	Pulmonary epithelial absorption. Increased alveolar blood flow results in rapid onset of action.	Inability to regulate dose
	Drug delivery to specific receptor sites of action (i.e., pulmonary: beta agonists)	Pulmonary epithelial irritation
	Rapid onset of action	Improper aerosol delivery
Topical	Highly lipid-soluble medications are absorbed through the epidermis into the systemic circulation.	Inability to regulate uptake and delivery
	Slow, timed-release pharmacologic effect	May require large body surface contact
	Sustained pharmacologic effect	
	Ease of use	

SUBCUTANEOUS. Subcutaneous administration is reserved for nonirritating medications. It offers a more rapid and superior absorption than oral administration. The quantity of medication absorbed depends on

- Surface area
- Local blood flow
- Drug solubility

A sustained effect after subcutaneous administration provided by a constant plasma level can be pharmacologically advantageous with drugs such as insulin.

INTRAMUSCULAR. Intramuscular injections afford sustained release and a more rapid pharmacologic effect. This increased bioavailability is directly proportional to blood flow of the muscular bed. Pharmacologic suspensions allow prolonged release. However, organic solvents such as propylene glycol used in the suspension of diazepam often result in erratic intramuscular absorption.

INTRAVENOUS. Intravenous administration of medications results in a rapid rise in the blood plasma level. The rapid onset of action is secondary to the direct deposition of pharmacologic agent into the bloodstream. Although this rapid onset of action is desirable, caution must be exercised during the administration of intravenous medications. Titration is required, and adequate time should be allowed to assess *individual* patient response.

INHALATIONAL. Medications may be absorbed through the pulmonary tract (atomized, aerosolized, metered-dose inhaler). The large pulmonary surface area allows pharmacologic agents to be readily absorbed. Alveolar blood flow closely couples cardiac output with resultant rapid uptake from the pulmonary epithelium. When used properly, metered-dose inhalers and aerosol delivery are efficacious for the delivery of pharmacologic agents to the systemic circulation.

TOPICAL. Topically administered medications must be lipid soluble, and the quantity absorbed is proportional to the body surface area exposed to the medication. Factors affecting delivery of topical medication to the circulation include the following:

- Hydrated skin (more permeable to drug than dry skin)
- Occlusive patch (timed-release patch)

Any activity that increases cutaneous blood flow will increase the uptake of topically administered medications. A complete review of the techniques of administration is given in Table 3–2.

DRUG DISTRIBUTION

Once the absorption phase is complete, several phases of pharmacologic distribution occur. The first phase of distribution is a result of cardiac output and regional blood flow. Organs with high blood flow, referred to as vessel-rich organs, receive the majority of the drug during this initial phase. These organs include the heart, brain, liver, lungs, and kidneys. Organ systems that are not considered in

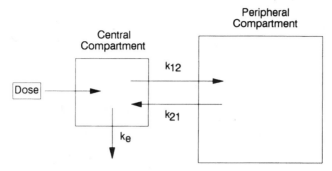

FIGURE 3-1. Two compartment pharmacokinetic model. K_{12} and K_{21} are rate constants that signify the intercompartmental transfer of drugs. K_e is the elimination rate constant for drug elimination from the body. (From Barash PG, Cullen B, Stoelting R. *Clinical Anesthesia*. 2nd ed. Philadelphia: JB Lippincott; 1992.)

the vessel-rich group require minutes to hours to attain equilibrium with pharmacologic agents. These organ systems include muscle, viscera, skin, and fat.

To understand basic pharmacokinetic principles, it is important to envision the body as composed of one or more compartments. Most drugs behave as though they have been distributed within two compartments, one central and the other peripheral. As illustrated in Figure 3-1, an initial drug dose is injected into the central compartment. After introduction into the central compartment, the drug disseminates to the peripheral compartment. The central compartment consists of intravascular fluid and organs in the vessel-rich group. The peripheral compartment consists of all other fluids and tissues of the body. Eventually, drugs return from the peripheral compartment to the central compartment for excretion and clearance.

METABOLISM

Metabolism and clearance of drugs from the systemic circulation rely on hepatic, biliary, pulmonary, and renal mechanisms. The goal of metabolic degradation is to transform active compounds into water-soluble, pharmacologically inactive substances. In some instances, the process of metabolism yields pharmacologically active metabolites (desmethyldiazepam during the metabolism of diazepam), which may prolong the drug's duration of action. Metabolic pathways in the liver responsible for biodegradation of pharmacologic compounds include oxidation, reduction, hydrolysis, and conjugation. These complex biochemical processes yield inactive pharmacologic compounds.

Hepatic Microsomal Enzyme System

Sites of drug metabolism include plasma, lungs, kidneys, gastrointestinal tract, and liver. The hepatic microsomal enzyme system lies in the smooth endoplasmic reticulum of the liver. The cytochrome P-450 enzyme system is located on hepatic microsomes. The degree of hepatic microsomal enzyme activity is determined ge-

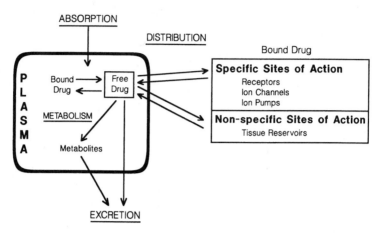

FIGURE 3–2.   Overview of the pharmacokinetic process: absorption, distribution, metabolism, and excretion. (From Miller R. *Anesthesia.* 4th ed. New York: Churchill Livingstone; 1994:94.)

netically. Aside from genetic predisposition to hepatic microsomal enzyme activity, certain medications may stimulate the cytochrome P-450 system. Prolonged barbiturate, benzodiazepine, or phenytoin use predisposes the patient to an increase in hepatic microsomal enzyme activity. This enhanced hepatic microsomal enzyme activity generally results in an increased medication requirement for the individual patient. As noted in the chapter on preprocedure assessment, it is important to ascertain a thorough medication history to assess for the presence of enzyme-inducing drugs.

EXCRETION

The kidneys are the major organ system for the excretion of drugs and metabolites. Renal excretion of pharmacologic agents or their metabolites depends on

- Glomerular filtration rate
- Active tubular secretion
- Passive tubular reabsorption

The clearance and excretion of drugs and metabolites require adequate renal function prior to the administration of sedative medications. Patients with suspected renal disease may require nephrology consultation with baseline testing (creatinine, BUN, etc.). A summary of the pharmacokinetic process is presented in Figure 3–2.

PHARMACODYNAMICS

As pharmacokinetics is the study of what the body does to a drug, pharmacodynamics is what the drug does to the body. Pharmacodynamics is the study of the effects of pharmacologic agents on the body.[4] Pharmacodynamics quantifies the chemical and physical interactions between the pharmacologic agent administered and the effects on target sites and actions of each drug. The pharmacodynamic effects associated with opioid use include the following:

* Analgesia
* Decreased gastrointestinal motility
* Dysphoria
* Euphoria
* Miosis
* Nausea
* Respiratory depression
* Sedation
* Suppression of opioid withdrawal
* Vomiting

RECEPTORS

Proteins compose one of the most important classes of pharmacologic receptors. A variety of receptor subtypes have been identified. These subtypes include the following:

* Hormone
* Growth factor
* Neurotransmitters
* Nucleic acid
* Opiate
* Gamma-aminobutyric acid (GABA) receptor complex

Fortunately, pharmacologic agents administered exert their actions on selective receptors to exert a specific drug response. Pharmacologic agents that bind to physiologic receptors to produce a specific effect are termed *agonists*.[5] Pharmacologic *antagonists* are agents that bind to physiologic receptors but have no pharmacologic effect.[5] Antagonists also inhibit the action of agonists. Agonist and antagonist actions are important in the autonomic nervous system. Many of the pharmacologic agents used to control heart rate (beta blockers) are antagonists. Alpha antagonists (phenoxybenzamine) antagonize alpha receptors and result in peripheral vasodilatation. Pharmacologic antagonists also include reversal agents (flumazenil [Romazicon], naloxone [Narcan]), which competitively bind to receptor sites to reverse the pharmacologic effects of medications administered. Examples of agonistic stimulation include beta stimulation (isoproterenol [Isuprel]) and alpha stimulation (phenylephrine [Neo-Synephrine]) to increase blood pressure.

Pharmacodynamic drug interactions may occur directly or indirectly at receptor sites. Many of the medications administered during conscious sedation act on individual specific receptor sites (opioids and benzodiazepines). Action on these receptor sites results in a synergism that provides analgesia and sedation. When one is considering pharmacodynamic principles, it is important to consider individual patient response coupled with varied drug dosages for individual patients during the administration of intravenous conscious sedation.

REFERENCES

1. Golembiewski J. Pharmacology of Neuromuscular Blocking Drugs and Intravenous Induction Agents. Anesthesia Today. Ohmeda, 1994;5:2.
2. Barash P, Cullen B, Stoelting R. *Clinical Anesthesia.* 2nd ed. Philadelphia: JB Lippincott; 1992:293.
3. Netter F. *Atlas of Human Anatomy.* Summit, NJ: Ciba-Geigy Corporation; 1993.
4. Schwinn D, Watkins W, Leslie J. *Basic Principles of Pharmacology. Anesthesia.* 4th ed. New York: Churchill Livingstone; 1994:57.
5. Hardman J, Limbird L. *Pharmacologic Basis of Therapeutics.* 9th ed. New York: McGraw-Hill; 1996.

Airway Management and Management of Respiratory Complications

CHAPTER 4

AMERICAN NURSE'S ASSOCIATION POSITION STATEMENT ON THE ROLE OF THE REGISTERED NURSE IN THE MANAGEMENT OF PATIENTS RECEIVING IV CONSCIOUS SEDATION

The registered nurse participating in the management and monitoring of the patient receiving conscious sedation understands the principles of oxygen delivery, respiratory physiology, transport and uptake, and demonstrates the ability to use oxygen delivery devices.

JCAHO MANUAL TX 78

General competency for the qualified individual managing the care of a patient receiving conscious sedation includes the ability to understand the principles of oxygen delivery, respiratory physiology, oxygen transport and oxygen uptake, and demonstrate the ability to use oxygen delivery devices.[1]

Respiratory insufficiency is a condition characterized by reduced gas exchange, which is inadequate to meet the body's metabolic demands. Use of sedative, hypnotic, and opioid medications in conjunction with pathophysiologic processes predisposes patients receiving intravenous conscious sedation to the development of respiratory compromise. Respiratory insufficiency may develop at any time during the procedure or in the postprocedure period. Attempts to decrease morbidity associated with the administration of intravenous conscious sedation are enhanced by identification of patients at risk of respiratory complications and optimization of preprocedure medical therapy (Chapter 2). The focus of this chapter includes a basic review of the anatomy of the airway, airway management, positive pressure ventilation, and use of oxygen-delivery devices. Prior to the administration of conscious sedation, registered nurses must be adept at airway management skills and treatment protocol used in the event of airway obstruction. These objectives may be accomplished by means of a thorough review of this chapter and practical clinical application. Preceptorship by an anesthesiologist, a certified registered nurse anesthetist, or a qualified airway management specialist also facilitates this learning process.

ANATOMY

To competently master airway management skills, it is important to understand the functional anatomy of the human airway. Air enters the pulmonary system through the nose, which has a bone and cartilage framework. The upper airway is defined as that portion above the vocal cords.

UPPER AIRWAY

The oral cavity consists of the tongue and teeth. The pharynx is a 13 cm tube that begins at the internal nares and consists of the tonsils, uvula, and epiglottic structure. The pharynx is divided into three parts:

1. *Nasopharynx:* The nasopharynx begins just posterior to the internal nasal cavity and extends to the soft palate. The nasopharynx contains the adenoids located at the posterior pharyngeal wall.
2. *Oropharynx:* The oropharynx begins at the soft palate and extends to the level of the hyoid bone. It contains the paired palatine and lingual tonsils. The oropharynx serves as both a respiratory and food passageway.
3. *Laryngopharynx:* The laryngopharynx begins at the level of the hyoid bone and diverges posteriorly to connect with the esophagus and anteriorly into

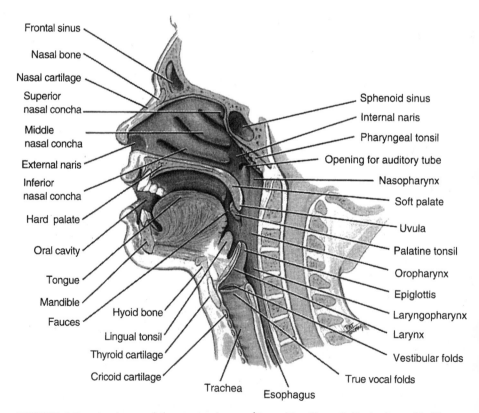

Frontal sinus

Nasal bone

Nasal cartilage

Superior nasal concha

Middle nasal concha

External naris

Inferior nasal concha

Hard palate

Oral cavity

Tongue

Mandible

Fauces

Hyoid bone

Lingual tonsil

Thyroid cartilage

Cricoid cartilage

Trachea

Esophagus

Sphenoid sinus

Internal naris

Pharyngeal tonsil

Opening for auditory tube

Nasopharynx

Soft palate

Uvula

Palatine tonsil

Oropharynx

Epiglottis

Laryngopharynx

Larynx

Vestibular folds

True vocal folds

FIGURE 4–1.   Anatomy of the upper airway. (From Nagelhout J, Zaglaniczny K. *Nurse Anesthesia.* Philadelphia: WB Saunders; 1997:709.)

the larynx. Like the oropharynx, the laryngopharynx also functions as a respiratory and gastrointestinal passageway.

Anatomy of the upper airway is depicted in Figure 4–1. The glottic aperture (glottis) is the opening to the larynx, which is covered by the epiglottis. The epiglottis is a large, leaflike structure with its stem attached anteriorly to the thyroid cartilage with no posterior attachment. The leaf portion of the epiglottis moves freely to prevent aspiration of gastric contents from the oropharynx into the trachea. During swallowing, the epiglottis covers the glottic opening. To avoid gastric acid aspiration and adhere to criteria for conscious sedation definition, the gag reflex must be maintained during the administration of sedative medications.

LOWER AIRWAY

The lower airway includes structures below the level of the vocal cords. The adult larynx (voice box) lies below the glottic opening anterior to the fourth through the sixth cervical vertebra.[2] The larynx is composed of three single and three paired cartilages. The three single cartilages include the

- Thyroid
- Cricoid
- Epiglottis

The three paired cartilages include

- Corniculate
- Cuneiform
- Arytenoid

Laryngeal cartilages are displayed in Figure 4–2. The thyroid cartilage (Adam's apple) comprises the anterior portion of the larynx. The cricoid cartilage is the single complete cartilaginous ring, which comprises the lower border of the larynx. Of the three paired cartilages, the arytenoid cartilages control vocal cord function through pharyngeal muscle movement.

The trachea (windpipe) is an air passageway, approximately 12 cm in length, which extends from the larynx to the fifth thoracic vertebra.[3] The trachea lies anterior to the esophagus and bifurcates into the right and left mainstem bronchi. The right and left bronchi progressively branch to eventually form the terminal bronchioles. The lungs consist of smooth muscle innervated by the autonomic nervous system. The lungs extend from the diaphragm to just above the clavicles and are housed within the rib cage. The function and purpose of the upper airway, larynx, trachea, and pulmonary circulation is to provide exchange of oxygen and carbon dioxide at the alveolar level. A primary concern of the physician and the registered nurse participating in the administration of conscious sedation is to maintain protective airway reflexes and the integrity of respiratory processes. As stated in Chapter 1, the goals and objectives of conscious sedation are not to produce unconsciousness or loss of the patient's protective airway reflexes. Because

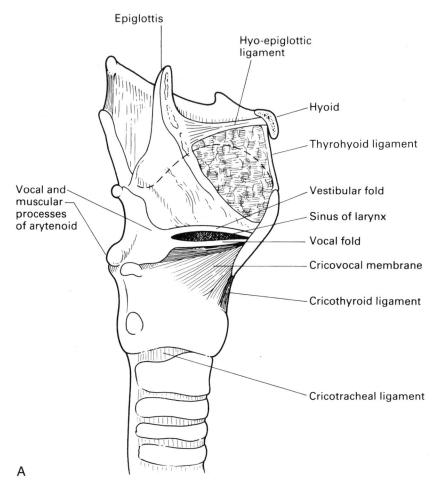

Epiglottis

Hyo-epiglottic ligament

Hyoid

Thyrohyoid ligament

Vocal and muscular processes of arytenoid

Vestibular fold

Sinus of larynx

Vocal fold

Cricovocal membrane

Cricothyroid ligament

Cricotracheal ligament

A

FIGURE 4–2. Laryngeal cartilages and membranes. **A,** The cartilages and ligaments of the larynx seen laterally.

of presence of disease processes, pharmacologic effects, and patient variability, protection of the patient's airway may become tenuous in some clinical situations. The focus of this chapter will be an early recognition, diagnosis, and intervention to alleviate airway obstruction.

EVALUATION OF THE AIRWAY

Diagnosis and intervention in the presence of respiratory distress is imperative. Equally important is the ability to identify patients who have the potential for difficult airway management. A comprehensive preprocedure physical assessment of the patient's airway includes oral cavity inspection, temporomandibular joint examination, physical characteristics, and application of the Mallampati airway classification system.

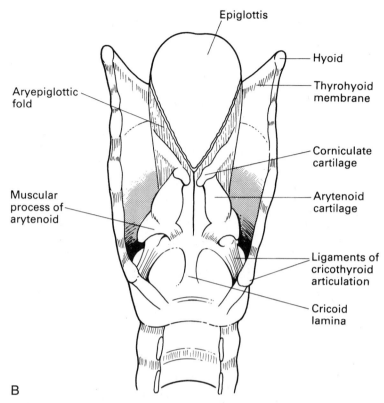

B

FIGURE 4–2.   *Continued.* **B,** The cartilages and ligaments of the larynx seen posteriorly. (From Ellis H, Feldman S. *Anatomy for Anaesthetists.* 6th ed. Cambridge, Mass: Blackwell Scientific Publications; 1993:32, 33.)

ORAL CAVITY INSPECTION

The oral cavity is assessed to identify loose, chipped, or capped teeth. Documentation of the presence of dental anomalies, crowns, bridges, and dentures should be documented before the start of the procedure. The oral cavity should be examined for the presence of tumors or obstruction of airflow.

TEMPOROMANDIBULAR JOINT EXAMINATION

Assessment of the temporomandibular joint is conducted with the patient's mouth opened wide. In the adult, the distance between the upper and lower central incisors is normally 4 to 6 cm.[3] The presence of a clicking sound, pain associated with opening of the mouth, or a reduced ability to open the mouth indicates reduced temporomandibular joint mobility. In the presence of respiratory distress, access to the patient's airway is reduced if mechanical conduits are required (oropharyngeal airways).

PHYSICAL CHARACTERISTICS

The following physical characteristics may indicate the potential for difficult airway management:

1. Hyponathic (recessed) jaw
2. Hypernathic (protruding) jaw
3. Deviated trachea
4. Large tongue
5. Short, thick neck
6. Protruding teeth
7. High arched palate

MALLAMPATI AIRWAY CLASSIFICATION SYSTEM

The Mallampati airway classification system, described in 1983, grades the degree of difficulty of endotracheal intubation from I to IV.[4] The examination is conducted with the patient in the sitting position. The patient's head is maintained in a neutral position and the mouth is opened 50 to 60 mm.[5] Classification of the patient's airway is based on a description of the anatomic area visualized. Figure 4–3 shows the Mallampati airway classification system.

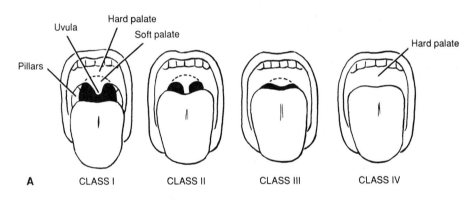

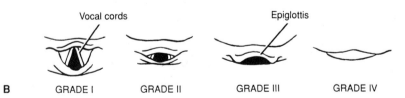

FIGURE 4–3.   Mallampati airway classification. A difficult orotracheal intubation (grade III or IV) may be predicted by the inability to visualize certain pharyngeal structures (class III or IV) during the preprocedure examination of a patient. (From Mallampati SR. Clinical signs to predict difficult tracheal intubation [hypothesis]. *Can Anaesth Soc J.* 1983;30: 316.)

AIRWAY MANAGEMENT

The pharmacologic effects associated with sedatives, hypnotics, and analgesics, particularly when combinations are used, result in a synergistic effect. This synergism, or the pharmacologic effects of individual medications, decreases oropharyngeal muscle tone. Decreased muscle tone may lead to upper airway obstruction. The impedance to air flow is secondary to impingement of the tongue and redundant tissue on the posterior pharyngeal wall. Signs and symptoms of airway obstruction include the following:

- Increased respiratory effort
- Sternal retraction
- Rocking chest motion (out of sync with respiratory effort)
- Inspiratory stridor (harsh, high-pitched inspiratory sounds)
- Hypoxemia
- Hypercarbia
- Absence of breath sounds

Skilled clinicians engaged in the administration of intravenous conscious sedation perform thousands of uneventful procedures yearly. When complications arise, however, the practitioner must immediately recognize the signs and symptoms of airway compromise and deal with them effectively. The focus of this chapter is to assist the clinician in rapid *diagnosis* and *intervention* in the presence of respiratory complications. Treatment modalities that result in effective ventilation follow.

UPPER AIRWAY OBSTRUCTION

As outlined earlier, the pharmacologic effect of intravenous sedatives may result in undesired side effects (respiratory depression, apnea, and the development of hypoxemia). Whether the problem is a central pharmacologic effect or a lack of sufficient oropharyngeal muscle tone, the clinician must restore air flow. When one is dealing with upper airway obstruction, initial interventions include the following:

- Auditory/tactile stimulation
- Head tilt
- Chin lift
- Jaw thrust
- Nasal/oral airway

As depicted in Figure 4–4, the goal of these interventions includes anterior displacement of the mandible and elevation of the base of the tongue off of the posterior pharyngeal wall to restore air flow.

Lateral Head Tilt

Patients receiving intravenous conscious sedation can be in a variety of positions during the procedure. The head tilt is a mechanical maneuver, depicted in

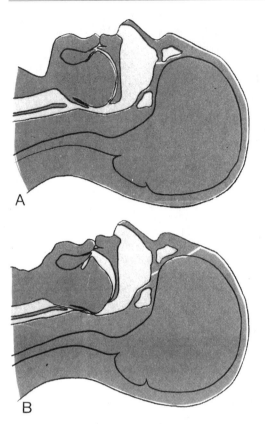

FIGURE 4–4. Normal vs. obstructed airway. **A,** The normal airway. The tongue and other soft tissues are forward, allowing an unobstructed air passage. **B,** The obstructed airway. The tongue and epiglottis fall back to the posterior pharyngeal wall, occluding the airway. Courtesy of V. Robideaux, M.D. (From Dorsch J. *Understanding Anesthesia Equipment.* 2nd ed. Baltimore: Williams & Wilkins; 1994:370.)

Figure 4–5, that moves the head from the neutral position to the side. This frequently results in tongue displacement from the posterior pharyngeal wall to the side of the oropharynx. Complete or partial relief of upper airway obstruction may occur after use of this maneuver.

Chin Lift

When the head tilt is unsuccessful, a chin lift may be used. The chin lift depicted in Figure 4–6 permits anterior movement of the mandible through superior displacement of the chin. Coupled with hyperextension of the head and neck, this maneuver results in anterior displacement of the tongue and relief of the airway obstruction.

Jaw Thrust

If stimulation, head tilt, and chin lift do not produce relief of airway obstruction, the patient is in a state of deep sedation or may have been induced into a state of general anesthesia. Unless the obstruction is relieved and air flow is restored, arterial oxygen desaturation will occur. The jaw thrust depicted in Figure 4–7 is a maneuver that requires the use of both hands. A jaw thrust provides significant anterior displacement of the mandible. Relief of airway obstruction by lifting the tongue off the posterior pharyngeal wall generally restores air flow.

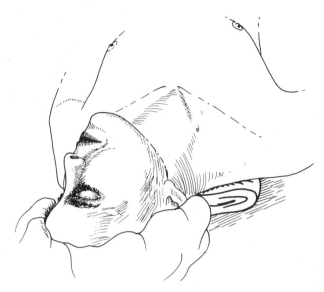

FIGURE 4–5.   Lateral head tilt maneuver. The lateral head tilt maneuver results in movement of the patient's head from the neutral position to the side. This maneuver may relieve minor upper airway obstruction. (From Butterworth J. *Atlas of Procedures in Anesthesia and Critical Care.* Philadelphia: WB Saunders; 1991:6.)

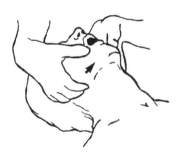

FIGURE 4–6.   Chin lift technique. Gentle superior movement of the mentum results in anterior displacement of the tongue, which can relieve upper airway obstruction. (From Chung D, Lam A. *Essentials of Anesthesiology.* 3rd ed. Philadelphia: WB Saunders; 1997: 163.)

Great care must be taken when performing this maneuver to prevent damage to the facial nerve. As depicted in Figure 4–8 the facial nerve runs behind the ramus of the mandible and fans out across the face. Damage to the facial nerve or its central pathway results in facial palsy.[6] In the unlikely event that these maneuvers do not relieve upper airway obstruction, use of a nasal or oral airway is required. Patients who require this invasive form of airway support do not meet the definition of conscious sedation. Airway obstruction not relieved by head tilt, chin lift, and jaw thrust may require immediate consultation by a certified registered nurse anesthetist or anesthesiologist for additional airway support.

Nasal Airway

When upper airway obstruction continues after the maneuvers just outlined, an airway conduit is required to physically displace the tongue. Nasal airways

84

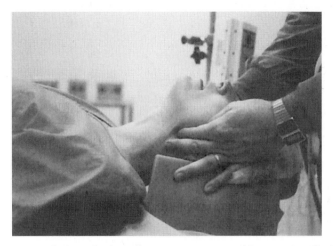

FIGURE 4–7. Jaw thrust. The jaw thrust maneuver provides anterior displacement of the mandible to elevate the tongue off the posterior pharyngeal wall. (From Nagelhout J, Zaglaniczny K. *Nurse Anesthesia*. Philadelphia: WB Saunders; 1997:710.)

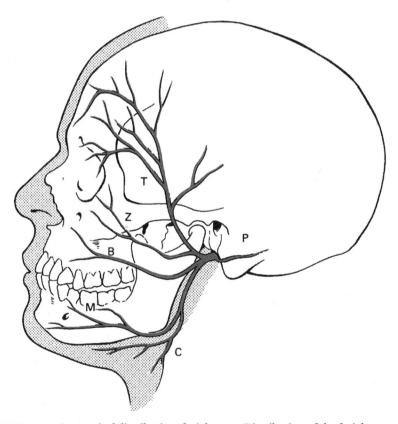

FIGURE 4–8. Anatomical distribution: facial nerve. Distribution of the facial nerve: T = temporal, Z = zygomatic, B = buccal, M = mandibular, C = cervical, P = posterior auricular branch. (From Ellis H, Feldman S. *Anatomy for Anaesthetists*. 6th ed. Cambridge, Mass: Blackwell Scientific Publications; 1993:284.)

TABLE 4–1. *Proper Oropharyngeal Airway Placement*

1. Carefully open the patient's mouth, exercising caution to prevent finger injury to the clinician or dental damage to the patient.
2. Once the mouth is open, insert the tongue blade into the posterior pharynx.
3. Insert the tongue blade toward the base of the tongue. Apply pressure with the tongue blade to displace the base of the tongue anteriorly.
4. Insert the oropharyngeal airway into the oropharynx. The oropharyngeal airway is designed to follow the natural curvature of the oropharynx. The tongue blade should expose a clear view of the posterior oropharynx. Do not force or blindly position the oropharyngeal airway. Malpositioning of the oropharyngeal airway can force the base of the tongue against the posterior pharyngeal wall, completely obstructing the airway.
5. Following insertion, verify that the tongue and lips have not been inadvertently positioned between the teeth.
6. It should be noted that a patient who tolerates the insertion of an oropharyngeal airway is deeply sedated, and at this point the practitioner is advised to consult an anesthesia practitioner to provide additional airway management assistance.

shown in Table 4–1 are generally tolerated much better than oral airways. Oral airways stimulate the gag reflex, with resultant vomiting or laryngospasm in lightly anesthetized patients. However, nasal airways are not without risks. Inherent risks associated with nasopharyngeal airway use include epistaxis, hypertension, and difficult placement in patients with nasal deformity. Epistaxis in the presence of respiratory distress results in blood in the oropharynx, which may stimulate laryngospasm or bronchospasm. Nasopharyngeal airways are not recommended in the presence of anticoagulants, CSF rhinorrhea, septal deformity, or nasal polyps, and they should not be forced in the presence of obstruction. Insertion of nasopharyngeal airways requires assessment of naris size. Nasopharyngeal airways come in an assortment of adult sizes:

- 6.0 mm
- 6.5 mm
- 7.0 mm
- 7.5 mm
- 8.0 mm

Sizes for nasopharyngeal airways indicate the internal diameter in millimeters. The larger the internal diameter, the longer the tube.[7] The nasopharyngeal airway must be long enough to physically displace the base of the tongue away from the posterior pharyngeal wall. Approximate length of the nasopharyngeal airway is measured from the tip of the naris to the lobe of the ear. Prior to insertion, the nasopharyngeal airway should be lubricated well. This can be accomplished with water-soluble lubricant, 2% lidocaine (Xylocaine) jelly, or 5% lidocaine ointment. Lubrication also helps decrease the incidence of epistaxis. During insertion (Fig. 4–9), the nasopharyngeal airway must not be forced. Gentle pressure may be used after initial insertion into the naris. *However, one should never force a nasopharyngeal airway that is impeded in the posterior nasopharynx.* The nasal airway must be inserted perpendicular to the face. Posi-

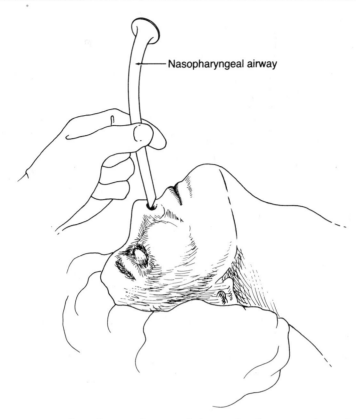

FIGURE 4–9.   Insertion of a nasopharyngeal airway. Gentle pressure is used to advance a well-lubricated nasopharyngeal airway into place. Excessive force must be avoided to prevent epistaxis. If excessive pressure is encountered on placement of the airway, one should withdraw and attempt placement on the opposite side. (From Butterworth J. *Atlas of Procedures in Anesthesia and Critical Care.* Philadelphia: WB Saunders; 1991:23.)

tioned properly, the nasopharyngeal airway provides a physical conduit for air passage.

Oral Airway

Just as a nasopharyngeal airway provides a mechanical passage for air flow, the oropharyngeal airway physically displaces the tongue off of the posterior pharyngeal wall. The oropharyngeal airway may stimulate vomiting if the gag reflex remains intact. Additional complications associated with insertion of an oropharyngeal airway include the following:

- Bradycardia secondary to vagal stimulation
- Retching with resultant hypertension and tachycardia
- Laryngospasm
- Dental damage
- Pharyngeal or lip lacerations

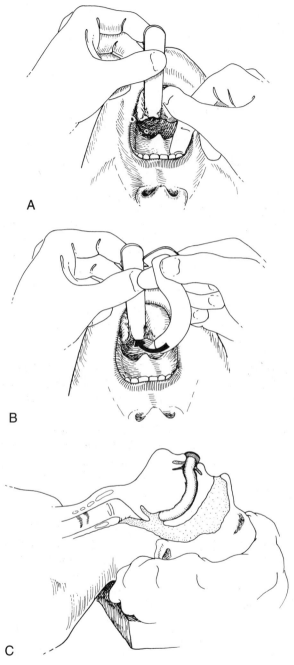

FIGURE 4–10.   Insertion of oropharyngeal airway. Proper insertion of an oropharyngeal airway to restore air flow requires careful placement of the airway into the posterior oropharynx. See Table 4–1 for proper placement procedure of an oropharyngeal airway. (From Butterworth J. *Atlas of Procedures in Anesthesia and Critical Care.* Philadelphia: WB Saunders; 1991:5, 16.)

When indicated, insertion of an oropharyngeal airway must be done carefully to avoid complications noted previously. Proper placement of an oropharyngeal airway, depicted in Figure 4–10, is outlined in Table 4–1.

Laryngospasm

Laryngospasm is a spasm of the laryngeal musculature. Often initiated by mucus, blood, or saliva irritating the vocal cords, results in complete or partial closure of the cords and inability of the patient to ventilate. Patients with total airway obstruction will often display "rocky" abdominal respirations with no air exchange. Initial treatment is positive pressure ventilation with 100% oxygen. A secure mask fit is required to generate positive pressure to break the spasm. If this maneuver is unsuccessful, an anesthesia provider or backup personnel should be summoned immediately. A nonparalyzing dose (approximately one tenth of the full intubating dose) of succinylcholine is given. Coupled with ventilatory support, relaxation of the skeletal muscles of the larynx generally ensues. If necessary, endotracheal intubation is employed as a last resort to break the laryngospasm.

EMERGENCY AIRWAY MANAGEMENT

MASK MANAGEMENT

Upper airway obstruction must be recognized promptly and treated effectively. Mechanisms to relieve upper airway obstruction must be provided in a systematic manner outlined in Figure 4–11. In the presence of respiratory depression or apnea, the registered nurse must be prepared to ventilate the patient with a positive pressure breathing device. If all maneuvers previously outlined fail to relieve upper airway obstruction and do not restore effective ventilation, then positive pressure mask ventilation should be instituted.

Commercially available bag valve mask devices are disposable systems for single patient use. Packaged with this system is *one* disposable mask for use with the bag valve device. It is important to note that many of the masks packaged with these units are large adult sizes. There are a variety of masks available for resuscitative procedures. The facial anatomy of each individual patient may be markedly different on the basis of patient weight, mandibular size, age, nutritional status, presence of facial hair, and dentition. Therefore it is important to select a mask of the proper size for the patient's use. To account for patient variability, disposable masks of several sizes must be available at each conscious sedation site. It is critical to have an assortment of masks available prior to the commencement of any conscious sedation procedure. A properly fitting mask should fit snugly between the bridge of the patient's nose, the mentum or the chin, and the medial aspects of the face. Masks that extend above the bridge of the nose, below the level of the mandible, or past the lateral aspects of the face are inappropriately sized. This results in ineffective positive pressure ventilation and the inability to generate positive pressure. Clear plastic masks currently available permit visual assessment of the oropharynx for

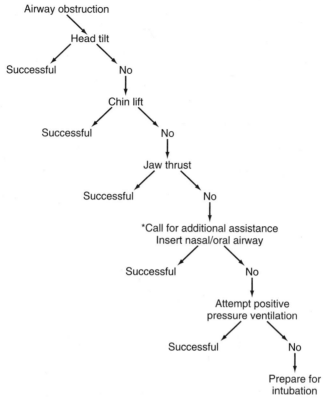

FIGURE 4-11. Conscious sedation airway obstruction algorithm. (© 1996, Specialty Health Consultants.)

the presence of vomitus. These masks are superior when compared to the black latex masks of earlier years, which prohibited visual inspection of the oropharynx.

To secure an appropriate mask fit, the mask must form an effective seal between the skin of the face and the polyvinylchloride mask. Once the mask has been properly positioned (Fig. 4-12), the third and fourth or fourth and fifth fingers (depending on the clinician's hand size) are placed on the mandible. This maneuver elevates the jaw and the base of the tongue off the posterior pharyngeal wall. On delivery of the first positive pressure ventilation, there should be chest rise and fall, breath sounds, and no air escape around the mask. If the patient remains apneic, positive pressure ventilation should ensue at a rate of 16 to 20 breaths per minute until additional assistance arrives. *Preparation for respiratory emergency* is required wherever the administration of conscious sedation is performed. When summoned, anesthesia personnel or the attending physician will need specific equipment and supplies to secure the airway and establish effective ventilation. Therefore it is important to maintain certain emergency airway equipment at each designated conscious sedation location.

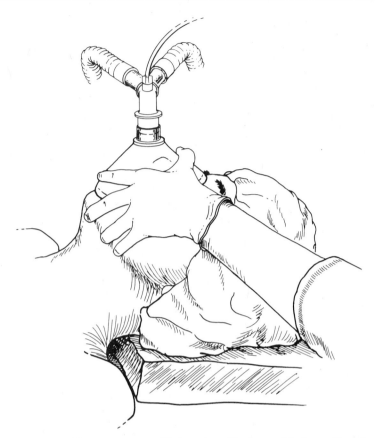

FIGURE 4–12.   Positive pressure ventilation. An effective seal is formed by placing the third, fourth, and fifth fingers below the mandible and exerting gentle pressure on the bridge of the nose. A proper mask fit does not allow oxygen to escape between the patient's face and the mask seal. Notice how the hands produce an effective mask seal and also extend the head to produce a patent airway. (From Butterworth J. *Atlas of Procedures in Anesthesia and Critical Care.* Philadelphia: WB Saunders; 1991:23.)

ENDOTRACHEAL TUBES

An assortment of endotracheal tubes must be kept on hand at all times for the variety of age groups receiving intravenous conscious sedation. Endotracheal tube sizes are designated in millimeters of internal diameter. Table 4–2 lists recommended endotracheal tube sizes on the basis of patient age. Figure 4–13 depicts a standard Murphy eye endotracheal tube.

STYLET

An endotracheal stylet (Fig. 4–14) is a polyvinylchloride or aluminum instrument that provides rigidity to the endotracheal tube. It enhances the clinician's

TABLE 4–2. *Recommended Sizes for Endotracheal Tubes*

AGE	ENDOTRACHEAL TUBE SIZE (INTERNAL DIAMETER, mm)
Newborn	3.0
6 months	3.5
18 months	4.0
36 months	4.5
5 years	5.0
6 years	5.5
8 years	6.0
12 years	6.5
16 years	6.5–7.0
Adult female	7.0
Adult male	8.0

ability to place the endotracheal tube in a variety of positions to aid in the intubation process. Stylets may be used for difficult intubation and allow direction of the endotracheal tube through the glottic opening. Stylets are available in malleable aluminum or metal with or without a rubberized cover. Adult and pediatric sizes are available, and the stylet should not extend past the tip of the endotracheal tube or into the Murphy eye. To facilitate the insertion and removal of stylets from endotracheal tubes, a water-soluble lubricant should be applied along its axis before insertion.

LARYNGOSCOPE HANDLE AND BLADE

The laryngoscope handle and blade are used to manipulate the oropharyngeal tissue and epiglottis. The blade provides the ability to visualize the glottic aperture and facilitate insertion of the endotracheal tube into the trachea. The laryngoscope handle (Fig. 4–15) serves a dual function. First, it acts as a power supply that is powered by nicad or alkaline batteries. Its second function is to act as a receptacle for the blade. A variety of blades are available for use with the handle. Selection of a blade depends on patient age, anatomic variabilities of the patient, and clinician preference. Age-appropriate selection of blades listed in Figure 4–16 should be maintained in each practice setting. In most adults, intubation can be done successfully with a Macintosh No. 3 blade or a Miller No. 2 blade. Having both readily available significantly enhances the clinician's ability to secure a patent airway.

MAGILL FORCEPS

Magill forceps are ancillary airway tools used to direct an endotracheal tube during nasotracheal intubation. Endotracheal tubes inserted for nasotracheal intubation hug the posterior pharyngeal wall and may require use of the Magill forceps to distally direct the tube anteriorly and through the glottic opening.

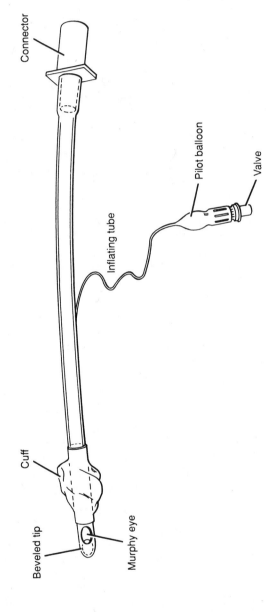

FIGURE 4-13. Murphy endotracheal tube. (From Morgan G, Mikhail M. *Clinical Anesthesiology.* 2nd ed. Stamford, Conn: Appleton & Lange; 1996:60.)

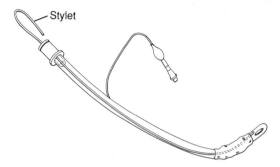

FIGURE 4–14.   Endotracheal tube stylet. Stylets should be well lubricated prior to insertion into the endotracheal tube. The stylet must be bent to prevent the proximal end from extending past the tip of the endotracheal tube. (From Morgan G, Mikhail M. *Clinical Anesthesiology.* 2nd ed. Stamford, Conn: Appleton & Lange; 1996:62.)

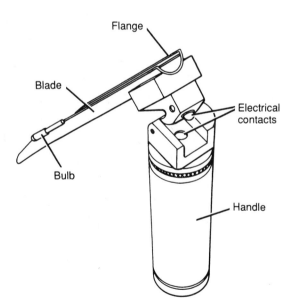

FIGURE 4–15.   Laryngoscope handle. (From Morgan G, Mikhail M. *Clinical Anesthesiology.* 2nd ed. Stamford, Conn: Appleton & Lange; 1996:60.)

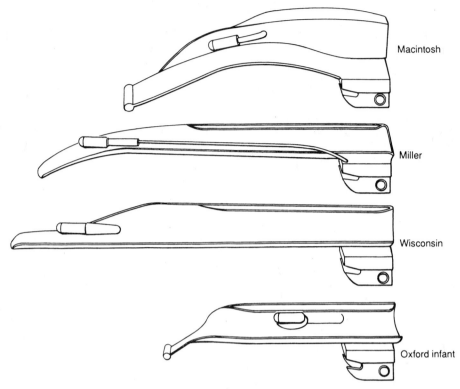

FIGURE 4–16.   Laryngoscope blades. (From Morgan G, Mikhail M. *Clinical Anesthesiology.* 2nd ed. Stamford, Conn: Appleton & Lange; 1996:61.)

SUCTION EQUIPMENT

A variety of suction equipment is currently available on the market. An ample supply of suction liners, filters, tubing, and suction tips must be readily available at each conscious sedation location. In areas where conscious sedation procedures are performed concurrently, one suction unit must be available for each patient. Yankauer suction tips aspirate large volumes of material from the oropharynx. They also offer the advantage of aspiration of larger particulate matter. Disadvantages associated with Yankauer suction tips include lip laceration, oropharyngeal damage, and dental trauma. No. 16 French suction catheters must be available to suction the oropharynx in the event of patients biting or clenching down. Advantages of No. 16 French suction catheters include insertion into small areas and the nasopharynx. Use of emergency airway equipment for respiratory resuscitation is dependent on clinician preference, the degree of respiratory distress, and the patient's anatomy. An ample supply of respiratory equipment must be kept on hand in all conscious sedation locations. Table 4–3 outlines *minimum* recommended emergency airway setup.

TABLE 4–3. *Minimum Recommended Emergency Airway Setup*

- Nasopharyngeal airways (age-appropriate sizes)
- Oropharyngeal airways (age-appropriate sizes)
- Tongue blades
- Lidocaine (Xylocaine) ointment or jelly and water-soluble lubricant
- Two laryngoscope handles
- Two MacIntosh blades (age-appropriate sizes)
- Two Miller blades (age-appropriate sizes)
- Spare blade lightbulbs
- Endotracheal tubes (age-appropriate sizes)
- Two stylets (adult and pediatric)
- Magill forceps (adult and pediatric)
- Suction units
- Yankauer suction tips
- No. 16 French suction catheters
- Supplemental oxygen E cylinders
- Oxygen
- Bag valve mask device
- Face mask (age-appropriate size)

OXYGEN DELIVERY DEVICES

Supplemental oxygen may be administered by a variety of methods. The primary goal of oxygen therapy is the prevention of hypoxia, hypoventilation, and respiratory depression. Table 4–4 shows oxygen systems available to deliver an enriched oxygen environment to the patient. *Because of the respiratory depressant effects associated with all sedatives, hypnotics, and analgesics, serious consideration should be given to the administration of supplemental oxygen to all patients receiving intravenous conscious sedation.*

NASAL CANNULA

Nasal cannulas are low-flow oxygen-administration systems that increase the patient's inspired oxygen concentration. Comfortable and inexpensive, they increase inspired oxygen concentration and allow the nasopharynx to serve as an oxygen reservoir. Inspired oxygen concentration increases 3% to 4% percent for each liter delivered through the nasal cannula.[8] Nasal cannulas are not recommended for flow rates exceeding 5 L/min. Flow rates greater than 4 L/min may lead to drying of mucous membranes, irritation, and bleeding.

OXYGEN FACE MASK

Simple oxygen face masks permit delivery of inspired oxygen of 40% to 60%. This increase in FiO_2 occurs secondary to increased reservoir space and oxygen

TABLE 4-4. *Methods of Oxygen Administration*

METHOD	FIO$_2$	FLOW (L/min)	COMMENTS
LOW-FLOW METHODS			
Nasal cannula (prongs)	0.24–0.40	5–6	Comfortable to wear, patient can breathe orally or nasally and still raise FIO$_2$; humidification unnecessary
Simple face mask	0.40–0.60	5–8	Adjustable to fit face; may be hot and uncomfortable for patients; poorly tolerated; potential for skin irritation from tight fit and oxygen contact
Face tent	0.30–0.55	4–10	Less confining, useful when extra humidity needed
Partial rebreathing mask	0.35–0.60	6–10	Mask with attached reservoir bag; no valves on mask (exhalation ports open)
HIGH-FLOW METHODS			
Nonrebreathing mask	0.40–1.00	6–15	Mask with reservoir bag; one-way valves on exhalation side ports of mask, one-way valve between mask and bag for inhalation
Venturi mask	0.24–0.55	2–14	Believed accurate delivery of desired FIO$_2$; may be less if patient is hyperpneic or unable to keep mask in position on face
T-piece or Brigg's	0.21–1.00	2–10	Used with endotracheal or tracheostomy tube; provides accurate delivery of desired FIO$_2$ and humidification; most often used when weaning patients from ventilator assistance before endotracheal tube removed
Mechanical ventilator	0.21–1.00	Direct from supply	Pressure, volume, flow, and oxygen percentage all adjustable

FIO$_2$ = Fraction of inspired oxygen concentration.
From Drain C. *The Post Anesthesia Care Unit.* 3rd ed. Philadelphia: WB Saunders; 1994:297.

flow. An FIO$_2$ of 40% to 60% depends on oxygen flow rate, the patient's inspiratory flow, and mask fit.

NONREBREATHING MASKS

A distinct advantage of the addition of a reservoir bag to the oxygen face mask is that it allows delivery of up to 100% oxygen when a tight face seal is assured.

Rebreathing is diminished through a combination of unidirectional valves and high inspiratory flow rates.

HUMIDIFIED OXYGEN

Humidified oxygen is indicated in the presence of increased pulmonary secretions, increased viscosity, and mobilization of secretions. The goal of humidification is to decrease viscosity and mobilize secretions by increasing water content in the alveoli. Humidification requires high flow rates to convert water to a vapor state.

MANUAL RESUSCITATIVE DEVICES: BAG VALVE DEVICE

It is important for the clinician participating in the administration of conscious sedation to ventilate patients both efficiently and effectively. As outlined earlier, the provider must be cognizant of airway obstruction and take definitive action when necessary. In the presence of apnea, hypoxemia, or respiratory distress, positive pressure ventilation must be used. In emergent situations the bag valve mask is the ventilation system of choice to deliver oxygen-enriched positive pressure ventilation to the patient. Manual resuscitative devices are known by a variety of names, including the following:

- Bag valve masks
- Bag valve resuscitative device
- Respiratory bags
- Self-inflating resuscitators

During the last several years, manual resuscitators have evolved from a multiuse patient device to a disposable resuscitator for single patient use. Advantages of bag valve masks include the following:

- They are inexpensive
- They allow an enriched oxygen environment
- They are mobile
- They are light in weight

The bag of the resuscitator is self-inflating and is coupled with a nonrebreathing valve to prevent rebreathing of exhaled gases. The American Society for Testing and Materials requires manual resuscitators to be equipped with a mechanism to increase inspired oxygen concentration.[9] When oxygen is delivered into the self-inflating bag, the inspired oxygen concentration increases. Some bags also have an additional reservoir, which allows an opportunity for oxygen to accumulate. Oxygen flows directly into the self-inflating bag when the refill valve opens. During a respiratory crisis, the oxygen flow rate should be 10 to 15 L in the adult patient.[10] Positive pressure ventilation requires the clinician to grasp the self-inflating bag in the middle with firm pressure and depress the bag to deliver an effective ventilation. If the patient is not completely apneic, the delivery of the manual ventilation should be synchronized with the inspiratory phase of the patient.

Complications associated with use of the bag valve mask devices are generally related to valve failure, with resultant rebreathing of expired gases and decreased F_{IO_2}. Additional complications include gastric insufflation secondary to attempted ventilation through a nonpatent airway. Since the advent of disposable single-use units, these complications occur with less frequency. A bag valve mask device that is self-inflating must be present with a backup source of oxygen available in each conscious sedation practice setting. The presence of a backup oxygen source (E cylinders) should be reserved in the event that the regular tank system or hospital pipeline system fails.

REFERENCES

1. Joint Commission for Accreditation of Healthcare Organizations. *1997 Accreditation Manual for Hospitals.* Oakbrook Terrace, Ill: The Commission; 1997:78.
2. Barash P, Cullen B, Stoelting R. *Clinical Anesthesia.* 2nd ed. Philadelphia: JB Lippincott; 1992:685.
3. Barash P, Cullen B, Stoelting R. *Clinical Anesthesia.* 2nd ed. Philadelphia: JB Lippincott; 1992:686.
4. Mallampati S. Clinical signs to predict difficult tracheal intubation. *Can Anaesth Soc J.* 1983;30:429–434.
5. Stoelting R, Miller F. *Basics of Anesthesia.* 3rd ed. New York: Churchill Livingstone; 1994:145.
6. Ellis H, Feldman S. *Anatomy for Anaesthetists.* 6th ed. Cambridge, Mass: Blackwell Scientific Publications; 1993:285.
7. Cummins R. *American Heart Association Advanced Cardiac Life Support.* Dallas: The Association; 1994:2.
8. Morgan E, Mikhail M. *Clinical Anesthesiology.* 2nd ed. Stamford, Conn: Appleton & Lange; 1996.
9. Dorsch J, Dorsch S. *Understanding Anesthesia Equipment.* 3rd ed. Baltimore: Williams & Wilkins; 1994:231.
10. Dorsch J, Dorsch S. *Understanding Anesthesia Equipment.* 3rd ed. Baltimore: Williams & Wilkins; 1994:234.

The ideal characteristics of injected pharmacologic agents to achieve the desired effects of conscious sedation (intact reflexes, patient cooperation, and reduced anxiety), include the following:

- Rapid onset of action
- Short duration of action
- Lack of cumulative effects
- Rapid recovery
- Minimal side effects
- Rapid metabolism to inactivate nontoxic metabolites
- Residual analgesia
- Increased patient satisfaction

Unfortunately, there is no one single pharmacologic agent or technique that satisfies all of these requirements. In an attempt to produce an amnestic, pain-free, sedated patient, a combination of medications is required. This combination of medications gives the clinician the ability to manipulate the patient's short-term memory and sense of time.[1] Through pharmacologic intervention, the patient's perception of time is altered and patient cooperation is enhanced. To successfully produce conscious sedation (drowsiness, nystagmus, slurred speech, relaxation, and anxiolysis) and minimize complications (respiratory distress, cardiovascular depression, and hypoxemia) requires an understanding of the pharmacologic agents used to produce conscious sedation. A complete pharmacologic profile of medications used to produce conscious sedation is provided in Appendix D. Table 5–1 outlines the advantages and disadvantages of pharmacologic combinations.

PHARMACODYNAMICS AND PHARMACOKINETICS

BENZODIAZEPINES

Pharmacodynamics

Benzodiazepines bind to specific receptor sites in the central nervous system, particularly in the cerebral cortex. Benzodiazepine receptor binding enhances gamma-aminobutyric acid (GABA) in the brain. Through this GABA interaction (Fig. 5–1), excitatory impulses are inhibited. Pharmacologic effects ranging from

99

TABLE 5–1.   *Pharmacologic Combinations*

Single pharmacologic agents may produce
- Adequate sedation in many cases
- Toxicity at increased doses
- Isolated pharmacologic effect (analgesia, amnesia)
- Cumulative effects

A **combination of pharmacologic agents** may produce
- Rapid recovery
- Decreased dosage requirement
- Unpredictable synergistic actions
- Increased likelihood of medication error with multiple injections

mild sedation to general anesthesia depend on the amount of medication administered. Benzodiazepines are used to achieve the following.

- Anxiolysis
- Sedation
- Hypnosis
- Anticonvulsion
- Skeletal muscle relaxation

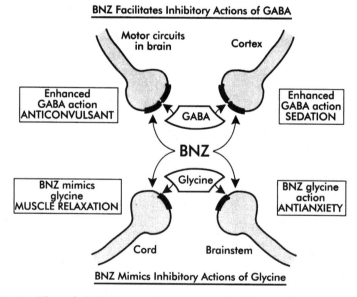

FIGURE 5–1.   Through GABA interaction, enhanced inhibition of neurotransmitters occurs, altering normal neuronal function in the central nervous system. (From Richter JJ. Current theories about the mechanisms of benzodiazepines and neuroleptic drugs. *Anesthesiology.* 1981;54:66.)

Pharmacokinetics

Benzodiazepines are administered in the following ways:

- Orally
- Intramuscularly
- Intravascularly

Benzodiazepines are lipid soluble and readily penetrate the blood-brain barrier. Metabolism of benzodiazepines occurs by means of hepatic metabolism and renal excretion.[2] Initially synthesized in 1959, diazepam is the prototype benzodiazepine with which all others are compared.[3] Classified as a long-acting benzodiazepine, intramuscular injections of diazepam are both painful and erratically absorbed.[4] Diazepam is well absorbed from the gastrointestinal tract. Peak plasma levels are achieved in 1 to 2 hours after oral administration and 1 to 2 minutes after intravenous administration. The initial metabolism of diazepam yields an active metabolite, desmethyldiazepam. Diazepam has a prolonged half-life (30 to 50 hours) when compared with its short-acting counterpart, midazolam (2 to 4 hours).[5] When compared with midazolam's water-soluble suspension, diazepam's propylene glycol suspension predisposes to venous irritation and phlebitis. The half-life associated with benzodiazepines is secondary to the degree of hepatic extraction and the volume of distribution. Excretion of benzodiazepines is dependent on renal clearance.

End-Organ Effects

CARDIOVASCULAR SYSTEM. Arterial blood pressure, cardiac output, and peripheral vascular resistance are slightly decreased with the administration of benzodiazepines.

RESPIRATORY SYSTEM. Benzodiazepines depress the ventilatory response to carbon dioxide. They are highly potent drugs, and even small doses may result in respiratory arrest, especially when given in conjunction with opioids. Careful titration and vigilance are required when these medications are administered.

CENTRAL NERVOUS SYSTEM. A reduction in cerebral blood flow, cerebral oxygen consumption, and intracranial pressure occurs with the administration of benzodiazepines. Benzodiazepines are effective in treating seizure disorders and are noted for their centrally mediated muscle relaxant properties. The anterograde amnesia, anxiolysis, and hypnosis provided by benzodiazepines are useful adjuncts during the administration of conscious sedation.

REVERSAL OF PHARMACOLOGIC EFFECT. The central nervous system and respiratory depressant effects of benzodiazepines may be reversed with the administration of flumazenil. A complete pharmacologic profile of flumazenil is given in Appendix D.

PRECAUTIONS. To avoid respiratory compromise or cardiovascular depression, caution must be exercised when benzodiazepines are administered to patients with the following conditions:

- Chronic obstructive pulmonary disease
- History of sleep apnea
- Cardiopulmonary depression
- Extremes of age
- Alcohol intoxication
- Morbid obesity
- Difficult airways
- Pathophysiologic disease process

OPIOIDS

Pharmacodynamics

The administration of opioids results in binding to specific opiate receptors located within the central nervous system. Opioids occupy mu, kappa, delta, and sigma receptor subtypes.

MU
1. Analgesia
2. Respiratory depression
3. Miosis
4. Decreased gastrointestinal motility
5. Euphoria
6. Suppression of opiate withdrawal

KAPPA
1. Analgesia
2. Respiratory depression
3. Miosis
4. Dysphoria

DELTA
1. Analgesia
2. Respiratory depression

SIGMA
1. Dysphoria
2. Hallucinations

The pharmacologic effects of opioids depend on the specific receptor subtypes stimulated. Opioids produce some degree of sedation; however, they are used mainly for their analgesic properties. Increased dosage of narcotics is associated with increased levels of sedation and the potential for severe respiratory depression.

Pharmacokinetics

Intramuscularly, intravenously, and orally administered opioids are readily absorbed to achieve effective plasma levels. Distribution characteristics are presented in Table 5–2. Opioids are metabolized by hepatic biotransformation. The

TABLE 5–2. *Distribution Characteristics of Opioids*

	MORPHINE	DEMEROL	FENTANYL	ALFENTANIL
Potency	1	0.1	75–125 × morphine's	$^1/_5$–$^1/_{10}$ of fentanyl's
Elimination half-life (minutes)	102–130	220–265	180–220	70–100
Protein binding	30%	64–82%	85%	90%
Heart rate	↓	↑	↓↓	↓↓
Mean arterial pressure	◆	◆	↓	↓↓
Ventilation	↓↓↓	↓↓↓	↓↓↓	↓↓↓
Cerebral blood flow	↓	↓	↓	↓
Cerebral metabolic rate of O_2	↓	↓	↓	↓
Intracranial pressure	↓	↓	↓	↓

◆ Decrease in MAP = Degree of histamine release.

extraction ratio depends on hepatic blood flow. Pharmacologic end products are excreted through the kidneys. Small fractions of opioids are excreted unchanged in the urine.

End-Organ Effects

CARDIOVASCULAR SYSTEM. Meperidine produces tachycardia because of its vagolytic effect. In comparison, morphine sulfate, fentanyl, sufentanil, and alfentanil produce vagally mediated bradycardia. Blood pressure may decrease because of bradycardia, decreased systemic vascular resistance, and alterations in the sympathetic nervous system. Meperidine and morphine sulfate release histamine, which may significantly decrease systemic vascular resistance and bronchoconstriction.

RESPIRATORY SYSTEM. Opioids depress respiratory rate and volume. $Paco_2$ and the apneic threshold for carbon dioxide are increased. Chest wall rigidity may occur with rapid administration of opioids. The incidence may be decreased through careful titration and slow injection of intravenous opioids.

CENTRAL NERVOUS SYSTEM. Opioids increase cerebral metabolic rate, cerebral blood flow, and intracranial pressure through respiratory depression and carbon dioxide retention. Additional central nervous system effects include the following:

- Analgesia
- Respiratory depression
- Drowsiness
- Sedation
- Euphoria
- Dysphoria
- Nausea and vomiting

REVERSAL OF PHARMACOLOGIC EFFECT. The central nervous system and respiratory depressant effects of opioids are reversed with the administration of naloxone (Narcan). Naloxone is a pure opioid antagonist, which competitively binds at the opiate receptors. A complete pharmacologic profile of nalaxone is featured in Appendix D.

PRECAUTIONS. Prior to the administration of intravenous opioids, extreme caution must be exercised in patients with the following:

- Chronic obstructive pulmonary disease
- History of sleep apnea
- Cardiopulmonary depression
- Extremes of age
- Alcohol intoxication
- Morbid obesity
- Difficult airways
- Pathophysiologic disease process
- Symptomatic bradycardia

BARBITURATES

Pharmacodynamics

Barbiturates suppress the reticular activating center (sleep-wake center) located in the brain stem and the cerebral cortex on a dose-dependent continuum.[6] However, the specific site of pharmacologic action is nonselective. Barbiturates are used for their sedative, hypnotic, and anticonvulsant properties. According to the total dose administered, barbiturates are capable of producing effects ranging from sedation to deep coma.

Pharmacokinetics

Barbiturates may be administered intravenously or rectally. Rectal administration is generally reserved for pediatric premedication. Intravenous use includes sedation, induction of general anesthesia, and barbiturate coma. Because of their high lipid solubility, barbiturates reach the brain within 30 seconds. Redistribution from the central compartment (intravascular fluid and highly perfused tissues: lungs, heart, brain, kidneys, liver) to the peripheral compartment (skeletal muscle, fat, bone) is responsible for the duration of action. Repeated doses of barbiturates result in a prolonged duration of action as the peripheral compartment becomes saturated. Metabolism of barbiturates requires hepatic oxidation. Once hepatic oxidation is complete, renal excretion is responsible for water-soluble metabolites.

End-Organ Effects

CARDIOVASCULAR SYSTEM. Hypotension, tachycardia, decreased systemic vascular resistance, and decreased venous return may occur with the administration of barbiturates. Cardiovascular changes associated with barbiturate administration are related to decreased cardiac output and reduced systemic vascular resistance. These effects are more pronounced in the hypovolemic patient.

RESPIRATORY SYSTEM. Decreased ventilatory response to oxygen and carbon dioxide occurs with the administration of barbiturates. Depression of the medullary respiratory center (hypoventilation and apnea) is associated with increased doses of barbiturates. Smooth muscle constriction may result in bronchospasm. Hiccoughs and tonic-clonic movements occur with the administration of methohexital, particularly after multiple cumulative doses.

CENTRAL NERVOUS SYSTEM. Barbiturates decrease cerebral metabolic rate, cerebral blood flow, and intracranial pressure by means of cerebral vasoconstriction. Small doses of barbiturates may cause a state of disorientation or excitement. Barbiturates do not have analgesic properties and appear to have an antianalgesic effect. Additional central nervous system effects include somnolence, agitation, confusion, nervousness, and anxiety.

PHARMACOLOGIC REVERSAL. Systemic pulmonary and cardiovascular support are required in the event of overdose. For respiratory depression, ventilation is required until recovery from pharmacologic effect.

PRECAUTIONS. Care should be taken in patients with the following conditions:

- Hepatic dysfunction
- Porphyria
- Cardiopulmonary depression
- Chronic obstructive pulmonary disease
- History of sleep apnea
- Extremes of age
- Alcohol intoxication
- Morbid obesity
- Difficult airways
- Pathophysiologic disease process

DISSOCIATIVE ANESTHESIA

Pharmacodynamics

Ketamine is a derivative of phencyclidine, which produces a dissociative state. In subanesthetic doses, ketamine provides profound analgesia. Ketamine "dissociates" the thalamus (sensory relay from the reticular activating system to the cerebral cortex) from the limbic system.[7] Characteristic appearance of the dissociative state include the following:

- Intense analgesia and amnesia
- Cataleptic state
- Nystagmus
- Open-eyed gaze

- Noncommunicative patient, although the patient gives the appearance of wakefulness
- Skeletal muscle movement

Pharmacokinetics

After intravenous administration, ketamine has a rapid onset and a short duration of action. Distribution half-life is approximately 10 to 15 minutes. Redistribution to the vessel-poor group (fat, skeletal muscle, bone) and biotransformation by the liver results in awakening. Biotransformation results in pharmacologic active metabolites (norketamine). Metabolites are excreted in the urine.

End-Organ Effects

CARDIOVASCULAR SYSTEM. Stimulation of the sympathetic nervous system increases heart rate, cardiac output, and arterial blood pressure. Increased myocardial oxygen consumption occurs in conjunction with these changes. Ketamine is contraindicated in patients with coronary artery disease, hypertension, congestive heart failure, or impaired myocardial performance.

RESPIRATORY SYSTEM. Ketamine produces bronchodilation and minimal reduction of ventilatory drive. Upper airway muscle tone is maintained, and airway reflexes remain intact. Salivary and mucous secretion is enhanced with ketamine administration. These effects may be counteracted with the administration of an antisialogogue (atropine, glycopyrrolate [Robinul]).

CENTRAL NERVOUS SYSTEM. Increased cerebral blood flow, cerebral oxygen consumption, and intracranial pressure occur as a result of cerebral vasodilation. Therefore ketamine use is contraindicated in patients with intracranial disease. Myoclonic activity is characteristic of ketamine administration. Emergence delirium and undesirable central nervous system side effects include visual and auditory illusions, dreams, and combativeness and may persist for 24 hours. Emergence delirium generally occurs as the patient is recovering from the pharmacologic effects of ketamine administration. Reassurance and provision of a quiet area in which to recover have been proposed to decrease the incidence of central nervous system excitation.

PHARMACOLOGIC REVERSAL. Systemic pulmonary and cardiovascular support are required in the event of overdose. For respiratory depression, ventilation is required until the patient recovers from pharmacologic effect.

PRECAUTIONS. Extreme caution is required in the presence of increased intracranial pressure, coronary artery disease, and hypertension.

LOCAL ANESTHETICS

Pharmacodynamics

Local anesthetics provide temporary loss of motor, sensory, and autonomic nervous system function. Local anesthetics generally consist of the following:

- A lipophilic group (benzene ring)
- A hydrophylic group (tertiary amine)
- An intermediate chain (ester or amide linkage)

However, they differ specifically with regard to

- Potency
- Time of onset
- Duration of pharmacologic effect
- Toxicity

Local anesthetics prevent the development of the action potential required for depolarization of nerve cells. For transmission of impulses to occur, movement of sodium and potassium ions is required. Depolarization occurs when sodium ions move from extracellular fluid to the intracellular space. Repolarization occurs when potassium ions move from the intracellular to the extracellular space. As depicted in Figure 5–2, by preventing development of an action potential, nerve conduction is impaired. Local anesthetics are classified as amides or esters. Amide local anesthetics include the following:

- Bupivicaine (Marcaine)
- Etidocaine (Duranest)
- Lidocaine (Xylocaine)
- Mepivicaine (Carbocaine)

Ester local anesthetics include the following:

- Chlorprocaine (Nesacaine)
- Cocaine
- Procaine (Novocain)
- Tetracaine (Pontocaine)

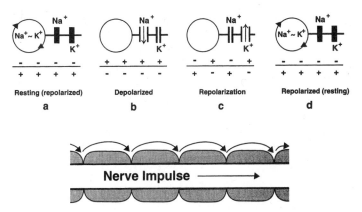

FIGURE 5–2.   Local anesthetic agents block the conduction of impulses along the nerve fiber. Local anesthetics make changes in the nerve membrane that prevent normal depolarization and repolarization of the nerve cell membrane. (From Chung DC, Lam AM. *Essentials of Anesthesiology.* 3rd ed. Philadelphia: WB Saunders; 1997:81.)

Pharmacokinetics

Local anesthetic absorption is dependent on a variety of factors:

- Increased vascularity at the injection site results in increased local anesthetic uptake
- Vasoconstrictors decrease rate of absorption
- Increased protein binding increases duration of action
- Increased lipid solubility increases potency

Ester local anesthetics are derived from para-aminobenzoic acid (PABA). Ester local anesthetics are metabolized by ester hydrolysis and pseudocholinesterase, which is found in the plasma.[8] Amide local anesthetics are metabolized by dealkylation and hydrolysis in the liver.[8] Local anesthetic potency is determined by lipid solubility. Protein binding determines the duration of effect as the highly bound local anesthetic remains in the lipoprotein of the nerve membrane for a longer duration. Commonly used local anesthetics for minor surgical and diagnostic procedures are listed in Table 5–3. At times, combinations of local anesthetics are used. This admixture of local anesthetics offers the clinician the beneficial pharmacologic effects of each local anesthetic selected.

Epinephrine may be added to local anesthetics to promote local tissue vasoconstriction. This vasoconstriction limits uptake into the tissue while prolonging the effects of the local anesthetic. The addition of epinephrine to the local anesthetic solution is contraindicated in the following patient populations:

- Those with unstable angina
- Those with cardiac dysrhythmias
- Infiltration into areas without adequate collateral blood flow (fingers, toes, etc.)
- Hyperthyroid patients
- Patients with uteroplacental insufficiency

End-Organ Effects

CARDIOVASCULAR SYSTEM. Intravenous injection of local anesthetics depresses the automaticity of the myocardium.[9] Myocardial contractility is reduced when local anesthetic concentration is increased. Decreased contractility is secondary to cardiac membrane changes and alterations in the response of the autonomic nervous system. Toxic manifestations associated with local anesthetic overdose include the following:

- Bradycardia
- Heart block
- Hypotension
- Cardiac arrest
- Circulatory collapse

Treatment of cardiovascular side effects associated with local anesthetic overdose includes the following.

TABLE 5–3. *Commonly Used Local Anesthetics*

LOCAL ANESTHETIC	CONCENTRATION (%)	DURATION (min)	DURATION WITH EPINEPHRINE (min)	MAXIMUM DOSE (mg)	MAXIMUM DOSE WITH EPINEPHRINE (mg)	ONSET	POTENCY	TOXICITY
Procaine (Novocain)	1	30–60 (short)	30–90	1000	Seldom used	Fast	Low	Low
Lidocaine (Xylocaine)	0.5–2	30–120 (moderate)	120–360	300	500	Rapid	Moderate	Moderate
Mepivicaine (Carbocaine)	0.5–1	45–90 (moderate)	120–360	300	500	Moderate	Moderate	Moderate
Bupivicaine (Marcaine)	0.25–0.5	120–240 (very long)	180–420	175	225	Slow	High	High
Chlorprocaine (Nesacaine)	1–2	30–45 (short)	30–90	800	1000	Very rapid	Low	Very low

- Administration of oxygen
- Airway support
- Circulatory support (volume expanders)
- Vasopressor and inotropes
- Advanced cardiac life support (ACLS) protocol implementation

Respiratory System. Apnea after the administration of local anesthetics may occur following specific nerve paralysis (phrenic, intercostal) or medullary center depression (retrobulbar block). Treatment of local anesthetic–induced respiratory center depression includes administration of oxygen, ventilation, and airway support.

Central Nervous System. The central nervous system is extremely sensitive to the excitatory effects of local anesthetic–induced toxicity. Neurologic signs and symptoms of local anesthetic–induced toxicity include the following:

- Agitation
- Numbness of the tongue and mouth
- Dizziness
- Visual disturbance
- Tinnitis
- Restlessness
- Slurred speech
- Irrational behavior
- Muscle twitching
- Apnea
- Convulsions

Central nervous system symptoms may range from mild complaints to life-threatening complications. As symptoms progress, tonic-clonic seizures, respiratory arrest, vomiting with aspiration, and loss of consciousness may ensue. Treatment of neurologic side effects associated with local anesthetic overdose include the following:

- Administration of oxygen
- Airway support and ventilation
- In the presence of seizures, small doses of benzodiazepines (1 to 2 mg midazolam [Versed], 5 to 10 mg diazepam [Valium]) or barbiturates (50 mg thiopental sodium [Pentothal Sodium]) may be used.

With proper selection of the local anesthetic combined with conscious sedation, most surgical and diagnostic procedures are performed uneventfully. As the registered nurse is cognizant of conscious sedation medications and mode of administration, the nurse too must be familiar with local anesthetics used for diagnostic or surgical procedures. Preparation for adverse effects associated with the administration of local anesthesia (seizures, cardiovascular depression) is required whenever local anesthetics are administered. Table 5–4 identifies medications and resuscitative equipment required in the event of a local anesthesia toxicity reaction.

TABLE 5–4. *Emergency Resuscitative Medication and Equipment for Local Anesthesia Toxicity Reaction*

- Benzodiazepine (midazolam or diazepam)
  or
  barbiturate (thiopental [Pentothal])
- Advanced Cardiac Life Support protocol medications
- Crash cart
- Oral airways
- Nasal airways
- Laryngoscope
- Endotracheal tubes
- Suction

TECHNIQUES OF ADMINISTRATION

When administered properly, the use of sedatives, analgesics, and tranquilizers provides a sedate patient with minimal side effects. The variety of sedative medications and modes of administration offer the physician and the registered nurse a wide range of options to achieve the goals and objectives of conscious sedation. Selection of any medication or administration by a particular technique is dependent on the patient's preprocedure physical status, the presence of pathophysiologic disease states, age, and the planned procedure. The medications that follow or particular techniques of administration are provided as a general guide to be used in consideration with the aforementioned variables.

SINGLE-DOSE INJECTION TECHNIQUES (TITRATION TO EFFECT)

Medications used for the administration of conscious sedation may be given in a variety of ways. As depicted in Figure 5–3, the single-dose injection technique uses individual medications titrated slowly to effect. To establish an analgesic base, opioids are often administered before benzodiazepines. Two to 3 minutes prior to the procedure, intravenous fentanyl, 1 to 2 µg/kg (titrated in 25 µg increments), alfentanil, 3 to 8 µg/kg (titrated in 125 µg increments), or meperidine 0.5 to 1 mg/kg (titrated in 25 mg increments) may be slowly administered to establish analgesia. Some clinicians prefer to administer narcotics by the intramuscular route. For intramuscular injection, the narcotic of choice is administered approximately 45 to 60 minutes before the scheduled procedure. Disadvantages associated with this technique include scheduling conflicts, injection into subcutaneous tissue, poor absorption, and the time required to monitor the patient after an opioid injection.

Combining medications (narcotics, benzodiazepines, and hypnotics) reduces total dosage through synergistic action, assists the clinician in the maintenance of conscious sedation parameters, and provides rapid patient recovery. In conjunction with the preexisting analgesia established with opioids, the addition of benzodi-

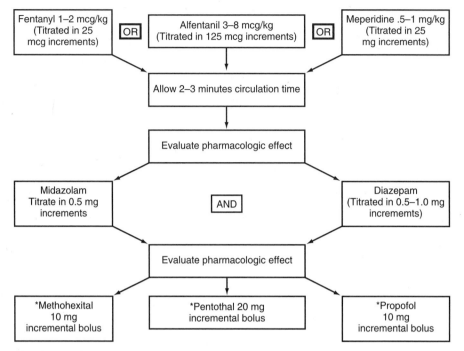

*Requires careful assessment and skill in administration technique to avoid deep levels of sedation, cardiopulmonary depression, or rapid oxygen desaturation.

FIGURE 5–3. Single-dose injection techniques.

azepines (midazolam in 0.5 mg increments or diazepam in 1 mg increments) titrated to an end point of nystagmus or slurred speech provides a sedate patient. To avoid cardiopulmonary depression, it is important to titrate medications slowly to the clinical end points outlined earlier. A complete pharmacologic profile for narcotics, benzodiazepines, and sedative hypnotic agents is outlined in Appendix D.

At times, small amounts of barbiturates or hypnotics are administered in addition to other agents to provide periodic increases in the depth of sedation. The addition of 10 mg boluses of methohexital, 20 mg boluses of thiopental, or 10 mg increments of propofol provides this deeper level of sedation. Propofol offers the distinct advantage of rapid awakening because of its short half-life, elimination, clearance, and antiemetic effect.

BOLUS TECHNIQUE

A popular technique used for oral surgery and gastroenterologic procedures is the bolus technique. Based on a predetermined dosage (mg/kg), the entire dose or a large percentage is administered in one single injection. The technique is particularly popular for administration of benzodiazepines. One advantage of this technique is its ability to provide a rapid therapeutic plasma level immediately before the procedure.

Disadvantages of bolus injection include respiratory depression, unconsciousness, chest wall rigidity, and cardiovascular depression. The bolus technique eliminates the safety features of slow titration, which assesses for patient response and clinical sedation end points (nystagmus, slurred speech). Despite the speed with which a desired plasma concentration can be achieved, the risks associated with the bolus technique may outweigh the potential benefits. Small incremental boluses offer the ability to produce therapeutic plasma levels slowly while potentially using less medication to produce the same pharmacologic effect.

CONTINUOUS-INFUSION TECHNIQUES

Continuous-infusion techniques permit a constant plasma level through a continuous infusion of medication. The continuous-infusion technique avoids the fluctuations in plasma levels associated with bolus techniques. Additional potential benefits include decreased recovery time, less drug administered, and minimized side effects. Careful titration based on predetermined clinical end points (nystagmus, slurred speech, sedation) allows the infusion to be discontinued at the conclusion of the procedure with a rapid return to an alert state. Continuous infusion techniques are popular with propofol administered at a micrograms per kilogram per minute administration rate (Table 5–5). Continuous-infusion techniques require a carrier intravenous solution with the continuous infusion piggybacked into the carrier solution. Extreme care must be exercised to avoid running the carrier solution at a keep-vein-open or slow rate, thereby allowing a buildup of the infusion into the venoset. Once the carrier fluid is opened, the patient receives a large bolus of medications and experiences the side effects associated with an overdose.

Regardless of the technique of administration, clinicians engaged in the administration of conscious sedation must appreciate the pharmacologic dynamics of medications used. Careful titration is warranted in all situations to prevent the development of deep sedation states, hypoxia, and cardiovascular depression.

TABLE 5–5. *Continuous-Infusion Technique*

- Initiate intravenous line with carrier solution (normal saline, Ringer's lactate, etc.)
- Establish narcotic base:
  Fentanyl, 1–2 µg/kg
    or
  Alfentanil, 3–8 µg/kg
- Sedation must be initiated slowly with a continuous-infusion technique to achieve the desired conscious sedation effect and to avoid cardiovascular and respiratory depression
- Begin administration of propofol (5 µg/kg/min)
- Infusion rate may be increased at 5 µg/kg/min intervals

Most patients exhibit clinical end points of conscious sedation (nystagmus, slurred speech) at dosage ranges of 5 to 40 µg/kg/min.

Dosage and rate of administration must be established slowly. Clinically relevant factors that decrease total dosage of medication administered include preprocedure patient status, age, presence of pathophysiologic disease, and desired level of sedation.

Clinician compliance with hospital conscious sedation policies, manufacturer's recommendations, Joint Commission on the Accreditation of Healthcare Organizations (JCAHO) requirements, and applicable state practice statutes is required to provide quality pharmacologic intervention for patients receiving conscious sedation.

REFERENCES

1. Spires G. The Big Mac, Conscious vs. Unconscious Sedation. Early Bird Symposium, 63rd AANA National Meeting. August, 1996.
2. Medical Economics. *Physician's Desk Reference.* 50th ed. Montvale, NJ: Medical Economics; 1996:2183.
3. Miller R, Stoelting R. *Anesthesia.* 4th ed. New York: Churchill Livingstone; 1994.
4. Davidson J, Eckhardt W, Perese D. *Clinical Anesthesia Procedures of the Massachusetts General Hospital.* 4th ed. Boston: Little, Brown; 1993:11.
5. White P. *International Anesthesiology Clinics: Anesthesia for Ambulatory Surgery.* Boston: Little, Brown; 1994;32:3.
6. Aldrete J, Stanley T. *Trends in Intravenous Anesthesia.* Chicago: Year Book Medical; 1980.
7. Morgan E, Mikhail M. *Clinical Anesthesiology.* 2nd ed. Stamford, Conn: Appleton & Lange; 1996:141.
8. Scott B. *Techniques of Regional Anesthesia.* Stamford, Conn: Appleton & Lange; 1989:15.
9. Morgan E, Mikhail M. *Clinical Anesthesiology.* 2nd ed. Stamford, Conn: Appleton & Lange; 1996:178.

Monitoring Modalities

CHAPTER 6

RECOMMENDED **AORN** PRACTICE III

The RN monitoring the patient's care should be clinically competent in the function and in the use of resuscitation medications and monitoring equipment and be able to interpret the data obtained from the patient.

JCAHO STANDARD **TX.2.3**

The patient's physiologic status is measured and assessed during the operative or invasive procedure.

Once the preprocedure assessment is completed, the patient is readied for the procedure. To avoid catastrophic mishaps and to comply with Joint Commission on Accreditation of Healthcare Organizations (JCAHO)- and Association of Operating Room Nurses (AORN)-recommended practice and specific state statutes, familiarity with monitoring equipment and interpretation of data is required. The monitoring process involves the following:

- Observation and vigilance
- Interpretation of data
- Initiation of corrective action when required

ELECTROCARDIOGRAM

The ECG is used during conscious sedation procedures to help in the detection of the following:

- Arrhythmias
- Myocardial ischemia
- Electrolyte disturbance
- Pacemaker function

ECG LEADS

The electrocardiogram reflects the electrical activity of the heart in graphic form. Electrodes pick up electrical signals generated by the heart's conduction system. Electrodes may be placed on the four limbs and six areas on the chest. ECG monitoring is useful in the detection of the pathophysiologic condition of the entire heart, cardiac rhythm disturbances, and conduction disorders. The majority of ECG monitors depict this electrical activity through a single lead. Lead position is determined by placement of the positive and negative electrode secured to the patient. The standard leads view the frontal plane of the heart through placement of a positive and a negative electrode. A difference in electrical potential is recorded in the left arm, the right arm, and the left leg.[1] Standard bipolar limb leads include the following:

- Lead I. Difference in electrical potential between the left arm and the right arm.
- Lead II. Difference in electrical potential between the left leg and the right arm.
- Lead III. Difference in electrical potential between the left leg and the left arm.

Figure 6–1 depicts the electrical potential for each bipolar limb lead.

Unipolar leads (Fig. 6–2) reflect the electrical potential between the designated extremity lead and a neutral electrical point at the center of the heart.[1] The three augmented leads view the heart in the frontal plane by means of the same three limbs in different combinations. The augmented or unipolar limb leads include the following:

- aVR. Augmented voltage of the right arm. The right arm is positive compared with the left arm and the left leg.

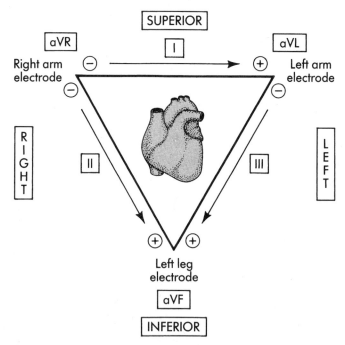

FIGURE 6–1.   Electrical potential for bipolar limb leads. (From Grauer K. *A Practical Guide to ECG Interpretation.* St. Louis: Mosby; 1992:14.)

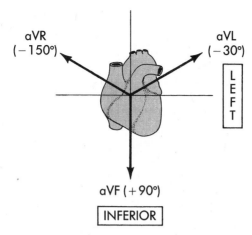

FIGURE 6-2. Electrical activity of unipolar limb leads. (From Grauer K. *A Practical Guide to ECG Interpretation.* St. Louis: Mosby; 1992:14.)

- aVL. Augmented voltage of the left arm. The left arm is positive compared with the right arm and the left leg.
- aVF. Augmented voltage of the left foot. The left foot is positive compared with the right arm and the left arm.

The unipolar precordial leads measure the heart's electrical activity in the horizontal planes.

- Leads V_1 and V_2 are placed over the right ventricle.
- V_3 and V_4 are placed over the interventricular septum.
- V_5 and V_6 are placed over the left ventricle.

Positioning of the precordial leads is depicted in Figure 6-3.

One lead (lead I, II, or III) of the standard bipolar limb leads is generally selected for procedural monitoring and recovery. Optimal ECG tracings depend on proper placement of two sensory electrodes and a ground or reference electrode. To obtain an accurate recording, gelled electrodes must be applied to clean, dry skin. For conscious sedation procedures, lead II is beneficial to detect the presence of arrhythmias. Lead II is useful in the detection of arrhythmias because of the increased visibility of the P wave in this lead. When indicated (coronary artery disease, angina, left ventricular dysfunction), lead V_5 is used to detect ischemia. Since a large portion of the left ventricle is located beneath the V_5 position, it is a useful lead in the detection of myocardial ischemia. An important rationale for use of the ECG is to assess for the presence of myocardial ischemia. Indicators for myocardial ischemia are depicted in Table 6-1. In situations that afford only three lead monitoring systems, a modified chest lead (MCL) may be used to monitor for the presence of myocardial ischemia. MCL electrode placement is depicted in Figure 6-4.

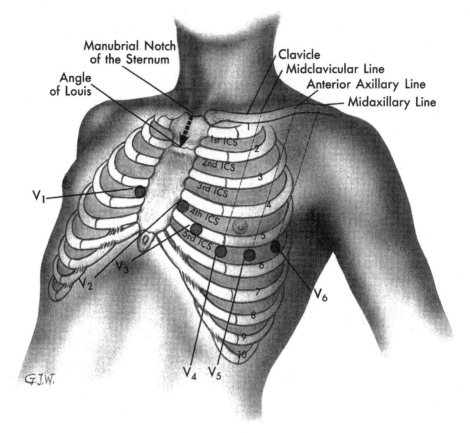

FIGURE 6–3.   Placement of the precordial leads. (From Grauer K. *A Practical Guide to ECG Interpretation.* St. Louis: Mosby; 1992:15.)

TABLE 6–1.   *Indicators of Myocardial Ischemia*

Another important rationale for utilization of the ECG is to assess for the presence of myocardial ischemia. Myocardial ischemic indicators include

ST SEGMENT ELEVATION
Acute myocardial infarction may be associated with ST segment elevation. ST segment changes may range from minor peaking or widening of the T wave to pronounced ST segment elevation. ST segment elevation is associated with acute ischemic injury.

ST SEGMENT DEPRESSION
Ischemia of the subendocardial layer of the myocardium results in ST segment depression. Ischemia is reflected as depression of the ST segment because the chest electrodes do not face the subendocardial layers of the heart.

T WAVE INVERSION
T wave inversion generally follows ST segment elevation and is associated with continued myocardial ischemia.

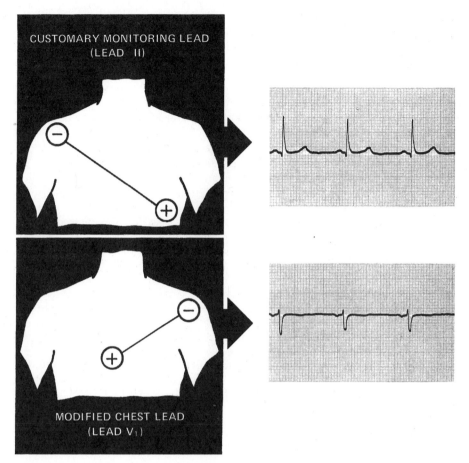

CUSTOMARY MONITORING LEAD
(LEAD II)

MODIFIED CHEST LEAD
(LEAD V₁)

FIGURE 6–4. MCL electrode positioning places the right arm lead under the left clavicle and the left arm in the V_5 position. The left leg lead is placed in the standard V_1 position. (From Meltzer L. *Intensive Coronary Care: A Manual for Nurses.* 4th ed. East Norwalk, Conn: Appleton & Lange; 1983:121.)

CARDIAC RHYTHM AND ARRHYTHMIAS

The cardiac cycle is associated with five distinct waves or deflections as defined in Table 6–2 and depicted in Figure 6–5. Figure 6–6 compares the cardiac cycle and electrocardiographic time measurements. Alterations or variations of this cardiac cycle may represent arrhythmias and lead to the associated symptoms presented in this chapter. Presentation of cardiac rhythms on pages 122 to 135 is intended as a basic review of common and life-threatening arrhythmias. It is strongly recommended that these materials be used as a reference tool and as a supplement to Advanced Cardiac Life Support (ACLS) training and treatment protocols. Although many state statutes require ACLS certification and many specialty organizations recommend ACLS training, it is not a uniform requirement in all facilities. As Dr. Richard Cummins, chairman of the Subcommittee on Ad-

TABLE 6–2.   *Cardiac Cycle*

P wave	Represents atrial depolarization and impulse generation from the SA node through the AV node.
PR interval	Represents the length of time required for the atria to depolarize and delay of the impulse through the AV junction. Normally measures 0.12 to 0.20 second.
QRS complex	Represents ventricular depolarization (phase 0 of the action potential). Q wave = first negative deflection after P wave. R wave = first positive deflection after P wave. The QRS normally measures 0.04 to 1 second. S wave = the negative deflection following the R wave.
ST segment	Represents early repolarization of the right and left ventricles. Begins at the end of the QRS complex and ends with onset of the T wave.
T wave	Represents ventricular repolarization. Peaked T waves are seen in patients with hyperkalemia.
QT interval	Represents total ventricular activity (depolarization and repolarization). Measured from the beginning of the QRS complex to the end of the T wave. Normally measures 0.36 to 0.44 second (varies with heart rate, age, and sex).

vanced Cardiac Life Support, states: *"ACLS is about preparing yourself to provide the best possible care for the most dramatic and emotional moment of a person's life."*[2] Therefore it is recommended that all team members participating in the administration of conscious sedation have ACLS certification and a working knowledge of treatment algorithms (see Appendix E).

Text continued on page 136

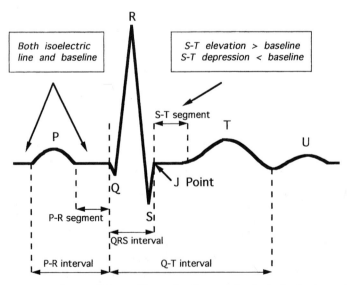

FIGURE 6–5.   Waveforms of the cardiac cycle. (From Atlee J. *Arrhythmias and Pacemakers.* Philadelphia: WB Saunders; 1996:108.)

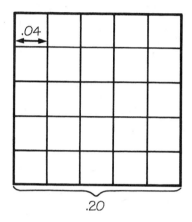

The small boxes represent 0.04 second. Each large box is made of five small boxes and represents 0.20 second.

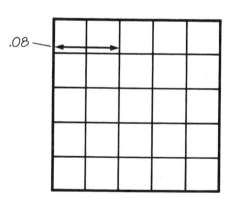

An event that takes 0.08 second would create a line two small boxes long.

FIGURE 6–6. The cardiac cycle and electrocardiograph time measurements. (From Cohn E, Gilroy-Doohan M. *Flip and See ECG*. Philadelphia: WB Saunders; 1996:44.)

Normal Sinus Rhythm (NSR)

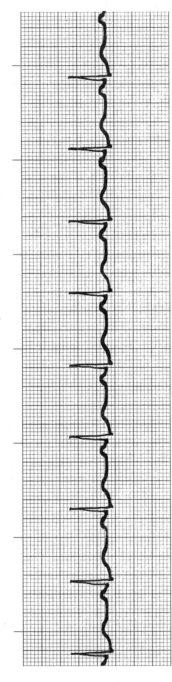

From Cohn E, Gilroy-Doohan M. *Flip and See ECG.* Philadelphia: WB Saunders; 1996:71.

Etiology: Each complex is complete and consists of one P wave, QRS complex, and T wave. There are no wide, bizarre, ectopic, late, or premature complexes.

Rate: 60 to 100 beats per minute

Rhythm: Regular

P waves: Uniform and upright in appearance. One P wave precedes each QRS complex, and the interval between P waves is constant.

PR interval: 0.12 to 0.20 second

QRS: 0.04 to 0.10 second

Treatment: None required

Sinus Tachycardia (ST)

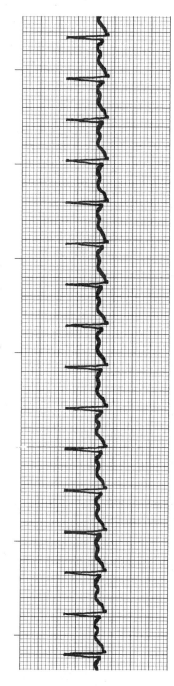

From Cohn E, Gilroy-Doohan M. *Flip and See ECG*. Philadelphia: WB Saunders; 1996:77.

Etiology: The SA node in the atria discharges at a rate greater than 100 beats per minute. Very rapid rates decrease cardiac output secondary to reduced cardiac filling. Factors that increase heart rate include fever, pain, hypoxia, sepsis, anxiety, myocardial ischemia, exercise, or increased sympathetic nervous system activity. Each complex is complete, consisting of a P wave, a QRS complex, and a T wave. The P wave may be buried in the previous T wave. There are no bizarre, wide, ectopic, early, or late complexes.

Rate: 100 to 160 beats per minute

Rhythm: Regular

P waves: Uniform and upright in appearance. One P wave precedes each QRS complex. 1:1 with QRS complex. The interval between P waves is constant.

PR interval: 0.12 to 0.20 second

QRS: 0.04 to 0.10 second

Comments: Normal response to increased demand for O_2 due to fever, pain, anxiety, hypoxia, congestive heart failure (CHF), fright, stress, etc.

Signs/Symptoms: In most cases, sinus tachycardia is asymptomatic. An attempt must be made to ascertain the underlying cause. Once recognized, treatment is directed at the causative factor (fever, anxiety, hypovolemia, etc.).

Treatment: Directed at correcting the underlying cause. *Fever:* ASA, acetaminophen, cooling. *Pain:* opioids, NSAIDs. *Hypovolemia:* volume infusion. *Medications:* reversal or washout.

Sinus Bradycardia (SB)

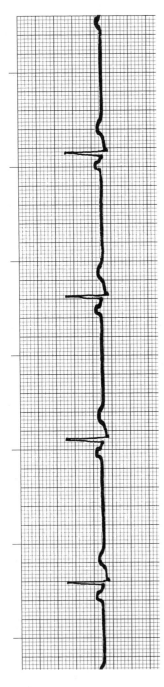

From Cohn E, Gilroy-Doohan M. *Flip and See ECG*. Philadelphia: WB Saunders; 1996:75.

Etiology: The SA node emits impulses at a rate less than 60 beats per minute. Each complex is complete, consisting of a P wave, a QRS complex, and a T wave. All intervals are within normal limits except heart rate. Parasympathetic dominance of the autonomic nervous system occurs. Sinus bradycardia is associated with pain, beta blockade, vagal stimulation, and myocardial infarction.

Rate: < 60 beats per minute

Rhythm: Regular

P waves: Uniform and upright in appearance. One P wave precedes each QRS complex. 1:1 with each QRS complex and the interval between the P waves is constant.

PR interval: 0.12 to 0.20 second

QRS: 0.04 to 0.10 second

Comments: Normal in conditioned athletes. May be due to a variety of factors, which include enhanced vagal tone, parasympathetic dominance of the autonomic nervous system, vomiting, straining, SA nodal

disease, increased intraocular pressure, or increased intracranial pressure. Often seen after acute inferior MI or in patients taking beta blockers, quinidine or verapamil, and some calcium channel blockers.

Signs/Symptoms: May be asymptomatic. Fatigue, hypotension, and syncope are associated with decreased cardiac output.

Treatment: Sinus bradycardia should be treated when signs and symptoms of decreased cardiac output occur (syncope, unconsciousness) or ventricular ectopy develops. If symptomatic:

- Assess airway
- Discontinue procedural or diagnostic stimulation (colonoscopy, endoscopy, hypoxia, etc.), which may correlate with the onset of bradycardia.
- The presence of severe pain may also enhance vagal tone. Stimulation may need to be decreased or discontinued, or additional analgesia may have to be administered. For additional treatment modalities, see ACLS Bradycardia Algorithm, Appendix E.

Sinus Arrhythmia (SA)

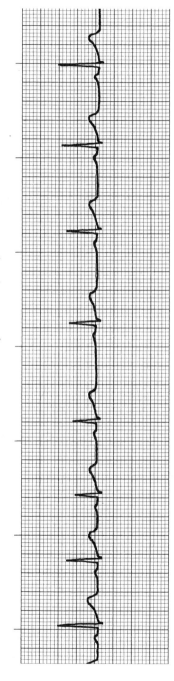

From Cohn E, Gilroy-Doohan M. *Flip and See ECG.* Philadelphia: WB Saunders; 1996:73.

Etiology: The SA node discharges at an irregular rate. The rate of discharge is influenced by the respiratory pattern and the degree of parasympathetic nervous system (vagal) control over the SA node. Each complex is complete, consisting of a P wave, a QRS complex, and a T wave. All intervals are within normal limits except the R-R interval.

Rate: Usually 60 to 100 beats per minute; however, the rate may be faster or slower. During inspiration the heart rate increases, while expiration produces a decrease in heart rate.

Rhythm: Irregular

P waves: Uniform and upright in appearance. One P wave precedes each QRS complex. The interval between P waves is not constant.

PR interval: 0.12 to 0.20 second

QRS: < 0.10 second

Comments: Common in children and physically fit adults. Reflex vagal stimulation is related to the normal respiratory cycle. Sinus arrhythmia is a natural variation caused by normal breathing.

Signs/Symptoms: The patient is generally unaware of the underlying rhythm. Although characterized by its irregularity, the rhythm possesses essentially normal waveform morphology.

Treatment: Generally, no treatment is required. Continued procedural and postprocedural monitoring as warranted by patient condition.

Premature Atrial Complexes/Contractions (PACs)

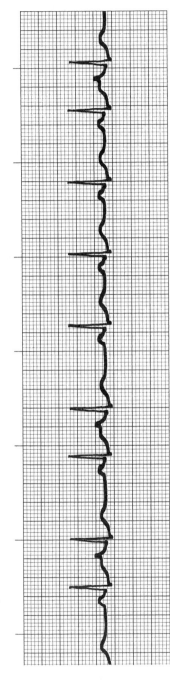

From Cohn E, Gilroy-Doohan M. *Flip and See ECG.* Philadelphia: WB Saunders; 1996:79.

Etiology: PACs occur secondary to irritable ectopic foci in the atrium discharging prior to the SA node. Isolated PACs are frequently inconsequential. An increase in the rate of PACs may signify impending atrial fibrillation or flutter secondary to irritability of the atrial musculature.

Rate: Usually normal, but varies depending on the number of extra atrial beats that are created and the rate of the underlying rhythm.

Rhythm: Irregular because of the PAC.

P wave: P wave of the early beat differs from the sinus P waves. The wave is premature and may be lost in the preceding T wave. 1:1 with the QRS complex.

PR interval: Varies from 0.12 to 0.20 second when the pacemaker site is near the SA node to 0.23 second when the pacemaker site is closer to the AV node.

QRS: Usually < 0.12 second but may be prolonged if underlying bundle branch block or aberrant conduction.

Comments: The most distinguishing feature of an ectopic beat aris-

ing in the atria (PAC) is that the configuration of the premature P wave differs from the other P waves. The P wave may also be obscured by the preceding T waves, particularly if the PAC occurs soon after the previous beat.

Signs/Symptoms: The patient may be unaware of the underlying rhythm. Premature atrial complexes are frequently diagnosed when ECG monitoring commences immediately prior to the procedure. Ingestion of caffeine, tobacco, or alcohol, hypoxia, anxiety, or atrial enlargement may elicit PACs.

Treatment: Identification of underlying cause. Rare PACs require no treatment. If PACs are increasing in frequency (> 6 per minute), it may be beneficial to complete the procedure as soon as feasible. Medical consultation may be indicated to prevent the development of atrial tachycardia or atrial fibrillation/flutter and to ascertain the cause of the atrial irritability. For additional treatment modalities, see ACLS Tachycardia Algorithm, Appendix E.

Supraventricular Tachycardia (SVT)

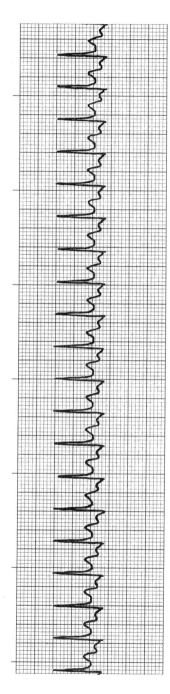

From Cohn E, Gilroy-Doohan M. *Flip and See ECG*. Philadelphia: WB Saunders; 1996:87.

Etiology: Like PACs, SVT occurs secondary to atrial irritability. SVT occurs at an atrial discharge rate between 150 and 250 beats per minute. Ectopic foci override the SA node with a corresponding ventricular response for each atrial impulse conducted.

Rate: 150 to 250 beats per minute

Rhythm: Regular

P waves: Atrial P waves differ from sinus P waves. P waves are generally identified at the lower end of the rate range but seldom are identified at rates > 200.

PR interval: Usually not measurable because the P wave is difficult to distinguish from the preceding T wave. If measurable, the PR interval is 0.12 to 0.20 second.

QRS: < 0.12 second but may be prolonged if bundle branch block or aberrant conduction.

Comments: Common causes are physical or psychologic stress, hy-

poxia, epinephrine in the local anesthetic solution, and excessive caffeine intake. Also may occur in patients with rheumatic heart disease, coronary artery disease, digitalis toxicity, and respiratory failure.

Signs/Symptoms: Because of decreased ventricular filling time, signs and symptoms of decreased cardiac output (hypotension, syncope) may occur. Sudden feelings of palpitations, lightheadedness, and severe anxiety are common. In patients with underlying heart disease, congestive heart failure, angina, or shock may occur as a result of decreased cardiac output. Myocardial oxygen consumption increases in response to the tachycardic state.

Treatment: Monitor patient for signs and symptoms of congestive heart failure or shock. *Stable:* Administer oxygen, establish intravenous line, vagal maneuvers, pharmacologic intervention. *Unstable:* Administer oxygen, intravenous medications. Additional treatment modalities are identified in ACLS Tachycardia Algorithm, Appendix E.

Atrial Flutter (A-Flutter)

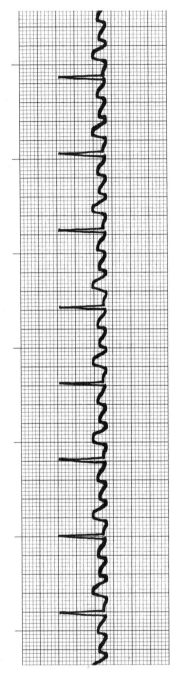

From Cohn E, Gilroy-Doohan M. *Flip and See ECG.* Philadelphia: WB Saunders; 1996:83.

Etiology: Atrial flutter occurs secondary to rapid ectopic atrial discharge at a rate of 250 to 350 beats per minute. Because of this rapid ectopic rate, the ventricle cannot respond to each impulse. However, the ventricle will selectively respond to impulses and contract. According to the number of atrial impulses discharged prior to ventricular contraction, atrial flutter is referred to as 2:1, 3:1, or 4:1 flutter.

Rate: Atrial rate is 250 to 350 beats per minute. Ventricular rate is variable, depending on conduction through to the ventricle.

Rhythm: Atrial rhythm is regular. Ventricular rhythm is usually regular with constant conduction ratio, but may be irregular.

P waves: Saw-toothed, "F" or "flutter waves".

PR interval: None, not measurable.

QRS: Usually 0.04 to 0.12 second but may be widened. Flutter waves are buried in the QRS complex.

Comments: Clinical significance of this rhythm depends on the ventricular response rate. The more rapid the rate, the more serious the dysrhythmia. Seldom occurs in the absence of organic heart disease. Seen in association with mitral or tricuspid valve disorders, digitalis toxicity, pericarditis, and inferior wall myocardial infarction.

Signs/Symptoms: The patient may report a sense of palpitations. If ventricular filling and coronary artery blood flow are compromised, symptoms of decreased cardiac output may become clinically evident.

Treatment: Hemodynamically stable patients generally require no initial treatment. Ventricular rates that are rapid may be terminated with cardioversion (50 watt seconds) digitalis or beta blockade. For additional treatment modalities, see ACLS Tachycardia Algorithm, Appendix E.

Atrial Fibrillation (A-Fib)

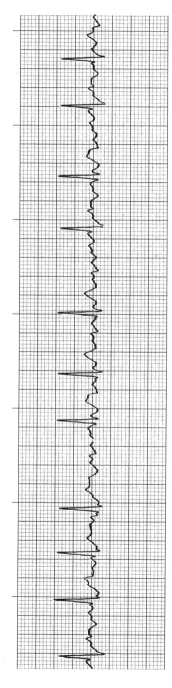

From Cohn E, Gilroy-Doohan M. *Flip and See ECG*. Philadelphia: WB Saunders; 1996:85.

Etiology: Rapid atrial ectopic foci discharge at a rate of 350 to 600. The atria fibrillate in an unsynchronized fashion. This fibrillation can result in a 20% to 30% reduction in cardiac output secondary to decreased diastolic filling time and loss of atrial contribution.

Rate: Atrial rate usually > 400. Ventricular rate variable: < 100 = controlled, > 100 = uncontrolled.

Rhythm: Atrial and ventricular rhythm is very irregular (regular, bradycardic ventricular rhythm may occur as a result of digitalis toxicity).

P waves: No identifiable P waves, erratic, wavy baseline.

PR interval: None

QRS: Usually 0.04 to 0.12 second

Comments: Erratic, wavy, chaotic baseline. Inefficient movement of blood in the atria predisposes the patient to stroke secondary to car-

dioemboli. May occur intermittently or as a chronic rhythm. Additional predisposing factors include myocardial infarction, chronic obstructive pulmonary disease, coronary artery disease, congestive heart failure, cardiac valve disorders, rheumatic heart disease.

Signs/Symptoms: Asymptomatic, or the patient may sense palpitations. If underlying heart disease exists, then signs of decreased cardiac output may be present. In patients with a history of coronary artery disease, angina may manifest as the primary patient complaint.

Treatment: Treatment is dependent on clinical presentation and ventricular rate. The goal of therapy is to convert to normal sinus rhythm, reduction of the ventricular rate to less than 100, and restoration of atrial kick. Additional treatment modalities are identified in the ACLS Tachycardia Algorithm, Appendix E.

129

Junctional Rhythm

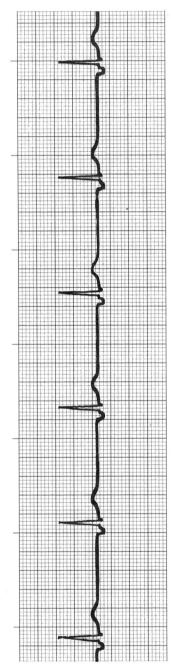

From Cohn E, Gilroy-Doohan M. *Flip and See ECG*. Philadelphia: WB Saunders; 1996:93.

Etiology: Junctional tissue surrounding the AV node will discharge when the intrinsic rate of the SA node or atria is less than 40 to 60 beats per minute.

Rate: 40 to 60 beats per minute.

Rhythm: *Atrial:* regular when present. *Ventricular:* regular.

P waves: May occur before, during, or after the QRS complex. If P waves are present, they are often inverted (retrograde) in lead II.

PR interval: Not measurable unless P wave precedes the QRS complex. When present, generally measures ≤ 0.12 second.

QRS: < 0.12 second

Comments: The presence of a junctional rhythm (at a rate of approximately 40 beats per minute) indicates that the SA node is no longer discharging or is firing at a rate of less than 40 beats per minute. A junctional rhythm is a safety mechanism that preserves the heart rate if higher pacemaker sites fail. The suppression of SA nodal discharge activity may permit lower pacemaker sites to develop. Junctional rhythm often results in response to excessive vagal activity. Additional factors include ischemic damage to the SA node and digitalis or quinidine toxicity.

Signs/Symptoms: A junctional rhythm seldom produces symptoms unless the rate is very slow (< 40 beats per minute).

Treatment: Generally, no special drug therapy is indicated. Atropine may be successful in increasing the discharge rate of the SA node. If the slow heart rate compromises circulation, a transvenous pacemaker may be required to increase the ventricular rate and cardiac output. If ventricular ectopy develops with a junctional rhythm, rate control (atropine, cardiac pacing) can be efficacious.

Premature Ventricular Contractions (PVCs)

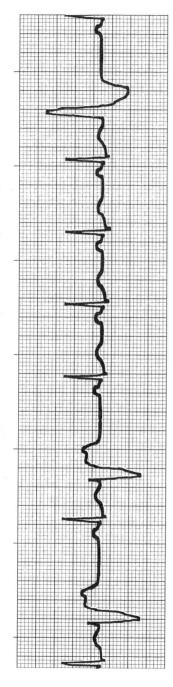

From Cohn E, Gilroy-Doohan M. *Flip and See ECG.* Philadelphia: WB Saunders; 1996:81.

Etiology: Discharge from an irritable ventricular focus prior to discharge of the next impulse from the SA node. The resultant wide, distorted, and bizarre ventricular complex is a result of ventricular contraction outside the normal conduction pathway.

Rate: Atrial and ventricular rate is dependent on underlying rhythm.

Rhythm: Irregular because of the premature ventricular complex.

P waves: There are no P waves associated with the PVC.

PR interval: None because the ectopic beat originates in the ventricle.

QRS: > 0.12 second. Wide and bizarre configuration is frequently in the opposite direction of the QRS complex.

Comments: PVCs are among the most common of all arrhythmias associated with acute myocardial infarction. PVCs signify ventricular irritability. PVCs are associated with hypoxia, electrolyte imbalance (hypokalemia), myocardial infarction, stress, chronic heart disease, and medication overdosage. It is important to treat the underlying cause, not merely the symptom (PVC). Complications associated with PVCs rest in their ability to initiate ventricular tachycardia or fibrillation.

Signs/Symptoms: Many patients are aware of PVCs and describe the sensation as "palpitations" or "skipping of the heart." When one is auscultating the heart or taking the pulse, a relatively long pause is noted immediately after the premature beat. This delay (complete compensatory pause) is characteristic and is particularly diagnostic of the arrhythmia.

Treatment: Treatment of PVCs should be considered if (1) they occur at a rate of > 6 per minute; (2) they are multifocal in appearance; (3) there are two or more in a row; or (4) an R on T phenomenon occurs (PVC falls on the T wave of the preceding beat).

Supportive care aimed at the cause of the PVCs. Treatment protocol during conscious sedation procedures requires airway assessment, procedural correlation, frequency of PVCs, and evaluation of the patient's pain threshold. For frequent PVCs (> 6 per minute), common causative factors must be ruled out. The administration of lidocaine, 1 to 1.5 mg/kg (at a rate of 50 mg/min) may decrease the incidence of PVCs for a brief period of time until additional studies may ensue.

Ventricular Tachycardia (V-Tach, Monomorphic VT)

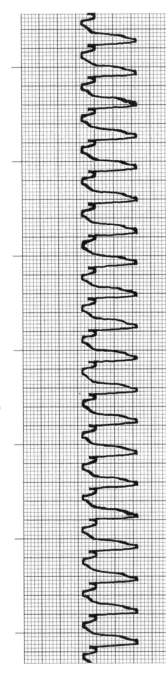

From Cohn E, Gilroy-Doohan M. *Flip and See ECG.* Philadelphia: WB Saunders; 1996:89.

Etiology: Ventricular tachycardia occurs when three or more PVCs occur at a rate greater than 100 beats per minute. These consecutive beats signify pronounced ventricular irritability. Persistent ventricular tachycardia leads to ventricular failure, cardiogenic shock, and decreased cardiac output and cerebral blood flow with resultant cerebral ischemia.

Rate: Atrial not discernible; ventricular 100 to 250 beats per minute.

Rhythm: Atrial not discernible, ventricular rhythm is essentially regular.

P waves: May be present or absent. If present, there is no set relationship to the QRS complexes. AV dissociation may be present during the ventricular tachycardia.

PR interval: None

QRS: > 0.12 second with a bizarre configuration. Often difficult to differentiate between the QRS complex and the T wave. Three or more PVCs occurring sequentially are referred to as a "run" of ventricular tachycardia.

Comments: May result in decreased cardiac output with potential deterioration to ventricular fibrillation. Often precipitated by R on T phenomenon, PVC, myocardial irritability due to acute myocardial infarction, coronary artery disease, congestive heart failure, or electrolyte imbalance. Development of ventricular tachycardia is also associated with toxicity from digitalis, quinidine, or procainamide.

Signs/Symptoms: If conscious, the patient may complain of palpitations, chest pain, or shortness of breath. If ventricular tachycardia is prolonged or sustained, signs and symptoms of decreased cardiac output generally occur.

Treatment: Conscious patients require lidocaine, 1 to 1.5 mg/kg, procainamide, or bretylium. Unconscious patients with no vital signs are treated as for ventricular fibrillation with serial defibrillation and cardiopulmonary resuscitation (CPR). For additional treatment modalities, see ACLS Pulseless Ventricular Tachycardia Algorithm, Appendix E.

Ventricular Fibrillation (V-Fib)

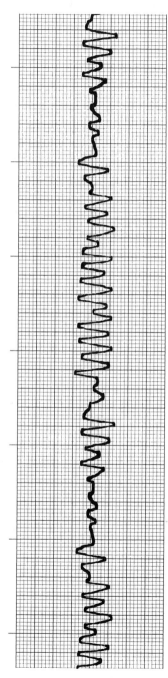

From Cohn E, Gilroy-Doohan M. *Flip and See ECG.* Philadelphia: WB Saunders; 1996:91.

Etiology: Ventricular muscle fibers, which normally contract as a single unit, lose this inherent ability. Individual ventricular muscle fibers are stimulated so rapidly that there is no recovery phase between ventricular contractions. Fibrillation is ineffective in moving blood out of the ventricles, and circulation stops. If not corrected immediately, death ensues within minutes.

Rate: Cannot be determined since there are no discernible wave forms or complexes to measure.

Rhythm: Rapid and chaotic, with no pattern or regularity.

P waves: Not discernible.

PR interval: Not discernible.

QRS: Not discernible.

Comments: Life-threatening arrhythmia. If not converted, causes death within minutes.

Signs/Symptoms: Unconsciousness, absence of pulse.

Treatment: Check vital signs; if none present, defibrillate immediately, begin CPR, establish intravenous line, institute ACLS protocol. For additional treatment modalities, see ACLS Ventricular Fibrillation Algorithm, Appendix E.

Asystole ("Flat Line")

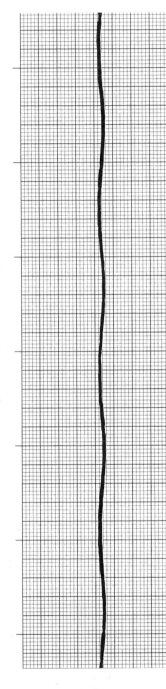

From Cohn E, Gilroy-Doohan M. *Flip and See ECG.* Philadelphia: WB Saunders; 1996:95.

Etiology: The absence of electrical impulse activity within the myocardium signifies massive myocardial ischemia. Development of asystole may be attributed to acute respiratory failure, myocardial rupture, or extensive ischemic damage.

Rate: None
Rhythm: None
P wave: None
QRS: None

PR interval: None
Comments: Always check "absence" of a rhythm in two leads and verification of lead placement.
Signs/Symptoms: Absence of pulse (check for carotid pulse), apnea, "no signs of life."
Treatment: CPR; again verify rhythm in two leads; consider other causes, pacing, and pharmacologic therapy. For additional treatment modalities, see ACLS Asystole Treatment Algorithm, Appendix E.

Pacemaker with Capture

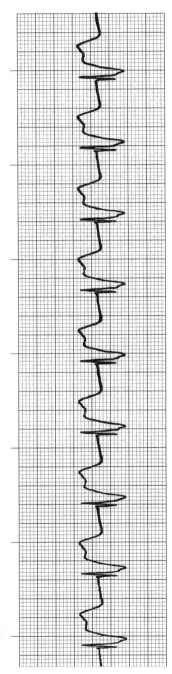

From Cohn E, Gilroy-Doohan M. *Flip and See ECG.* Philadelphia: WB Saunders; 1996:105.

Etiology: Cardiac pacemakers deliver an electrical stimulus to the heart with resultant electronic depolarization and cardiac contraction.

Rate: Overdrive pacing is used occasionally for severe tachycardia. Demand pacing is activated if the heart drops below a preset rate.

Rhythm: A variety of rhythms may occur in patients with pacemakers

P waves: May be present or absent. P waves may or may not be associated with the QRS complex. Functional pacemakers produce spikes followed by a wide QRS complex and T wave.

Comments: A variety of pacemakers for use:

- Transcutaneous: through the skin

- Transvenous: tip of venous catheter in the right ventricle, right atrium, or both
- Transthoracic: through the anterior chest wall into the heart
- Epicardial: on the surface of the heart
- Permanent: surgically implanted inside the heart

Signs/Symptoms: Patients presenting for pacemaker insertion may have a compromised hemodynamic profile.

Treatment: Indications for pacemaker insertion include complete heart block, sick sinus syndrome, and symptomatic bradycardia.

BLOOD PRESSURE MONITORING (NONINVASIVE)

The manual blood pressure cuff applied externally provides an estimation of systolic and diastolic blood pressure. Systolic blood pressure is ascertained once the first Korotkoff sound is detected. Korotkoff sounds are a result of turbulent blood flow detected during deflation of the blood pressure cuff. Diastolic blood pressure is ascertained when the Korotkoff sounds change or disappear. Oscillotonometers are small microprocessor units that measure systolic (SBP), diastolic (DBP), and mean arterial pressure (MAP).[3]

$$MAP = (SBP + [2 \times DBP]) \div 3$$

Cuff oscillations are obtained through the sensing unit at approximately 3 mm Hg increments. The sensory unit directly measures mean blood pressure by maximal changes in cuff pressure during the deflation phase of the cycle. Nursing implications related to automated blood pressure cuffs are listed in Table 6–3.

HYPOTENSION

Significant hypotension is defined as a decrease in systemic arterial blood pressure of 20% to 30%.[4] Hypotension may be caused by a variety of factors, including the following:

- Hypovolemia
- Myocardial ischemia
- Pharmacologic agents
- Acidosis
- Parasympathetic stimulation (pain, vagal response)

Definitive treatment for hypotension includes the following:

- Administration of oxygen
- Administration of fluid challenge (300 to 500 ml of crystalloid)
- Correction of acidosis or hypoxemia

TABLE 6–3. *Nursing Considerations: Automated Blood Pressure Cuffs*

- Requires several cardiac cycles to adapt to respiratory patterns and motion artifact.
- Erratic cuff movement alters the accuracy of pressure output.
- Inappropriate cuff size = erroneous readings:
  - Narrow cuffs = elevated readings
  - Wide cuffs = decreased readings
- Appropriately sized blood pressure cuffs should fit approximately two thirds of the extremity or offer a width that is approximately 20% greater than the diameter of the limb.
- Vascular congestion may occur when frequent blood pressures are cycled.
- To avoid low readings for manual cuffs, recommended inflation rate is 3 to 5 mm Hg per second.
- One layer of Webril may be used to protect friable skin (geriatric patients) against abrasion and bruising without greatly influencing the accuracy of cuff pressure.

- Relief of myocardial ischemia
- Titration of sympathomimetic medications:
  - Beta agonists (ephedrine)
  - Alpha agonists (phenylephrine)
  - Alpha and beta agonists (epinephrine)
- Titration of inotropic agents:
  - Dopamine
  - Calcium chloride

In the presence of hypotension, it is important to arrive at a timely diagnosis. Close communication is required of all team members to identify and treat the underlying causative factor.

HYPERTENSION

As outlined in Chapter 2, hypertension is defined as a systolic blood pressure greater than 160 mm Hg or a diastolic blood pressure greater than 95 mm Hg.[5] To prevent complications, hypertension must be treated in a timely fashion. Hypertension increases bleeding, predisposes the patient to hemorrhage, leads to cardiac arrhythmias, and increases myocardial oxygen consumption. Activation of the sympathetic nervous system (alpha and beta agonist stimulation) results in increased systemic vascular resistance and heart rate. Identification of the cause of hypertension is required to effectively return the blood pressure to baseline or normal values:

- Fluid overload requires diuresis
- Noxious stimuli require analgesia or discontinuation of stimuli
- Sympathetic nervous stimulation may require alpha and beta blockade
- Myocardial ischemia may require nitrates and analgesia

PULSE OXIMETRY

The advent of pulse oximetry in the 1980s has provided the clinician with a simple, safe, and inexpensive method to assess patient oxygenation. Pulse oximetry is now widely accepted as an assessment tool to decrease the incidence of unrecognized hypoxic events. Pulse oximetry provides a noninvasive, continuous monitoring parameter to assess the percent of oxygen combined with hemoglobin. Oxygen saturation is recorded as an SpO_2 parameter. Ninety-eight percent of oxygen is transported throughout the body in combination with hemoglobin, whereas 2% is dissolved in plasma. The oxyhemoglobin dissociation curve depicted in Figure 6–7 assists the clinician in determining the correlation between oxygen saturation and PO_2. Hemoglobin saturation is determined by a light-absorbence technique with pulse oximeter technology. Examination of the oxyhemoglobin dissociation curve reveals the *development of hypoxia at an SaO_2 of 90%, which equals a PO_2 of 60 mm Hg*. Severe hypoxemia develops when SaO_2 decreases to 75% with a resultant PO_2 of 40 mm Hg. The height and slope of the curve depend on a variety of factors (Table 6–4). Factors that shift the curve to the left result in a decreased release of oxygen at the tissue level. Factors that shift the curve

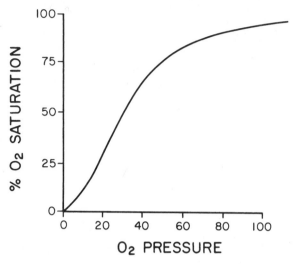

O₂ PRESSURE

FIGURE 6–7.   Oxyhemoglobin dissociation curve. The relationship between oxygen saturation and P_{O_2} is important in clinical practice. A general rule of thumb equates

P_{O_2} (mm Hg)	40	50	60
Saturation (%)	70	80	90

(From Lake C. *Clinical Monitoring.* Philadelphia: WB Saunders; 1991:587.)

TABLE 6–4.   *Factors Affecting Hemoglobin-Oxygen Affinity*

CAUSES OF INCREASED OXYGEN AFFINITY
Hypothermia
Respiratory alkalosis
Metabolic alkalosis
Decreased 2,3-diphosphoglycerate (2,3-DPG)
Decreased serum phosphate
Anemia
Hypothyroidism

FACTORS THAT DECREASE OXYGEN AFFINITY
Fever
Respiratory acidosis
Metabolic acidosis
Increased 2,3-DPG
Steroid administration
Hyperaldosteronism
Hyperthyroidism
Polycythemia

From Lake C. *Clinical Monitoring.* Philadelphia: WB Saunders; 1991:589.

TABLE 6–5. *Optical Plethysmography and Spectrophotometry Technology*

Optical plethysmography uses light absorption to reproduce waveforms produced by pulsatile blood flow. Changes that occur in the absorption of light due to vascular bed changes are reproduced by the pulse oximeter as plethysmographic waveforms. Spectrophotometry is the scientific technology that uses various wavelengths of light to perform quantitative measurements of light absorption through given substances.

to the right result in an increase in the amount of oxygen released at the tissue level. During conscious sedation procedures it is important to understand the principles of pulse oximetry in order to recognize the development of hypoxic episodes and to take corrective action when required.

OXYGEN TRANSPORT

The arterial system carries oxygen to the tissue and is dependent on a balance between oxygen supply and tissue oxygen demand. Hypoxia occurs when oxygen demand exceeds oxygen supply. An adequate balance is provided by maintenance of

- Adequate blood oxygen
- Adequate hemoglobin content to carry oxygen
- Adequate cardiac output to transport oxygen
- Appropriate tissue utilization of oxygen

PULSE OXIMETRY TECHNOLOGY

Pulse oximetry combines the principles of optical plethysmography and spectrophotometry to ascertain hemoglobin oxygen saturation. The technology of optical plethysmography and spectrophotometry is outlined in Table 6–5. As depicted in Figure 6–8, pulse oximeters use two light-emitting diodes (LEDs), which

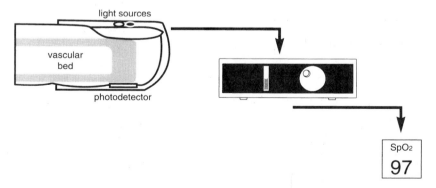

FIGURE 6–8. Pulse oximeter technology. Two light-emitting diodes measure the intensity of transmitted light across the vascular bed. (Courtesy Nellcor, Inc., Pleasanton, California.)

are placed opposite each other across an arterial vascular bed. These LEDs measure the intensity of transmitted light across the vascular bed. The critical feature of pulse oximetry is that it measures the difference in the intensity of light absorption at each wavelength caused by oxygenated and deoxygenated hemoglobin. The signal is then transmitted to the pulse oximetry unit for determination of arterial hemoglobin oxygen saturation. Pulse oximeters come in a variety of types, which include adhesive sensors (adult, neonatal, infant, pediatric, and adult nasal) and reusable sensors (adult, adult/neonatal, pediatric/infant, reflectance, multisite, and ear clip) (Fig. 6–9). Sensors are chosen according to the patient's body weight, exposed site of application, patient activity level, and expected duration of patient monitoring. Factors that contribute to pulse oximetry interference are shown in Table 6–6.

DOCUMENTATION AND RECORD KEEPING

RECOMMENDED AORN PRACTICE VI

Documentation of patient care during conscious sedation/analgesia should be consistent with AORN "Recommended Practices for Documentation of Perioperative Nursing Care" wherever conscious sedation/analgesia is administered.

The purpose of the medical record (see Conscious Sedation Flowsheet, pp 146–147) is to provide a legible, complete record of patient care during the administration of the conscious sedation procedure. The record should be

- Neat
- Accurate
- Clear
- Concise

The conscious sedation flowsheet should provide proof of continuous care reflective of medical and nursing standards of care. The components of the conscious sedation flowsheet include the following:

- Date
- Patient name
- Physical characteristics (age, height, weight)
- Premedication
- Medications
- Allergies
- Preprocedure vital signs
- Monitors used

- Airway management
- Medications administered
- Administration of reversal agents
- Graphic flowchart for vital signs
- Intravenous solutions administered
- Estimated blood loss (if applicable)
- Attending physician
- Nurse's signature
- Procedure start and stop time

Incorrect notations may be changed in the medical record as follows:

- Lining out the original notation
- Insertion of the correct data
- Initialing the change
- The original entry must remain legible

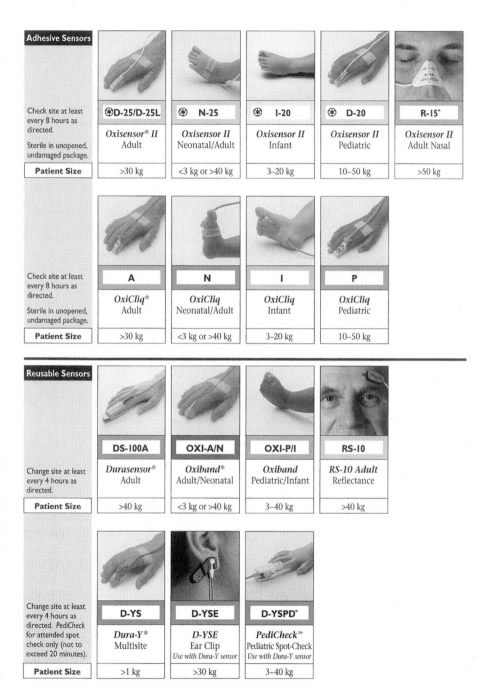

Adhesive Sensors					
Check site at least every 8 hours as directed. Sterile in unopened, undamaged package.	⊕D-25/D-25L	⊕ N-25	⊕ I-20	⊕ D-20	R-15*
	Oxisensor® II Adult	*Oxisensor II* Neonatal/Adult	*Oxisensor II* Infant	*Oxisensor II* Pediatric	*Oxisensor II* Adult Nasal
Patient Size	>30 kg	<3 kg or >40 kg	3–20 kg	10–50 kg	>50 kg
Check site at least every 8 hours as directed. Sterile in unopened, undamaged package.	A	N	I	P	
	OxiCliq® Adult	*OxiCliq* Neonatal/Adult	*OxiCliq* Infant	*OxiCliq* Pediatric	
Patient Size	>30 kg	<3 kg or >40 kg	3–20 kg	10–50 kg	
Reusable Sensors					
Change site at least every 4 hours as directed.	DS-100A	OXI-A/N	OXI-P/I	RS-10	
	Durasensor® Adult	*Oxiband®* Adult/Neonatal	*Oxiband* Pediatric/Infant	*RS-10 Adult* Reflectance	
Patient Size	>40 kg	<3 kg or >40 kg	3–40 kg	>40 kg	
Change site at least every 4 hours as directed. *PediCheck* for attended spot check only (not to exceed 20 minutes).	D-YS	D-YSE	D-YSPD*		
	Dura-Y® Multisite	*D-YSE* Ear Clip *Use with Dura-Y sensor*	*PediCheck™* Pediatric Spot-Check *Use with Dura-Y sensor*		
Patient Size	>1 kg	>30 kg	3–40 kg		

FIGURE 6–9. Nellcor Sensor Family Selection Guide. (Courtesy Nellcor, Inc., Pleasanton, California.)

TABLE 6–6. *Pulse Oximeter Interference*

FACTOR	RATIONALE	CORRECTIVE ACTION
Motion	Motion at the sensor site may result in light absorption alterations that mimic pulsatile blood flow. Pulse rate and SpO_2 values ascertained by the pulse oximeter may be inaccurate.	Application of an adhesive sensor to a less active site
Low perfusion	Weak pulsatile activity may result in little or no increase in light absorption. If pulsatile flow is not identified, there may be no SpO_2 reading, and the pulse oximeter may read "pulse search."	The signal is enhanced once the underlying cause of the low perfusion state is corrected. Use of a low perfusion sensor (nasal sensor) may enhance signal acquisition. This nasal sensor measures oxygen saturation of the anterior ethmoid artery.
Venous pulsation	In the presence of elevated venous pressure (right-sided heart failure, tightly applied sensors, presence of a tourniquet), peripheral venous blood may become pulsatile. Therefore the pulse oximeter may reflect an SpO_2 value lower than true arterial saturation.	No additional tape should be applied to the sensor; oximeter probe should not be placed distal to blood pressure cuffs, pressure dressings, tourniquets, A-lines, or invasive catheters.
Ambient light interference	Ambient light (sunlight, infrared warming lights, phototherapy, fluorescent, and surgical lights) may alter pulse oximeter readings. In the presence of this ambient light, the photodetector of the pulse oximetry unit may detect incoming optical signals in addition to vascular bed signals.	In the presence of excessive ambient light, sensors must be shielded (blankets, drapes, etc.).

Optical shunt	Optical shunting occurs in the presence of misplaced or inappropriately applied sensors. Light from the LED reaches the photodetector without passing through the vascular bed.	Proper sensor selection and application avoid optical shunting.
Edema	In the presence of significant edema, light from the LED sensor may be scattered through the edematous tissue.	Every attempt should be made to position the sensor on nonedematous application sites. In the presence of significant peripheral edema, the nasal sensor or forehead reflectant sensor may be used.
Anemia	Severe anemia values below 5 g/dl are unable to provide reliable information.	Restoration of hemoglobin greater than 5 g/dl.
Intravascular dyes	Intravascular dye injection (methelyne blue, indigo carmine, and indocyanine green) can cause sudden and temporary decreases in oxygen saturation immediately after injection. These alterations in SaO_2 readings occur because of dyes that are known to absorb light in a region of one of the wavelengths of light used in pulse oximetry technology.	Preparation for a momentary drop in the pulse oximeter requires use of subjective observation skills (skin color, nailbeds, blood color, etc.)
Nail polish	Certain nail polishes, particularly blue, green, black, and brownish red, may interfere with the actions of pulse oximetry. Red nail polish is not known to interfere with the action of pulse oximetry.	Several fingernails should have nail polish routinely removed prior to conscious sedation procedures and application of the SaO_2 probe.

The medical record is considered a legal document that *may not be altered in any manner other than listed on p 140. Spoilation of medical records refers to the illegal alteration, destruction, or removal of the medical record.* Any attempt to tamper with or alter the patient's medical record may be viewed as evidence that supports a defendant's cause.

CONSCIOUS SEDATION FLOWSHEET (pp 146–147)

NAME, DATE, PHYSICAL CHARACTERISTICS

Basic patient identification information is initially recorded on the conscious sedation flowsheet and includes the patient's name, address, hospital administrative identification number, etc. Physical characteristics (height, weight) may be recorded on the flowsheet or placed in the preprocedure patient assessment form.

PREMEDICATION, MEDICATIONS, ALLERGY STATUS

Any premedication that has been administered should be documented on the patient's flowsheet before the procedure. The effect of the sedative should be noted and is characteristically recorded as cooperative, calm, sleeping, etc. The time of administration of the premedication should also be noted. Patient medications are recorded on the conscious sedation flowsheet with last dose administered noted before the procedure. Allergy status should also be recorded on the flowsheet. The patient's allergies should be documented, and an attempt should be made to elicit the type of reaction (hives, gastrointestinal upset, etc.) recorded on the flowsheet.

Preprocedure vital signs or the first set of vital signs obtained immediately before the procedure should be recorded on the conscious sedation flowsheet. Although these initial vital signs may be falsely elevated because of anxiety, they provide a baseline prior to the diagnostic or surgical procedure. Monitors used and site of application are recorded before the procedure. The site of intravenous catheter insertion and the size of the catheter should be recorded. Type and amount of intravenous solution administered must be recorded and should be totaled at the conclusion of the procedure. A column for blood loss (if applicable) allows an accurate mechanism for postprocedure assessment.

Medications used during the procedure are recorded on the graphic flowsheet. Depending on the pharmacologic technique used, medications are recorded in incremental doses or continuous infusion. Total dose administered should be tallied and recorded in a total dose column. If reversal agents are required to counteract the pharmacololgic effects of sedative medications, dosage and time of administration must be recorded. Information on time of administration and total dose of reversal agent used assists the clinician with postprocedure monitoring and discharge planning.

GRAPHIC FLOWSHEET

A graphic flowsheet for vital signs provides a quick reference and history of the patient's cardiovascular stability throughout the procedure. Vital signs recorded every 5 minutes provide an accurate reflection of cardiovascular parameters. In addition to the notation of cardiovascular parameters, it is important to identify the patient's level of consciousness. In 1994, Clark outlined the Conscious Sedation Scale.[6] As depicted on the conscious sedation flowsheet, the scale provides documentation of the degree of sedation by means of a numerical rating system. Five variables that reflect degrees of sedation are scored. Optimal sedation score ranges from 8 to 10. Providing a detailed description of these five variables, the patient's level of consciousness and condition throughout the procedure is summarized. This concise assessment demonstrates adherence to the goals and objectives of conscious sedation outlined in Chapter 1 by regulatory bodies, state statutes, and professional organizations. Finally, the flowsheet should be signed by the nurse involved in direct patient care. Additional information recorded on the conscious sedation flowsheet includes name or signature of the attending physician, diagnosis, procedure, and start and stop time.

SUMMARY

Patients receiving conscious sedation are monitored on a continuous basis. Although vital sign parameters are recorded at regular intervals, subjective and objective monitoring is conducted on a continuum. Clinical correlation of presenting symptoms is essential for effective assessment, diagnosis, and intervention when indicated. Monitoring parameters outlined in this chapter are effective tools to use in conjunction with nursing assessment strategies. Recommended (professional organization) and required (state statute, hospital policy) monitoring must be congruent with institutional and personal philosophy to promote quality patient care. Faulty equipment requires intervention. Rescheduling of procedures may be inconvenient and costly. However, in the presence of malfunctioning equipment, it is the definitive option. Monitoring alarms and alarm limits are designed to provide patient safety. Before the commencement of any procedure, the patient monitors should be turned on and the alarm parameters activated. Alarm limits should not be so broad that dangerous clinical situations are ignored. Parameters must not be so narrow that they cause undue stress to the patient or clinician throughout the procedure. Initial alarm limits may be set approximately 20% above or below the patient's preprocedure baseline vital signs. Disabling of alarms is a dangerous trend in medicine and may lead to devastating complications. Effective monitoring of the patient receiving conscious sedation includes the use of ECG, noninvasive blood pressure (NIBP), pulse oximetry, and the implementation of critical nursing assessment skills to provide safe, effective quality patient care.

Conscious Sedation Flowsheet

Date	Unit	Procedure	MD	Consent: ☐ Yes ☐ No

Allergies				

IV START
Time _____ Site _____ Size _____

IV DISCONTINUED
Time _____ Condition _____

IV FLUIDS	Totals Infused
Time	
Type	
Blood Products	

Instruments		

INDICATE TIME M.D. STARTS/STOPS PROCEDURE WITH*

Time																
220																
210																
200																
190																
180																
170																
160																
150																
140																
130																
120																
110																
100																
90																
80																
70																
60																
50																
40																
R																
T																
SaO$_2$																

LEGEND:
V = Systolic BP
∧ = Diastolic BP
● = Pulse
* = See Comments
— = Negative or Not Reassessed

Specimen: _____

Cautery Type: _____

Grounding Pad: ☐ Yes ☐ No
Site: _____

Dilation Type: _____

O$_2$ Appliance: 1. Cannula 2. Mask
O$_2$ Liter Flow: _____
ECG: 1. NSR 2. Consistent w/Baseline 3.Other
Pulses: ☐ Pedal ☐ Radial   Rt. _____ Lt. _____
☐ Doppler: 0-None +1-Weak +2-Normal +3-Bounding

DISCHARGE

LOC:
☐ Awake ☐ Drowsy
☐ Consistent with Baseline
☐ Other _____

PROCEDURE RECALL
0. Total _____ Score _____
1. Limited
2. No Recall

DISCHARGE CRITERIA
☐ Ambulatory/Steady Gait
☐ Ambulatory/Min. Support
☐ Wheelchair ☐ Cart
☐ Min. or No Nausea/Vomiting
☐ Wound Site _____

DISCHARGE
Time: _____
Accompanied by:
☐ Relative ☐ Alone
☐ Friend ☐ Staff
☐ Other _____

CONSCIOUS SEDATION SCALE

Emotional Affect:
- 0. Anxious/Uneasy
- 1. Calm/Tolerant
- 2. Unresponsive/Flat

LOC:
- 0. Alert or Awakening
- 1. Follows Commands/Intermittent Arousal
- 2. Unresponsive

Vital Signs:
- 0. Increase/Requires Intervention
- 1. Within Acceptable Limits
- 2. Decrease/Requires Intervention

Physical Reaction To Procedure:
- 0. Resistive or Intense Response
- 1. Tempered or Intermittent Response
- 2. No Response

Totals Sedation Scale (Optimal 3-5)

MEDICATIONS

Route	Drug	Increment	Dosage					

Initials

Destination:
- ☐ Home   ☐ Unit
- ☐ Other _____

DISCHARGE INSTRUCTIONS

Reviewed, Understanding
Verbalized, Printed Information

Given:
- ☐ Yes   ☐ N/A   Initials _____
- ☐ Report to Floor
- To: _____

Patient Identification

Patient Care Standards

Initials _____ Signature _____

Initials _____ Signature _____

65-95400
PSHP #233
1/97 A 4-022

Courtesy Poudre Valley Hospital, Fort Collins, Colorado.

REFERENCES

1. Grauer K. *A Practical Guide to ECG Interpretation.* St. Louis: Mosby; 1992.
2. Cummins R. *Advanced Cardiac Life Support.* Dallas, Tex: American Heart Association; 1994.
3. Morgan G, Mikhail M. *Clinical Anesthesiology.* 2nd ed. Stamford, Conn: Appleton & Lange; 1996:73.
4. Morgan G, Mikhail M. *Clinical Anesthesiology.* 2nd ed. Stamford, Conn: Appleton & Lange; 1996:800.
5. Larson P. Evaluation of the patient and preoperative preparation. In: *Clinical Anesthesia.* 2nd ed. Philadelphia: JB Lippincott; 1995:550.
6. Clark B. *A New Approach to Assessment and Documentation of Conscious Sedation During Endoscopic Examinations.* Society of Gastroenterology Nurses and Associates, April, 1994.

Specific Patient Populations
GERIATRICS AND PEDIATRICS

All patients scheduled for conscious sedation procedures require careful titration of medications and vigilant care. Two patient populations that require particular attention are geriatric and pediatric patients. Inherent risks associated with the administration of conscious sedation to geriatric and pediatric patients require heightened practitioner awareness before the start of the procedure. This chapter will focus on the anatomic and physiologic differences, preprocedure assessment, and pharmacologic considerations of the pediatric and geriatric patient populations.

GERIATRICS

Gerontology is the study of the effects of time on human development, specifically the study of the aged. The geriatric patient population currently composes approximately 12% of the U.S. population. A currently accepted definition of the beginning of old age is 65 years. However, the patient's functional age is more important than his or her chronologic age. A decline in organ system function accompanies the aging process. This progressive decline in organ function is responsible for the *physiologic* aging process. Aging is associated with progressive decreases (1% to 1.5% per year) in function of major organ systems. Table 7–1 identifies the physiologic aspects associated with the aging process.

Administration of conscious sedation to the geriatric patient must focus on proper preprocedure preparation strategies (Chapter 2) to identify the presence of concomitant disease, prescribed treatment protocol, and effectiveness of therapy. A careful review of the cardiopulmonary system to identify coronary artery disease, hypertension, prior myocardial infarction, chronic obstructive pulmonary disease, or central nervous system dysfunction is required. Changes in mentation, delirium, or confusion require preprocedure investigation to ascertain whether these neurologic findings are recent or represent a chronic disease state. Careful titration and reduced doses of medications are required to avoid the development of deep sedation states, prolonged recovery, and cardiovascular depression. Decreased gastroesophageal sphincter tone, decreased laryngeal reflexes, and the physiologic changes associated with the aging process listed in Table 7–1 preclude the use of deep sedation states in the geriatric population.

GERIATRIC PHARMACOLOGIC CONSIDERATIONS

The following physiologic changes lead to increased sensitivity to pharmacologic agents in the geriatric patient population.

149

- Decreased renal and hepatic blood flow
- Decreased hepatic microsomal enzyme activity
- Decreased protein binding
- Decreased basal metabolic rate

These physiologic alterations result in the following pharmacokinetic changes:

- Prolonged medication half-life
- Cumulative pharmacologic effect
- Decreased plasma clearance

Pharmacokinetic alterations associated with the aging process require practitioner awareness to prevent the development of deep sedative states and prolonged recovery periods. Conscious sedation medications administered to the geriatric patient should be given incrementally in small divided doses. Adequate time must be allowed to establish pharmacologic effect. Decreased cardiac output prolongs circulation time and the ability to rapidly achieve therapeutic plasma concentrations. Disorientation or delirium during the administration of conscious sedation requires careful evaluation to rule out the presence of respiratory

TABLE 7-1. *Physiologic Effects of the Aging Process*

BODY COMPOSITION • ↑ Proportion of body fat • ↓ Skeletal muscle mass • ↓ Intracellular fluid	**NEUROLOGIC SYSTEM** • ↓ Cerebral blood flow • ↓ Cerebral oxygen uptake • ↑ Sensitivity to central nervous system depressant drug
CARDIOVASCULAR SYSTEM • ↓ Tissue elasticity, which results in increased blood pressure • ↑ Systolic blood pressure secondary to ventricular hypertrophy and decreased arterial wall compliance • ↓ Cardiac output by 1% for each year after 30 • Cardiac dysrhythmias secondary to degenerative changes of the cardiac conduction system • ↓ Baroreceptor activity	**RENAL SYSTEM** • ↓ Glomerular filtration rate (1% to 1.5% per year) • ↓ Creatinine clearance • ↓ Tubular function (excretion) **HEPATIC SYSTEM** • ↓ Hepatic blood flow • ↓ Microsomal enzyme activity • ↓ Albumen leads to decreased plasma protein binding with resultant increased available free drug
PULMONARY SYSTEM • ↓ Total lung capacity • ↓ Vital capacity • ↓ FEV_1 • ↑ Residual volume • ↑ Dead space • ↓ Pao_2 • Altered ventilation response to hypercapnia and hypoxia	**ENDOCRINE SYSTEM** • ↓ Basal metabolic rate, 1% per year after age 30 • Glucose intolerance **AIRWAY** • Laryngeal and pharyngeal reflexes are diminished • Inadequate mask fit for positive pressure ventilation • ↓ Neuronal function

depression (obstruction, hypoxia, and hypercarbia). At times, geriatric patients demonstrate confusion and disorientation when combinations of opioids, benzodiazepines, and sedative hypnotics are administered. Immediate reaction may lead the clinician to the supposition that the patient needs additional sedation. In many cases, however, confusion, delirium, and agitation are indicators that the patient's level of sedation may be too deep. Patients exhibiting these characteristics should not receive additional sedation. Time should also be allotted for the patients to return to the awake state. In the presence of respiratory distress or cardiovascular depression, benzodiazepine or opiate reversal agents may be ordered by the attending physician.

PHARMACOLOGIC PROFILE

A complete profile of each pharmacologic classification and reversal agent is presented in Chapter 5 and Appendix D.

Benzodiazepines

Geriatric patients are particularly vulnerable to the sedative effects associated with the administration of benzodiazepines.[1,2] Dosage reduction of 30% to 50% may be required when benzodiazepines are administered to the geriatric patient. The sedative effects of benzodiazepines are enhanced by decreased hepatic microsomal enzyme activity and renal clearance. Considerations with the administration of benzodiazepines include careful titration, decreased total dose, and the use of benzodiazepines with inactive metabolites (midazolam).

Opioids

Decreased protein binding and reduced pharmacologic clearance, coupled with an increased volume of distribution, may result in a prolonged duration of action and an enhanced pharmacologic effect. These variations also result in significant respiratory and cardiovascular depression in the geriatric patient population. The addition of opioids in the presence of benzodiazepines produces a pronounced synergistic effect. Respiratory depression is a common complication associated with the combination of benzodiazepines and opioids.

Sedative Hypnotics

Decreased total dosage of propofol is required in the geriatric patient population. Reduced clearance, coupled with altered pharmacokinetics, requires careful titration. Specific gerontologic considerations include small (10 mg) increments of propofol administered slowly. Reduced cardiac output in the geriatric patient population requires several minutes after the administration of each medication dose to allow sufficient circulation time and to assess full pharmacologic effect.

Barbiturates

Reduced pharmacologic clearance, higher plasma concentration, and a prolonged duration of action require a decrease in the total dosage of barbiturates in the geriatric patient population. When required to increase the depth of sedation, thiopental (10 to 20 mg increments) or methohexital (10 mg increments) may be slowly administered. Decreased cardiac output and prolonged circulation time in the geriatric patient require that these incremental doses of medications be administered slowly over several minutes.

AIRWAY EVALUATION

During conscious sedation procedures, management of the geriatric patient's airway may prove particularly challenging. Redundant oropharyngeal tissue in the edentulous state may result in upper airway obstruction. Loss of bony jaw structure distorts the face, which may make it difficult to ventilate the patient or deliver positive pressure ventilation. An oropharyngeal or nasopharyngeal airway may be required to function as a mechanical conduit to maintain airflow.

PSYCHOLOGIC WELL-BEING

It is important to incorporate the psychologic well-being of the geriatric patient when providing conscious sedation services. Many geriatric patients are acclimated to a specific daily routine. Administration of conscious sedation for a diagnostic or minor surgical procedure removes the patient from this specific pattern of behavior. Physical limitations (hearing, vision loss) and lack of autonomy may lead to increased levels of frustration and feelings of confusion. The practitioner engaged in the care of this patient population requires slow diction, assessment of specific patient needs, and dissemination of information. Most geriatric patients do not respond well to fast-paced, disorganized practice settings. Through identification of specific patient needs, a thorough preprocedure assessment, and timely explanation of the planned procedure, many geriatric patients tolerate the administration of conscious sedation without incident.

PEDIATRICS

Pediatrics is the study of medical science related to the care of children and their specific disease states.[3] Although conscious sedation is not a popular pediatric technique in the operating room, it is used on a wide scale for diagnostic and scanning procedures. The preparation, practice, and administration of conscious sedation to the pediatric population carries with it additional practitioner responsibilities. Guidelines for monitoring and managing pediatric patients during and after sedation for diagnostic and therapeutic procedures have been published by the American Academy of Pediatrics Committee on Drugs and are featured in Appendix F. When dealing with the pediatric population, it is important *not to envision the child as a small adult.* Treating a child as a "small adult" may inevitably lead to errors in medication dosage, fluid administration, and resuscitative measures. The pediatric population is identified as

- Neonates (< than 30 days)
- Infants (1 to 12 months)

- Children (1 to 12 years of age)
- Adolescents (13 to 19 years of age)

The remainder of this chapter will address the anatomic/physiologic variations, preprocedure assessment, and pharmacologic techniques to safely provide conscious sedation to the pediatric patient population.

ANATOMIC AND PHYSIOLOGIC DIFFERENCES

Cardiovascular

Because of the pediatric patient's limited stroke volume, cardiac output is rate dependent. Stroke volume is limited as a result of poor left ventricular compliance of the underdeveloped left ventricle. The parasympathetic nervous system is particularly active in the pediatric patient. Hypoxia, respiratory obstruction, and pain result in an exaggerated parasympathetic nervous system reaction with resultant bradycardia. Deep sedation, respiratory obstruction, or painful procedures may result in rapid respiratory and cardiovascular decompensation in the pediatric patient. Pediatric cardiovascular parameters are shown in Table 7–2.

Respiratory System

Newborn infants are particularly vulnerable to airway obstruction and the development of hypoxia because of the following characteristics:

- Obligate nose breathing
- Large tongues
- Short neck
- Small mandible
- Redundant upper airway lymphoid tissue

To meet an increased oxygen demand, alveolar ventilation is increased in neonates. Children have an increased metabolic rate, which equates with a higher oxygen demand requiring 6 to 8 ml/kg/min, compared with 3 to 4 ml/kg/min of oxygen consumption in the adult.[4] Therefore, in the presence of respiratory obstruction, hypoxemia develops much more rapidly. Respiratory rate approaches adult values by adolescence. Anatomic and physiologic pulmonary considerations include a cartilaginous chest wall, decreased functional residual capacity, and immature alveolar development. Ineffective ventilation results from chest wall col-

TABLE 7–2. *Pediatric Cardiovascular Parameters*

AGE (y)	WEIGHT (kg)	HEART RATE	SYSTOLIC BLOOD PRESSURE	DIASTOLIC BLOOD PRESSURE
Neonate	3	100–160	55–70	40
1	6–10	100–140	70–100	60
3	10–15	84–115	75–110	70
5	18	80–100	80–120	70
Adult	70	80	120	80

lapse associated with the infant's pliable rib cage and reduced oxygen reserve. Periods of apnea are not well tolerated in the pediatric age group. Signs of respiratory obstruction or depression require immediate intervention to avoid desaturation and hypoxia.

Fluid Replacement

Careful attention to body fluid homeostasis is important in the pediatric patient. The kidney reaches normal function by 6 to 12 months of age. Before this maturation process, renal function is characterized by a decreased glomerular filtration rate, decreased sodium excretion, and decreased creatinine clearance. It is important to calculate pediatric fluid replacement and to administer the proper volume required for the pediatric patient population. Hourly fluid maintenance is accomplished with a balanced salt solution (lactated Ringer's or 0.45% normal saline solution) at a rate of 4 ml/kg/h for the first 10 kg of body weight, 2 ml/kg/h for the next 10 kg of body weight, and 1 ml/kg/h for every kilogram of body weight thereafter.[5] An example of maintenance fluid replacement is outlined in Table 7–3. Use of a pediatric burette (Fig. 7–1) or minidrip Venoset chamber (Fig. 8–2) assists in the prevention of volume overload from the inadvertent infusion of large amounts of intravenous fluids.

When used (on the basis of pediatric pharmacologic conscious sedation technique), an intravenous line is established in the pediatric patient. Prior to insertion of the intravenous catheter, local anesthetic cream may be applied at least 1 hour before insertion of the intravenous catheter. EMLA cream (Astra Pharmaceuticals) is a local anesthetic emulsion that contains lidocaine 2.5% and prilocaine 2.5%. When EMLA is applied to intact skin with an occlusive dressing, dermal analgesia occurs. This analgesia is secondary to the release of local anesthetic infiltration into the epidermal and dermal layers of the skin. The local anesthetic action is directed at the dermal pain receptors and nerve endings. EMLA cream should not be administered to patients less than 12 months of age.

NPO Status

Pediatric patients do not tolerate hypovolemia. Hypovolemia occurs in the pediatric patient without reflex tachycardia. When preparing and scheduling pediatric patients for conscious sedation procedures, it is important that the physician, procedure unit personnel, and parents be cognizant of NPO restrictions. Optimally, procedures on pediatric patients should be scheduled as early in the

TABLE 7–3. *Hourly Maintenance Fluid Calculation*

29 kg child presenting for the administration of IV conscious sedation		
1st 10 kg	→ × 4 ml =	**40 ml**
2nd 10 kg	→ × 2 ml =	**20 ml**
Remaining 9 kg → × 1 ml =		**9 ml**
Weight = 29 kg		
Maintenance		**69 ml/h**

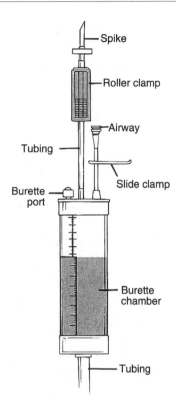

FIGURE 7-1. Pediatric burette. (From Booker M, Ignatavicius D. *Infusion Therapy.* Philadelphia: WB Saunders; 1996:57.)

morning as possible. When this is not feasible, it is important for the pediatric patient to have clear liquids up to 3 to 4 hours before the procedure to prevent dehydration.[6] Inpatient preprocedure orders should specifically state time of procedure and specify no solid foods after midnight. Clear liquids (no milk, breast milk, or pulp juices) may be administered 3 to 4 hours before the procedure.[7] To prevent the development of dehydration and minimize the risk of gastric acid aspiration, parents of outpatients need specific preprocedure NPO instructions and must demonstrate an understanding prior to leaving the physician's office, hospital, or procedure unit. Pediatric NPO guidelines are identified in Table 2–16. Therefore, through enhanced communication, realistic scheduling, and parent cooperation, the pediatric patient arrives in a proper state of hydration prior to the planned procedure.[8]

PEDIATRIC AIRWAY SUPPORT

Several anatomic and physiologic pediatric variations provide a challenge to the caregiver during intervention or management of the pediatric airway. Anatomic and physiologic variations that may impede respiration and result in rapid development of hypoxemia include the following:

- Reduced upper and lower airway diameter
- Large tongue

TABLE 7-4.   *Signs and Symptoms of Pediatric Airway Compromise*

• Inspiratory stridor	• Restlessness
• Hoarseness	• Use of intercostal muscles
• Croup	• Agitation
• Crowing	• Tachypnea

• Cephalad larynx
• Short, stiff epiglottis

These anatomic and physiologic differences have a significant impact in the management of the pediatric airway. Airway obstruction results from relaxation of the oropharyngeal musculature, a misplaced oropharyngeal airway, or a large tongue. Airway edema associated with prolonged or difficult intubation results in decreased airway diameter and impedes air flow and gas exchange. One millimeter of edema in an infant's airway results in a 75% decrease in the cross-sectional diameter of the airway, accompanied by a significant reduction in air flow.[9] Signs of pediatric respiratory compromise are listed in Table 7-4. Signs of decreased tracheal lumen (croup, inspiratory stridor, tachypnea, nasal flaring) may constitute a respiratory emergency that requires immediate intervention to restore air flow. Treatment of respiratory compromise is dependent on the magnitude of obstruction and includes the following:

• Attempts to clear obstruction: head tilt, jaw thrust, mandibular thrust
• Administration of high-humidity oxygen
• Intubation if these measures fail to relieve obstruction

When required, insertion of an endotracheal tube may be particularly difficult in the pediatric patient. The large tongue, cephalad positioning of the larynx, and stiff U-shaped epiglottis make endotracheal tube placement difficult. The large tongue often obscures or obliterates visualization of the pediatric larynx, while isolation of the epiglottis with the laryngoscope blade may be technically difficult for the clinician. In the event of a pediatric airway emergency, the clinician with the most experience or skill should manage the patient's airway. Vigorous manipulation of the pediatric airway by an inexperienced clinician will most likely result in the patient's demise. Gentle, precise maneuvers to relieve obstruction by the skilled clinician are required to alleviate obstruction and restore air flow. If obstruction occurs during conscious sedation procedures, a gentle jaw thrust with one or two hands should be used to clear the patient's airway and restore air flow. If the chin lift does not relieve the pediatric airway obstruction, additional maneuvers outlined in Table 7-5 may be used. It is important to apply gentle, sustained pressure with one or two fingers when managing the pediatric airway. The pediatric airway requires *gentle* manipulation to restore air flow.

In the presence of an acute respiratory crisis, an appropriate selection of pediatric-sized endotracheal tubes must be readily available (Table 4-3). Selection of the endotracheal tube is based on the formula in Table 7-6.

The presence of pediatric emergency airway equipment is required in all conscious sedation practice settings where pediatric procedures are performed.

TABLE 7–5.   *Pediatric Airway Obstruction Maneuvers*

- Head tilt
- Chin lift
- Mandibular thrust
- Attempt positive pressure ventilation
- Placement of oropharyngeal or nasopharyngeal airway

If above measures fail, intubation with an age-appropriate endotracheal tube may be required.

TEMPERATURE REGULATION

During the administration of conscious sedation, it is important to maintain the patient's body temperature. The procedure room should be kept warm, and the child should be covered. When compared with the adult patient, cooling in this patient population is due to the larger body surface area per kilogram. Factors that enhance pediatric cooling include the following:

- Cold procedure room
- Exposed body parts
- Administration of room temperature IV fluid
- Administration of dehumidified oxygen

Pediatric patients maintain body temperature by metabolizing brown fat, crying, and shivering. Shivering increases total body consumption by 300% to 500%.[10] In procedures that require body exposure, the patient should be kept covered until commencement of the procedure. The administration of humidified oxygen, application of warming blankets, and limited body exposure decrease the incidence of hypothermia in the pediatric patient population.

PREPROCEDURE ASSESSMENT

Preprocedure assessment and admission of the pediatric patient to the procedure area or physician's office provide the clinician an excellent opportunity to establish rapport with the parents and the patient. The patient's history is obtained in a parent interview. In addition to information outlined in Chapter 2, additional variables that require assessment in pediatric practice include the following:

- Recent upper respiratory infection, asthma (reactive airway disease)
- Presence of congenital anomalies

TABLE 7–6.   *Pediatric Endotracheal Tubes: Children > 2 Years of Age*

$$\frac{16 + \text{Age in years}}{4} = \text{Internal diameter tube size}$$

Example: 4-year-old patient

$$16 + 4 = \frac{20}{4} = 5 \text{ mm ETT}$$

- Recent exposure to communicable diseases
- Presence of esophageal reflux (risk of aspiration)
- Presence of neurologic disease (increased intracranial pressure)

Once a medical history is obtained from the parents, a physical examination should be conducted on the child. Assessment of physical development, heart rate, breath sounds, and dentition should be evaluated by the clinician. Age-appropriate rapport is accomplished by explaining, demonstrating, or identifying components of the procedure and by use of monitoring devices. During the preprocedure assessment, the attending physician and the registered nurse participating in the patient's care should answer all of the parent's questions in a relaxed, confident manner. Appearing rushed, hurried, or inattentive reduces parent confidence and limits rapport that has been developed. Methods to develop rapport with the child are based on the child's developmental stages and are highlighted in Table 7–7.

TABLE 7–7.   *Developmental Mechanisms of Pediatric Patient Rapport*

AGE	DEVELOPMENTAL STAGE	MECHANISMS OF PAIN CONTROL	CHARACTERISTICS OF PAIN RESPONSE
Infant (1–12 mo)	Trust vs. mistrust	Cuddling Sucking Parental presence	Generalized body response (tensing, stiffening) Crying Facial tension Cannot anticipate impending pain
Toddler (1–3 y)	Autonomy vs. shame and doubt	Parental presence Allow objects of security (blankets or toys) Clearly delineate end of procedure (all done, no more, etc.)	Crying Physical resistance to stimulus
Preschool (2–5 y)	Initiative vs. guilt	Teach and explain prior to procedure Positive reinforcement Parental presence Use of storytelling, books	
School-age (5–12 y)	Industry vs. inferiority	Teach and explain prior to procedure Positive reinforcement Parental presence	
Adolescent (13–19 y)	Identity vs. role diffusion	Teach and explain prior to procedure Specific information related to all aspects of procedure and recovery Use of music	

PEDIATRIC SEDATION TECHNIQUES

As depicted in Appendix F practice patterns have been published by the American Academy of Pediatrics Committee on Drugs, as well as JCAHO requirements for pediatric patients receiving sedation.[11,12] The goal of any pediatric pharmacologic technique in infants and children is to reduce movement during diagnostic procedures. Selection of sedative technique is varied in pediatric practice. Attempts to produce the ideal sedative (i.e., one that is easy to administer, reliable, effective, reversible, and inexpensive) have resulted in the numerous sedative techniques reported in the literature. Chloral hydrate has long been a popular pediatric sedative. However, a variety of sedative combinations have recently been reported in the literature. Glaser et al. reported, in the *Journal of Neuroradiology,* a study of 462 infants and children who were sedated with thiopental sodium instilled into the distal rectum.[13] Prior to the instillation of thiopental, all children were NPO and sleep deprived before the imaging study. Thiopental sodium was administered in an initial dosage of 25 mg/kg into the distal rectum. If the child was awake 20 minutes later, a second dose of 15 mg/kg was administered. No dose greater than 40 mg/kg was administered to any child. Success was defined as adequate sedation to complete the requested examination without the need for a return visit to the radiology department. Specific advantages cited in this study included a 96% success rate. Disadvantages cited in the study included a prolonged duration of action when the medication was stored in fat tissue. Proximal rectal administration resulted in portal drainage and hepatic inactivation. Rectal irritation and diarrhea were also noted with the administration of thiopental.

Pohlgeers et al. compared the combination of fentanyl and diazepam for pediatric conscious sedation.[14] Diazepam, 0.1 mg/kg, given IV over 2 minutes, was administered to a total maximum dose of 10 mg. Fentanyl, 2 µg/kg, was then administered IV over 1 to 2 minutes. A period of 1 to 2 minutes elapsed before the administration of fentanyl. If required, additional doses of fentanyl were titrated to a maximum total dose of 5 µg/kg over a 1-hour period. Specific advantages of this technique include production of a calm, drowsy patient for planned orthopedic procedures in an outpatient emergency room facility. Specific disadvantages include an 11% incidence of SaO_2 below 90%. Recommendations by the authors include an initial dose of less than or equal to 2 µg/kg of fentanyl titrated to effect in order to avoid decreased oxygen saturation.

Weber et al. report, in a research-based protocol, the use of intranasal midazolam compared with traditionally administered chloral hydrate given in a dose of 80 mg/kg. In the control group a significant number of children vomited the initial dose or were awake and crying when transported for examinations.[15] Calculation of a supplemental dose of chloral hydrate was difficult in the presence of vomiting coupled with time lost in returning the child to the patient unit for the administration of additional sedation. This study further cited a retrospective audit of 63 children who received chloral hydrate, indicating a 23% failure to sedate with one dose of chloral hydrate. A 30% failure rate was also noted with administration of the supplemental dose of chloral hydrate in the dosage range of 20 mg/kg. When required to supplement chloral hydrate, the addition of intranasal

TABLE 7–8.   *Oral, Intramuscular, and Intravenous Sedation Techniques in Pediatrics*

DRUG	USUAL DOSE
ORAL	
Chloral hydrate	25–50 mg/kg (for small infants up to 12 mo)
	25–75 mg/kg (for children older than 12 mo)
Ketamine	5–10 mg/kg (above 1 y)
Midazolam	0.5–1.0 mg/kg orally
	0.2–0.3 mg/kg intranasally (above 1 y)
Fentanyl (Oralet)	5–15 μg/kg transmucosally (for children weighing more than 15 kg)
INTRAMUSCULAR	
Ketamine	2–5 mg/kg
Midazolam	0.08 mg/kg
Pentobarbital	4–5 mg/kg (injection can be painful)
DPT cocktail	
Meperidine	2 mg/kg
Promethazine	1 mg/kg
Chlorpromazine	1 mg/kg
INTRAVENOUS	
Pentobarbital	2.5 mg/kg; may repeat up to 7.5 mg/kg; watch for apnea
Methohexital	0.5–1.0 mg/kg; may repeat as needed; watch for apnea
Midazolam	0.08 mg/kg; may follow with infusion at 0.04–0.12 mg/kg/h
Propofol	1–2 mg/kg; may follow with infusion at 4–8 mg/kg/h
Ketamine	0.5–1.0 mg/kg; may repeat as needed
Fentanyl	0.5–2.0 μg/kg

From Twersky R. *The Ambulatory Anesthesia Handbook.* St. Louis: Mosby; 1995:348–349.

midazolam resulted in an 80% success rate, with no hypoxemia, bradycardia, or excessive sedation noted. Commonly used pediatric conscious sedation medications and doses are outlined in Table 7–8.[16] Whatever pharmacologic technique is selected, pediatric sedation uses medications to reduce painful stimuli and anxiety. The ideal conscious sedation technique attempts to produce a motion-free study or diagnostic procedure. Through selection of a pharmacologic technique based on the patient's condition and procedural requirements, many pediatric patients tolerate the administration of sedation without incident.

DISCHARGE CRITERIA

Once the procedure is concluded, it is important to allow the child to recover in a closely monitored patient care area. Pediatric discharge criteria are similar to adult discharge criteria and include the following:

- Return of consciousness
- Ability to sit upright without assistance (appropriate to developmental level)

- Easily arousable, reflexes intact
- Appropriate responses to environmental stimuli
- Stable vital signs (within 10% to 15% of preprocedure baseline)
- Absence of or minimal nausea or vomiting
- Adequate state of hydration
- Presence of minimal discomfort
- Adequate respiratory rate and volume with no signs of respiratory embarrassment

REFERENCES

1. Scholer S, Schafer D, Potter J. The effect of age on the relative potency of midazolam and diazepam for sedation in upper gastrointestinal endoscopy. *J Clin Gastroenterol.* 1990;12:145.
2. McLeskey C. *Geriatric Anesthesiology.* Baltimore: Williams & Wilkins; 1997:134.
3. Thomas C. *Taber's Cyclopedic Medical Dictionary.* 6th ed. Philadelphia: FA Davis; 1983.
4. Lister G. Oxygen delivery in lambs: cardiovascular and hematologic development. *Am J Physiol.* 1979;237:H668.
5. Morgan E, Mikhail M. *Clinical Anesthesiology.* 2nd ed. Stamford, Conn: Appleton & Lange; 1996.
6. Patel R, Hannallah R. *International Anesthesiology Clinics: Anesthesia for Ambulatory Surgery.* Pediatric Anesthesia Techniques. Boston: Little, Brown; 1994;32:3.
7. Cote C. *Anesthesia: Pediatric Anesthesia.* 4th ed. New York: Churchill Livingstone; 1994:2108.
8. Twersky R. *The Ambulatory Anesthesia Handbook.* St. Louis: Mosby; 1995:146.
9. Bell C, Hughes C, Oh T. *The Pediatric Anesthesia Handbook.* St. Louis: Mosby; 1991: 131.
10. Gaba D, Fish K, Howard S. *Crisis Management in Anesthesiology.* New York: Churchill Livingstone; 1994:165.
11. American Academy of Pediatrics, Committee on Drugs. Guidelines for Monitoring and Management of Pediatric Patients During and After Sedation for Diagnostic and Therapeutic Procedures. *Pediatrics.* 1992;89:1110.
12. *JCAHO Comprehensive Accreditation Manual for Hospitals.* Oakbrook Terrace, Ill: Joint Commission on Accreditation of Healthcare Organizations; 1997.
13. Glaser C, Stark J, Brown R, et al. Rectal thiopental sodium for sedation of pediatric patients undergoing MR and other imaging studies. *J Neuroradiol.* 1995;16:111.
14. Pohlgeers A, Friedland L, Jones L. Combination fentanyl and diazepam for pediatric conscious sedation. *Acad Emerg Med.* 1995;2:879.
15. Weber E, Holida D, Moore M. New routes in pediatric sedation: a research based protocol for intranasal midazolam. *J Nurs Care Qual.* 1995;10:55.
16. Twersky R. *The Ambulatory Anesthesia Handbook.* St. Louis: Mosby; 1995:348.

Intravenous Insertion Techniques

PRINCIPLES OF IV THERAPY

The purpose of intravenous cannulation is to provide direct vascular access for administration of medications and supplemental fluid during conscious sedation procedures. Intravenous access provides immediate uptake and distribution of conscious sedation medications as well as a lifeline in the event of patient decompensation or crisis. Placement of the intravenous cannula is critical to the success of the planned procedure. Whenever there is doubt regarding successful cannulation or possible infiltration, the clinician should err on the side of caution and replace the catheter.

IV INSERTION TECHNIQUES

Supplies and equipment are assembled before the application of a tourniquet and selection of a vein. Supplies and equipment required for intravenous insertion are listed in Table 8–1. Intravenous solutions have been available in plastic containers since 1971.[1] Plastic containers displayed in Figure 8–1 offer the following advantages when compared with glass containers:

- They do not require that air be admitted to the system for fluid to flow.
- They do not require vented intravenous administration sets.
- They use atmospheric pressure to collapse the container as the intravenous solution flows into the patient.
- They do not break or rupture during routine use.

A variety of administration sets are currently available for use. Administration sets are selected on the basis of the following criteria:

- Length
- Location of access ports
- Size of drop chamber: microdrip vs. macrodrip (Fig. 8–2)
- Type of flow regulator (Fig. 8–3)
- Connectors

Once supplies and equipment are prepared, the patient is assessed for identification of a vascular access site. Veins generally used for peripheral cannulation are depicted in Figure 8–4. Selection of a vein for vascular access depends on a number of variables, which include surgical site, patient positioning, diagnostic

TABLE 8–1. *Intravenous Insertion Supplies*

- Disposable gloves
- Alcohol swabs/antiseptic solution
- Tourniquet
- Selection of IV catheters
  - 16 gauge
  - 18 gauge
  - 20 gauge
  - 22 gauge
- 1% lidocaine
- Local anesthesia (EMLA) cream for pediatric patients
- Adhesive/paper tape
- Tuberculin syringe with 25- or 30-gauge needle for local anesthetic injection
- Assortment of syringes: 3 ml, 5 ml, 10 ml
- Intravenous tubing (Venoset, minidrip, macrodrip)
- Extension tubing
- Intravenous solutions (Ringer's lactate, normal saline, dextrose)
- Sterile dressings

---

procedure, patient status (inpatient vs. outpatient), postprocedure activity level, and anticipated length of time that intravenous access is required. Previous mastectomy, lymph node dissection, or the presence of renal access grafts are contraindications for vascular access in the affected extremity or surgical side.

Inpatients receiving prolonged intravenous fluid therapy benefit from intravenous insertion at the most distal portion of the upper extremity. Advantages

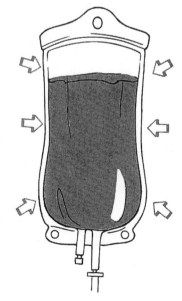

FIGURE 8–1. Plastic intravenous solution containers. Outside atmospheric pressure collapses plastic intravenous containers, which have been commercially available since 1971. (From Booker MF, Ignatavicius DD. *Infusion Therapy: Techniques and Medications.* Philadelphia: WB Saunders; 1996:46.)

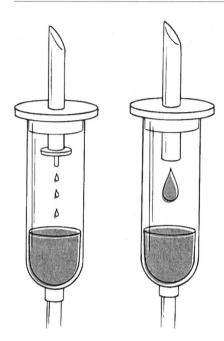

FIGURE 8–2.   Administration Venoset drip chambers. **A,** Minidrip. **B,** Macrodrip. (From Booker MF, Ignatavicius DD. *Infusion Therapy: Techniques and Medications.* Philadelphia: WB Saunders; 1996:51.)

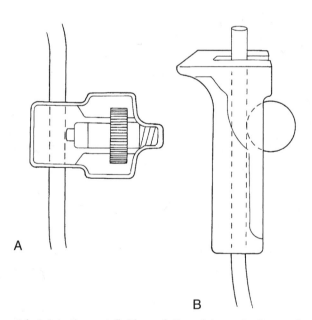

FIGURE 8–3.   Administration set fluid regulating clamps. **A,** Screw clamp. **B,** Roller clamp. (From Booker MF, Ignatavicius DD. *Infusion Therapy: Techniques and Medications.* Philadelphia: WB Saunders; 1996:51.)

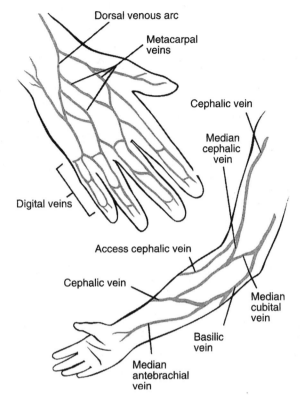

FIGURE 8–4.   Peripheral vein cannulation sites. Peripheral veins appropriate for vascular access in older children and adults. (From Booker MF, Ignatavicius DD. *Infusion Therapy: Techniques and Medications.* Philadelphia: WB Saunders; 1996:97.)

and disadvantages of peripheral vein selection are listed in Table 8–2. The catheter selected for intravenous cannulation for short-term care should be ³⁄₄ to 1 inch (2 to 2.5 cm) in length with a 20- or 22-gauge diameter.[2] However, larger-gauge catheters may be required to facilitate hydration or for specific patient procedures. Application of a tourniquet approximately 6 inches above the insertion site (Fig. 8–5) distends the peripheral blood vessels. Periodic clenching of the patient's hand distends the vessel more fully. Warm cloths and rubbing of the extremity provide vasodilation and venous filling in patients who are peripherally vasoconstricted. Prior to insertion the area should be cleansed in a circular fashion (Fig. 8–6) with a 2 to 2.5 inch radius from the intended insertion site. The cleansing agent (iodine, alcohol) is allowed to air dry to provide antibacterial action.

When a local anesthetic is used to anesthetize the skin, it should be injected superficially. A small intradermal skin wheal (0.1 ml of plain lidocaine, 30-gauge needle) anesthetizes the local tissue. Care must be taken not to insert the local needle deeply into the skin, or venous perforation and hematoma formation may occur. Once the area has been localized, traction on the vein is applied by the nondomi-

TABLE 8–2. *Advantages and Disadvantages of Peripheral Vein Selection*

Site	Advantages	Disadvantages
Basilic	Largest vein; straight pathway in upper arm and thorax	May be located too far to the posterior side for sterile procedure and routine care; may only be able to palpate a short segment
Median	Communicates with larger basilic; easily accessible for insertion and routine care	
Median cubital		
Median basilic	Joins with larger basilic; easily accessible for insertion and routine care	Valve may be located at junction with basilic, causing obstruction to cannula advancement
Median cephalic	Easily accessible	Valve may be located at junction with basilic, causing obstruction to cannula advancement; terminates in smaller cephalic; may not be present in some patients
Accessory cephalic	Easily accessible for insertion and routine care	Valve may be located at junction with cephalic, causing obstruction to cannula advancement; terminates in smaller cephalic; may not be present in some patients
Cephalic	Easily accessible for insertion and routine care; easy palpation and visualization above and below antecubital fossa	Smaller than basilic; pathway in upper arm and thorax is variable and unknown

From INS (Intravenous Nurses Society). *Intravenous Therapy: Clinical Principles and Practice.* Philadelphia: WB Saunders; 1995:101.

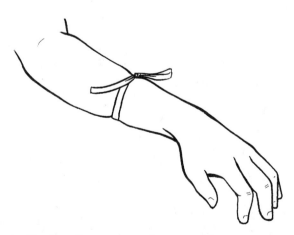

FIGURE 8–5. Application of venous tourniquet provides venous engorgement prior to intravenous cannulation. (From Booker MF, Ignatavicius DD. *Infusion Therapy: Techniques and Medications.* Philadelphia: WB Saunders; 1996:115.)

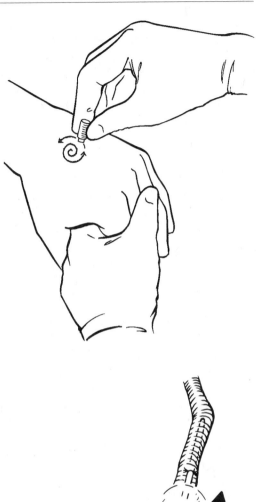

FIGURE 8-6. Preparation of intravenous cannulation site. Prior to vascular access, cleansing agent is applied in a circular fashion within a 2-inch radius and permitted to dry. (From Booker MF, Ignatavicius DD. *Infusion Therapy: Techniques and Medications.* Philadelphia: WB Saunders; 1996:116.)

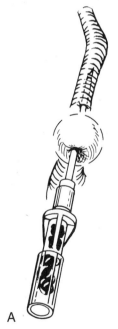
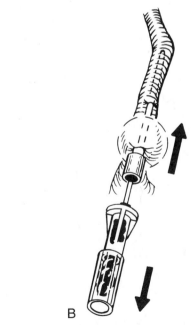

A   B

FIGURE 8-7. Presence of venous flash with advancement of catheter. **A,** Venous access is ascertained with the presence of a flash followed by **(B)** advancement of the catheter into the peripheral blood vessel. (From Butterworth J. *Atlas of Procedures in Anesthesia and Critical Care.* Philadelphia: WB Saunders; 1991:72.)

nant hand to secure or anchor the vein. This prevents the vein from "rolling" and excessive movement when one is preparing to insert the intravenous catheter.

When the appropriately sized intravenous catheter is selected, it should be inserted through the small skin wheal of local anesthesia. The needle is then advanced at a 30- to 40-degree angle in the direction of the vein to be cannulated. Once a "flash" or blood is noted in the catheter chamber (Fig. 8–7), the needle should be advanced slightly (several millimeters). This maneuver assures that the plastic catheter is situated in the vein and not positioned superficially over the vein. At this point, extreme care must be taken not to advance the needle through the back wall of the vein. Malpositioning of the catheter may result in local tissue trauma, hematoma formation, and a nonfunctional intravenous site. If the attempt to secure an intravenous line is unsuccessful, it is beneficial to leave the plastic catheter in place while an attempt is made at another intravenous access to avoid hematoma formation. After venous access is established, the unsuccessful intravenous catheter may be removed. Pressure is then applied for several minutes to decrease the incidence of ecchymosis and hematoma formation.

Once the intravenous line is established (presence of a "flash"), the caregiver advances the catheter with the index finger of his or her dominant hand or opposite hand. Either technique is acceptable for positioning the intravenous catheter into the vein. The Venoset is then connected with pressure applied between the male Venoset connector and the female catheter receptacle. Firm pressure should be applied at this junction to avoid unintentional disconnect. It is important to secure the catheter and tubing with a sterile dressing, tape, or transparent dressing. Transparent dressings afford direct visualization of the intravenous site. Redness, swelling, edema, or leakage around the site may be evaluated directly through the presence of the clear tegaderm dressing.

COMPLICATIONS OF INTRAVENOUS CATHETER INSERTION

Local complications associated with intravenous catheter insertion include infiltration, extravasation, phlebitis, hematoma formation, catheter embolism, local infection, and venous irritation. Local and systemic complications associated with intravenous therapy are listed in Table 8–3.

INTRAVENOUS FLUIDS

Intravenous fluid replacement may be accomplished with crystalloid solutions during the administration of conscious sedation. Intravenous solutions maintain fluid and electrolyte balance. Body fluids are divided into intracellular and extracellular fluids. Intracellular fluids are contained within the cells of the body. Extracellular fluid is divided into three compartments:

- Interstitial
- Intravascular
- Transcellular

TABLE 8–3. *Intravenous Therapy Complications*

COMPLICATION	ETIOLOGY	SIGNS/SYMPTOMS	TREATMENT	PREVENTION
LOCAL COMPLICATIONS				
Infiltration	Infusion of seepage of intravenous fluid into extravascular tissue caused by partial or complete venous access dislodgment	Decreased infusion rate Localized edema Complaints of burning, pain, and tenderness at IV site	Remove catheter Application of warm, moist heat to enhance fluid absorption	Stabilize catheter insertion site Avoid catheter insertion at points of flexion Frequent assessment of catheter site
Extravasation	Accidental administration of medication or solution, which results in tissue destruction (dopamine, diazepam)	Patient complaint of: • Stinging or localized burning at the catheter insertion site • Swelling • Localized tissue destruction (blister formation)	Stop the infusion Related to the amount of concentration of the medication or solution Physician notification Catheter remains in place	Monitor insertion site frequently Stabilize catheter insertion site Administer IV push medications via a free-flowing intravenous insertion site
Phlebitis	Inflammation along the course of the vein. Contributing factors in the development of phlebitis include • Insertion technique • Type of medication • Catheter size and length	Pain at the catheter site Red, inflamed "knotty" cord-like vein Temperature	Catheter removal Warm compresses	Change catheter site every 48–72 hours Use of large veins when irritation solutions (highly osmolar) are used Strict aseptic handling of catheter during insertion
Hematoma formation	Leakage of blood into the surrounding tissue	Bruising around the intravenous insertion site Pain at the site	Removal of catheter Application of direct pressure at insertion site Warm soaks applied if hematoma site is stable	Selection of small-gauge catheter Careful advancement of catheter parallel to patient's skin

Table continued on following page

169

TABLE 8–3. *Intravenous Therapy Complications Continued*

COMPLICATION	ETIOLOGY	SIGNS/SYMPTOMS	TREATMENT	PREVENTION
Local infection	Contamination at the intravenous insertion site secondary to a break in aseptic technique	Red, swollen, warm area or presence of purulent exudate at the insertion site	Catheter removal Catheter tip may be sent for culture Site is cleansed with antibacterial solution and covered with a sterile dressing	Strict aseptic technique Change of infusion containers after a minimum of 24 hours Venoset change every 48–72 hours
Catheter embolization	A piece of the intravenous catheter breaks off and floats freely in the blood vessel. Embolization can occur when the needle is reinserted into the catheter and advanced once a flash has been obtained.	Cardiovascular compromise: • Hypotension • Tachycardia • Cyanosis Pain along the vein	Catheter removal Tourniquet placement proximal to the insertion site Radiograph to locate catheter tip Surgical excision of catheter tip	Never reinsert the needle into the catheter during jelco catheter insertion During medication administration, use the shortest needle to puncture the injection port (1 inch)
SYSTEMIC COMPLICATIONS				
Systemic infection/sepsis	Pathogenic organism entrance into the systemic circulation. Results from poor aseptic technique, contaminated solution, or catheter insertion.	Early: Fever Chills Headache Malaise Late: Cardiovascular collapse Death	Change entire infusion system Notify physician Obtain cultures as ordered	Strict adherence to aseptic technique Change of infusion containers at a minimum of every 24 hours Venoset change every 48–72 hours

Air embolism	Air entrains into the systemic circulation. Entrainment may occur secondary to empty solution container, air in Venoset, tubing, and loose intravenous connections.	Chest/shoulder pain Back pain Dyspnea Hypotension Cyanosis	Position patient on left side in the Trendelenburg position to contain air in right atrium Notify physician Administer oxygen Cardiovascular support as ordered	Use of Luer-Lok connectors Careful monitoring of IV volume infused Use of electronic control device to detect presence of air
Circulatory overload	Excess fluid within the circulatory system at a rate greater than the patient's cardiovascular system can accommodate	Shortness of breath Rales on auscultation Engorged neck veins Dependent edema	Reduce IV flow rate Administer oxygen, monitor vital signs as ordered Administration of diuretics as ordered	Monitor intake and output
Allergic reaction	A localized or systemic reaction to an allergen	Skin wheal Redness, edema Hypotension, tachycardia Bronchospasm Wheezing Cardiovascular collapse	Remove allergen Redress with hypoallergenic tape If medication is suspected allergen, discontinue medication Systemic treatment is dependent on presenting symptoms and includes administration of: • Oxygen • Antihistamines • Epinephrine • Steroids	Careful preprocedure assessment to elicit allergy status Assessment for medication cross-reaction

Interstitial fluid is located between cells, whereas intravascular fluid lies within blood vessels or plasma. Transcellular fluid is secreted by epithelial cells and constitutes cerebrospinal fluid, intraocular fluid, and digestive fluids. Factors that have an impact on intravascular fluid replacement include the presence of concomitant disease states (hypertension, dehydration), intraprocedure fluid losses, and the patient's cardiovascular status. In emergency situations, restoration of intravascular volume restores plasma volume and optimizes cardiac output to ensure adequate tissue oxygen delivery.

Crystalloid solutions are generally selected according to their osmolality. *Osmolality* is a term used to identify the number of particles in a liter of solution. Measured in milliosmoles per liter (mOsm/L), the osmolality of the extracellular fluid is determined by measuring solute concentration of the blood (normal serum osmolality equals 280 to 300 mOsm). Electrolyte solutions (crystalloid) are capable of conducting an electrical charge. Cations (potassium, sodium) maintain a positive charge, and anions (chloride) produce a negative charge. Major body fluid electrolyte concentrations and their function are identified in Table 8–4.

The tonicity of crystalloids is also a major factor in the selection of intravenous fluids. Crystalloid solutions are therefore divided into the following classifications:

- Hypotonic: Lower osmotic pressure than plasma
- Isotonic: Same osmotic pressure as plasma
- Hypertonic: Greater osmotic pressure than that of plasma

TABLE 8–4. *Major Body Fluid Electrolyte Concentrations and Functions*

ELECTROLYTE	SERUM CONCENTRATION (mEq/L)	MAJOR FUNCTIONS
Sodium (Na^+)	136–145	Maintenance of plama osmolarity Generation and transmission of action potentials Maintenance of acid-base balance Maintenance of electroneutrality
Potassium (K^+)	3.5–5	Regulation of intracellular osmolarity Maintenance of membrane electrical excitability Maintenance of plasma acid-base balance
Calcium (Ca^{2+})	4.5–5.5 8–10.5 mg/dl	Cofactor in blood-clotting cascade Excitable membrane stabilizer Provision of strength and density to teeth and bones Essential element in contractile processes in cardiac, skeletal, and smooth muscle
Chloride (Cl^-)	96–106	Maintenance of plasma acid-base balance Maintenance of plasma electroneutrality Formation of hydrochloric acid

From Keyes J. *Fluid, Electrolyte, and Acid-Base Regulation.* 2nd ed. Belmont, Calif: Wadsworth; 1990. Copyright 1990 Wadsworth Publishing Co.

TABLE 8–5. *Composition of Common Intravenous Solutions*

SOLUTION	SUGAR (g/L)	Na+	Cl−	K+	Ca++	TONICITY
		(mEq/L)				
0.9% saline		154	154			Isotonic
0.45% saline		77	77			Hypotonic
5% dextrose in water (D5W)	50					Isotonic
10% dextrose in water (D10W)	100					Hypertonic
5% dextrose in 0.45% saline	50	77	77			Hypertonic
5% dextrose in 0.225% saline	50	38.5	38.5			Isotonic
Ringer's solution		147	156	4	4	Isotonic
Lactated Ringer's solution		130	109	4	3	Isotonic

Adapted from Luckmann J. *Saunders Manual of Nursing Care.* Philadelphia: WB Saunders; 1997.

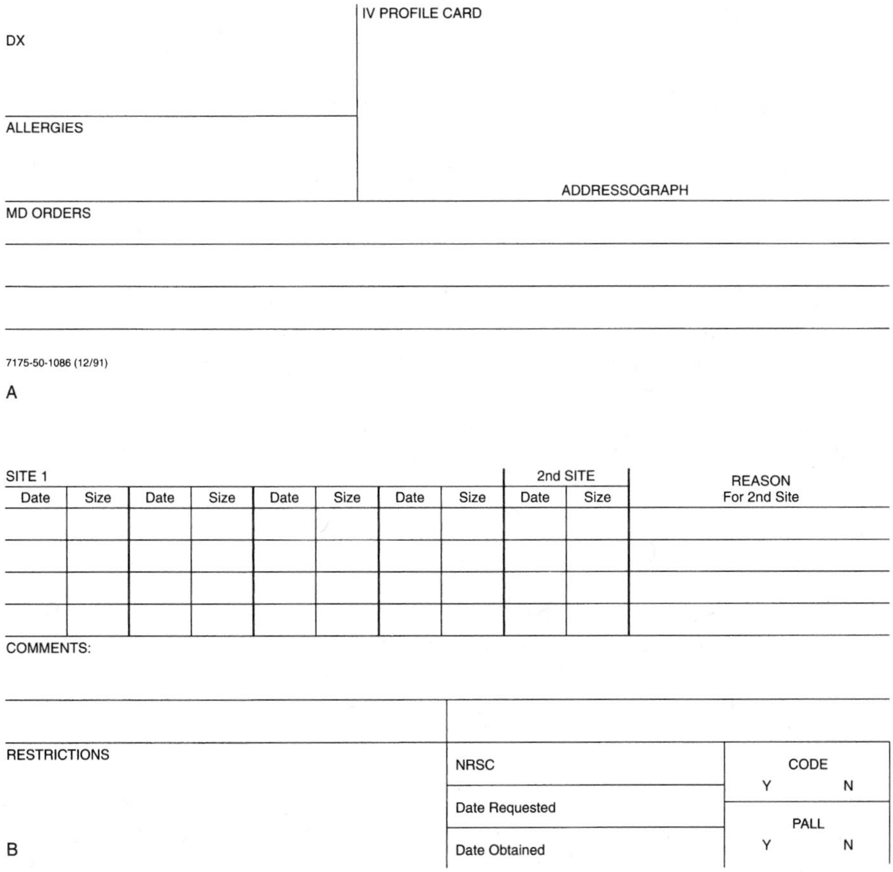

IV PROFILE CARD

DX

ALLERGIES

ADDRESSOGRAPH

MD ORDERS

7175-50-1086 (12/91)

A

SITE 1								2nd SITE		REASON For 2nd Site
Date	Size	Date	Size	Date	Size	Date	Size	Date	Size	

COMMENTS:

RESTRICTIONS	NRSC	CODE
		Y N
	Date Requested	PALL
B	Date Obtained	Y N

FIGURE 8–8.   Intravenous profile card for peripheral catheter care. **A,** Front. **B,** Back. (From INS [Intravenous Nurses Society]. *Intravenous Therapy: Clinical Principles and Practice.* Philadelphia: WB Saunders; 1995:25.)

YEAR: 19 DATE:								
TIME:								
NEW START								
O.R./E.R. START								
RESTART								
I.V. ACCESS FOR:								
FLUIDS								
MEDS VIA HEP LOCK								
BLOOD/COMPONENTS								
ACCESS ONLY								
CONVERT I.V. TO HEP LOCK								
FLUSHED W./SALINE & HEPARIN								
REASON FOR D.C.:								
ROUTINE SITE ROTATION								
PHLEBITIS: GRADE								
INFILTRATED								
OCCLUDED								
LEAKING								
POSITIONAL								
MEDIC START								
DR. ORDERS								
CATHETER D.C.'d INTACT?								
HOT PACKS APPLIED								
DEVICE/BRAND:								
GAUGE								
LENGTH								
# ATTEMPTS								
LIDOCAINE 1% S.C.								
SKIN PREP:								
ALCOHOL/BETADINE								
INSERTION SITE:								
DRESSING TYPE								
CHANGES:								
DRESSING								
TUBING								
FILTER								
SITE INSPECTION								
? PROBLEMS OBSERVED:								
COMMENTS:								
Pump Set-up								
Lab Draw								
INFUSION CONTROL DEVICE:								
PT. ED. VERBAL/BOOKLET								
NURSE INITIALS								

INTRAVENOUS NURSING CARE PLAN
(circle all that apply)

Date Care Plan Initiated:
SHORT TERM GOAL
(initial 72 hrs.): Establish I.V. access for: fluids, drugs, chemotherapy, blood/components, hyperalimentation, access only H.L.

LONG TERM GOAL (beyond 72 hrs.): Maintain safe access until physician discontinues.

POTENTIAL PROBLEMS: Phlebitis, occlusion, infiltration, limited access, confusion, electrolyte imbalance, circulatory overload, transfusion reaction, drug extrav. with tissue damage, sepsis, air embolism.

PLAN: AVI pump for accuracy, daily site check, tubing/filter chge. q 24-72 hrs., long-term cannula, 2nd line for incomp. drugs, restart PRN

ACTION: PCA set-up & instruc. with return demo., PIC line per physician order, intracath, landmark, S.C. line per physician, Infus-A-Port

OUTCOME: Completion of therapy; pt. discharged; cannula in place for: home, ECF.

COMMENTS:_____
PHYSICIAN CONTACTED_____ DATE:_____
INTRAVENOUS NURSE:_____

FIGURE 8-9. Intravenous therapy nursing care plan. (From INS [Intravenous Nurses Society]. *Intravenous Therapy: Clinical Principles and Practice.* Philadelphia: WB Saunders; 1995:464.)

With the administration of hypotonic solution (0.45% saline), cells begin to swell. As hypotonic solution is added to the extracellular fluid, the osmolality decreases, forcing water to enter the cells in an area of higher osmolality. Hypertonic solution (3% saline) increases osmolality of the surrounding extracellular fluid and forces water to leave the cell and enter the extracellular fluid with resultant cellular shrinkage. Isotonic solutions (0.9% normal saline, lactated Ringer's) produce no osmosis or change in osmolality of body fluids. Isotonic solutions are generally the crystalloid of choice for intravenous maintenance during the administration of conscious sedation. The infusion of isotonic solutions results in equal distribution throughout the extracellular compartment since the tonicity is similar to plasma (300 mOsm). The composition of various intravenous solutions is given in Table 8–5.

Before discharge, ambulatory care patients should have the intravenous catheter removed. Firm, consistent pressure is applied for 5 to 10 minutes after catheter removal. A 4 × 4 or 2 × 2 inch reinforcement dressing applied with tape provides additional pressure after discharge. Patients should be instructed to remove the gauze once they are at home and replace it with a Band-Aid. This additional reinforcement may decrease the incidence of hematoma formation. In-house patients or patients who require prolonged intravenous therapy require peripheral catheter care. Nursing documentation of patients with peripheral catheters is summarized in Figure 8–8. Documentation of intravenous cannulation required on the intravenous conscious sedation flow sheet or medical record includes the following:

- Identification of intravenous insertion site
- Catheter gauge
- Number of attempts
- Intravenous infusion infused

A nursing care plan for peripheral catheter care is presented in Figure 8–9.

REFERENCES

1. Booker M, Ignatavicius D. *Infusion Therapy: Techniques and Medications.* Philadelphia: WB Saunders; 1996:46.
2. Booker M, Ignatavicius D. *Infusion Therapy: Techniques and Medications.* Philadelphia: WB Saunders; 1996:103.

CHAPTER 9

Locations and Specific Conscious Sedation Procedures

Intravenous conscious sedation may be administered in a variety of settings:

- Critical care units
- Emergency rooms
- Operating room suites
- Outpatient ambulatory care centers
- Physicians' offices and diagnostic centers
- Radiology suites
- Pain management centers
- Gastroenterology suites
- Bronchoscopy suites

The administration of intravenous conscious sedation outside the operating room suite may be particularly challenging to the provider. The clinician may be called upon to administer sedation in areas where space is limited. In certain circumstances, access to the patient may be limited. To perform radiologic or diagnostic procedures, illumination may be reduced, which presents an environmental hazard. Vigilant assessment of respiratory status is required for all patients receiving intravenous conscious sedation, particularly in poorly illuminated areas. As mandated by JCAHO, state statute, and recommended practice, the prudent practitioner realizes that, regardless of the practice setting, the requirements for intravenous conscious sedation remain the same.

RADIOLOGY

Procedures performed in the radiology department include invasive and noninvasive studies. Registered nurses may be required to administer intravenous conscious sedation for patients scheduled for magnetic resonance imaging (MRI), computed tomography (CT scan), angiography, embolization, arteriography, and radiation therapy. The administration of intravenous conscious sedation for radiologic procedures may be warranted secondary to invasive manipulation, injection of contrast material, and intraprocedural monitoring of unstable patients. Recommendations for prevention of burns associated with the use of monitoring equipment during magnetic resonance procedures are presented in Table 9–1.

TABLE 9-1. *Recommendations for the Prevention of Burns Associated with the Use of Physiologic Monitoring Equipment During MRI Procedures*

1. Use only monitoring equipment that has been tested and determined to be MR-compatible.
2. Permit only individuals who have been properly trained for work on the MR system and properly trained to operate monitors to be responsible for patients in the MR environment.
3. Check the integrity (e.g., cracking, fraying, etc.) of the electrical insulation of each monitoring lead, cable, or wire before using the device during an MRI procedure.
4. Remove all electrically conductive material from the bore of the MR system that is not required for the MRI procedure (i.e., unused surface coils, cables, etc.).
5. Keep all electrically conductive material(s) that must remain in the bore of the MR system from directly contacting the patient by placing thermal and/or electrical insulation (including air) between the conductive material and the patient. For example, place ECG leads underneath the patient comfort pads and/or use additional foam pads between the patient and cables to prevent direct contact with the patient's tissue.
6. Keep electrically conductive material (ECG leads, cables, etc.) that must remain within the bore of the MR system from forming large-diameter, conductive loops (remember, the patient's tissue may be involved in the formation of the conductive loop).
7. Position all cables to prevent "cross points." A cross point is the point where a cable crosses another cable, a cable loops across itself, or a cable touches either the patient or sides of the magnetic bore more than once.
8. Do not cross cables inside or outside of the bore of the magnet of the MR system (note that loops can be closed, U-shaped, or S-shaped).
9. Position all ECG cables so that they exit down the center of the patient table of the MR system.
10. Position the patient so that there is no direct contact between the patient's skin and the bore of the magnet of the MR system.
11. Use only MR system manufacturer-approved ECG wires, leads, and electrodes and appropriate application techniques.
12. Do not position conductive leads or cables across a metallic prosthesis.
13. Remove any monitor that does not appear to be operating properly during the MRI procedure.
14. Discontinue the MRI procedure immediately if the patient reports feeling warm or hot.
15. Follow the instructions for proper operation of the monitoring equipment provided by the manufacturer of the device.

From Shellock F, Lipczak H, Kanal E. Monitoring patients during MR procedures: a review. *Appl Radiol.* February 1995.

CONTRAST MEDIA

Contrast media is frequently used in the radiology suite to enhance visualization of specific anatomic areas. Nurses providing procedural patient care must be prepared to recognize and participate in the treatment of an allergic reaction to contrast media. Approximately 5% to 8% of patients receiving intravenous contrast media experience an allergic reaction to the dye.[1] A variety of factors influence the risk of systemic reaction:

- Speed of injection (slow vs. fast)
- Type of dye used
- Total dose administered
- Anatomic site (coronary/cerebral)
- Known allergy to shellfish

Manifestations of allergic reaction include the following:

- Nausea
- Vomiting
- Flushing
- Chills
- Urticaria
- Bronchial constriction
- Seizures
- Hypotension
- Cyanosis
- Anoxia
- Pulmonary edema
- Angina
- Dysrhythmias

According to the severity of presenting symptoms, treatment includes administration of oxygen and fluids and the institution of ACLS protocol. Epinephrine, aminophylline, atropine, diphenhydramine, and methylprednisolone have been used in the past. Dosage and route of emergency medication administration are dependent on presenting symptoms.

Iodine is a component of contrast media. Patients with a history of iodine, shellfish, or seafood allergy are at increased risk of developing an adverse reaction to contrast media. Patients receiving intravenous contrast media may become anxious or nauseated, complain of chills, or display changes in mentation. These symptoms are secondary to a transient increase in serum osmolarity produced by administration of the intravenous contrast media.[2] Contrast material is hypertonic (1400 to 1500 mOsm).[2] After initial administration of contrast media, there is a brief period of hypertension and increased cardiac filling pressure. As the dye begins the excretion process, equilibration with the extracellular fluid generally ensues within 10 to 15 minutes followed by a transient diuresis. The introduction of reduced osmolality contrast media has reduced the incidence of nausea, vomiting, pain on injection, and cardiovascular symptoms.

CARDIAC CATHERIZATION

Several procedures may be performed under conscious sedation in the cardiac catheterization laboratory or cardiology suite:

- Cardiac catheterization
- Electrophysiologic studies
- Ablation procedures
- Pacemaker insertion
- Automatic implantable cardioverter-defibrillator (AICD) insertion
- Transesophageal echocardiography

Before initiating conscious sedation in the cardiology suite, it is important to obtain adequate preprocedure assessment of the cardiac patient. The degree of cardiovascular impairment must be ascertained prior to the administration of medications to provide optimal sedation, avoid overdose, and prevent unexpected drug interactions.

OPERATING ROOM

Nurses engaged in the administration of intravenous conscious sedation within the operating room frequently have adequate sedation supplies and resuscitative equipment available. Oxygen is administered by means of piped-in oxygen flowmeters or a flowmeter attached to the anesthesia machine. Suction and emergency resuscitative medications and equipment (laryngoscope, airway supplies, defibrillator) are readily available in the immediate area. Generally, anesthesia personnel are immediately available in the operating room environment to respond to untoward patient reactions and emergent complications associated with the administration of intravenous conscious sedation. Monitoring equipment (ECG, blood pressure, and pulse oximetry) is also readily available within the surgical suites. Proper inservicing is required prior to the use of monitoring equipment. Effective postprocedure monitoring may be provided by postanesthesia care unit personnel, or the patient may be returned to the ambulatory surgery area for postprocedure monitoring. Regardless of the postprocedure recovery site, patients must meet *standardized institutional criteria* (Table 10–5) before discharge (outpatients) or transfer of care (inpatients). *Discharge criteria must be the same for all areas within the institution.*

AMBULATORY SURGICENTERS

Ambulatory surgicenters may use operating room suites or ancillary areas for conscious sedation procedures. As outlined earlier, operating room suites are generally well equipped to monitor patients receiving intravenous conscious sedation. Ancillary areas (holding areas, endoscopy suites) must be properly equipped and adhere to monitoring and resuscitative equipment requirements for patients receiving conscious sedation. Postprocedure monitoring may be provided by ambulatory care nurses involved with the conscious sedation procedure or in a separate postprocedure recovery room.

TABLE 9–2.   *Contents of Oxygen Cylinders Commonly Used for Medical Purposes*

TANK SIZE	DIMENSIONS (inches)	SERVICE PRESSURE (psig)	CONTENTS (liters)
B	3½ × 13	1900	200
D	4½ × 17	1900	400
E	4¼ × 26	1900	660
H	9¼ × 51	2200	6900

EXAMPLE:
1. 1 full E cylinder = 660 L O_2
   Patient receives 3 L/min for 60 minutes.
   180 L used of full oxygen E tank.
2. Emergency resuscitation
   Bag valve mask = 10 L/min:
   66 minutes of use in a full E cylinder.

OFFICES

Conscious sedation performed in physicians' offices presents additional challenges to the clinician. *Required monitoring, emergency resuscitative equipment, and medications must be present to satisfy minimal state practice requirements and the recommended practices of professional organizations.*[3,4] Practitioners and clinicians administering conscious sedation in isolated settings (outside hospital facilities, surgicenters, etc.) should be particularly skilled in airway management and resuscitative care should an emergent situation arise. An ample supply of oxygen must be readily available. In the absence of an oxygen pipeline system, the physi-

TABLE 9–3.   *Medical Gas Cylinder Handling Procedures*

1. Do not allow valves, fittings to come into contact with grease, oil, or solvents.
2. Store tanks in a cool, dry place. *Never* expose to heat. Do not store near radiators or furnaces or in overheated rooms.
3. Secure connections when changing cylinders to prevent inadvertent emptying into the atmosphere.
4. Adapters to change outlet size must not be used.
5. When oxygen is not in use, the cylinder valve should be closed. Hand tightening is adequate to close the cylinder valve. *Do not overtighten.*
6. Maintain valve protection caps for oxygen cylinders not in use. These devices protect the fragile outlet valve.
7. Secure cylinders properly when in use or in storage. Cylinders should be secured to a wall with a chain mechanism to prevent tipping. Oxygen is stored under pressure; therefore damage to the outlet valve could result in the tank becoming a dangerous projectile if the tank is not secured properly.
8. Use a tank-transport cart to move tanks. Do not drag, roll, or slide tanks.
9. Markings and labeling must not be defaced.

NOTE: If you have any questions regarding safe storage, transport, or use of medical cylinders, contact your service representative or medical gas distributor.

cian and the nurse must be cognizant of the quantity of oxygen available for routine administration and emergency use. Table 9–2 identifies the contents of commonly used oxygen cylinders for medical purposes. Table 9–3 identifies safe handling procedures for gas cylinders.

PAIN MANAGEMENT CENTER

An increased awareness and understanding of pain physiology has led to the proliferation of therapeutic intervention in the management of acute and chronic pain syndromes. Conscious sedation is often used during the administration of diagnostic and therapeutic procedures. Common diagnostic and therapeutic interventions are identified in Table 9–4. Patients presenting for pain management procedures may provide additional challenges to the clinician for a variety of reasons. The difficulty of assessment and diagnosis of pain disorders, the presence of acute and chronic pain syndromes, and variations in the psychologic, social, and environmental characteristics of the patient preclude the routine administration of pain-management services. Individual patient variations must be considered and addressed before the procedure. The administration of chronic opioid or sedative medications required for preprocedure pain relief generally results in increased requirements of conscious sedation medications throughout the procedure. Pain associated with specific nerves or anatomic areas requires additional time to position and adequately protect the patient during the procedure. Members of the multidisciplinary team caring for the patient with acute or chronic pain syndromes must document specific patient care requirements, which must be considered prior to the commencement of any procedure.

TABLE 9–4. *Pain Management Techniques*

I. DIAGNOSTIC BLOCKS	Celiac plexus block
Zygapophyseal (facet) facet	Superior hypogastric block
Sacroiliac joint	Ganglion block
Selective nerve root block	Sacroiliac joint block
Dorsal primary ramus nerve block	Epidural blood patch
Costovertebral	Epidural steroids
Peripheral nerve block	Transforaminal steroids
Differential spinal	Interlaminar steroids
	Neurolytic procedures
II. DIAGNOSTIC INFUSION	• Chemolysis
Lidocaine	• Cryotherapy
Fentanyl	• Radio frequency ablation
Thiopental	Motor point block
Phentolamine	• Phenol
	• Alcohol
III. DIAGNOSTIC AND THERAPEUTIC	Indwelling epidural catheter
PROCEDURES	Intrathecal catheter
Stellate ganglion block	Indwelling interpleural catheter
Lumbar sympathetic block	Spinal cord stimulator
Thoracic sympathetic block	

BRONCHOSCOPY SUITE

Bronchoscopy is often performed in a designated area (bronchoscopy or pulmonary suite). Bronchoscopy permits direct or indirect visualization of the upper airway, trachea, and pulmonary tree. Specific patient considerations include preprocedure cardiopulmonary assessment and evaluation of the patient's airway for anomalies. The presence of reduced pulmonary reserve or documented upper airway anomalies may predispose the patient to the development of respiratory distress during the procedure. Adequate topical anesthesia is critical to the success of the procedure. The application of topical anesthesia requires several minutes to reach maximal effectiveness. Postprocedure considerations include nothing by mouth until the gag reflex has returned and observation for signs and symptoms of local anesthesia toxicity (Chapter 5).

GASTROENTEROLOGY SUITE

Conscious sedation is administered for gastroenterologic procedures, including upper endoscopy, colonoscopy, and endoscopic retrograde cholangiopancreatography. Gastroenterology procedures are frequently performed in designated gastrointestinal suites, ambulatory care centers, or physicians' offices. Required monitoring, emergency resuscitative equipment, and medications must be present to satisfy minimal state practice requirements and recommended practices of professional organizations. Patients presenting for gastroenterology procedures are frequently anxious and elderly and may have a significant medical history. The administration of conscious sedation requires careful titration, critical assessment, and the ability to rapidly intervene in the event of respiratory or physiologic compromise. *Practitioners and clinicians administering conscious sedation in isolated settings (outside hospital facilities, surgicenters, etc.) should be particularly skilled in airway management and resuscitative care should an emergent situation arise.* In the presence of reduced room illumination frequently required for the procedure, accessory lighting or a flashlight must be readily available for periodic patient assessment.

CONSCIOUS SEDATION PROCEDURES

The remainder of this chapter details specific considerations associated with a variety of conscious sedation procedures.

Angiography/Embolization

Description: Injection of contrast media in isolated blood vessels to identify stenotic lesions, malformations, etc.

Indications: Visualization of vasculature of the viscera, extremities, and major vascular structures: aorta, femoral artery.

Estimated Time: 30 to 60 minutes.

Considerations: Use of local anesthesia for catheter placement is required prior to injection of the contrast media. Conscious sedation medications should be administered 3 to 5 minutes prior to the injection of a local anesthetic. Injection of contrast media may produce pain or nausea during administration. Adequate hydration is re-quired to assist in the excretion of the osmotic load. Cerebral angiography/embolization procedures may be painful, and supplemental analgesia may be required. Neurologic assessment is required during the procedure; therefore deep sedation is contraindicated.

Postprocedure Considerations: Postprocedure assessment is dependent on the anatomic area and presenting symptoms. Patients must be monitored after the procedure until all discharge criteria are met.

Nursing Diagnoses: Potential for hemodynamic compromise; impaired level of consciousness; potential for bleeding.

Anorectal Surgery

Description: Exposure and ligation of hemorrhoids. Opening and drainage of an anal fistula tract, or excision and removal of anal lesions.

Indications: Hemorrhoidectomy; anal fistulotomy; anal fistulectomy; anal warts.

Estimated Time: 30 to 60 minutes, depending on the pathologic condition.

Considerations: Superficial anorectal surgery may be performed with the patient under conscious sedation. Infected areas do not absorb local anesthetic medications well. Therefore it is difficult to achieve adequate anesthetic activity in the infected area. Administration of a local anesthetic to external hemorrhoids, lesions, etc. may produce a vagal episode in some patients (young, anxious, or in the presence of concomitant disease states). Treatment of vagal episodes includes

- Administration of oxygen
- IV fluid bolus (300 to 500 ml)
- Atropine 0.5 to 1 mg
- Positioning of patient with head down (Trendelenburg)

These procedures are frequently performed with the patient in the lateral or prone position. It is important to titrate the effects of sedation to a clinical end point of conscious sedation (nystagmus, slurring of speech) and avoid heavy sedation. Deep sedation may lead to airway compromise in a patient whose airway is not easily accessible.

Postoperative Considerations: Postprocedure pain may be severe once the local anesthetic has worn off. Rather than waiting for the local anesthetic effects to dissipate, patients may benefit from the early administration of analgesic medications. Because of the pain associated with the procedure and the administration of oral opioids for postprocedure pain management, patients may require a stool softener. To avoid postprocedure vagal episodes, adequate pain management is required before the patient is discharged.

Nursing Diagnoses: Alterations in gastrointestinal function; alteration in comfort level; impaired ventilation associated with patient positioning.

Arteriovenous Access for Hemodialysis

Description: An arteriovenous (AV) fistula is created by anastomosing a vein to an artery. Prosthetic grafts and veins may be used to create the AV fistula. Conscious sedation may be administered prior to the localization of the wrist or forearm area. Forearm grafts require local anesthesia injection into four different areas to create the AV loop between the radial or ulnar artery and the antecubital or brachial vein.

Indications: Vascular access for chronic renal dialysis patients.

Estimated Time: 45 minutes to 3 hours. Is dependent on the status of the veins, arteries, and desired location of the graft.

Considerations: Creation of an AV fistula with use of conscious sedation is possible. Patients presenting for fistula formation are generally extremely sick. Chronic hypertension, pulmonary edema secondary to fluid overload, uremic pleuritis, electrolyte disturbances, cardiomyopathy, and chronic anemia are associated with chronic renal disease. Particular attention to laboratory values is warranted prior to the procedure:

- Creatinine
- Potassium
- Hemoglobin
- ECG
- Chest x-ray

Intravenous access may be particularly difficult to establish. The intravenous line for sedation should not be started in the operative arm. An intravenous line for the administration of sedation should use a microdrip chamber with a low solute solution (0.5% to 0.25% saline). Patients should not be overhydrated during these procedures. Minimal intravenous fluids (50 to 75 ml) are generally all that is required to infuse sedative medications, heparin, or protamine as requested by the physician. The surgeon generally requests heparin prior to the anastomosis and may request protamine at the completion of the procedure. Protamine should be administered slowly (no more than 5 mg/min). Each 1 mg of protamine reverses 90 units of heparin. The surgeon will inform you how much protamine to administer. It is imperative to administer the protamine slowly. Hypotension, cardiovascular collapse, and cardiac arrest have been associated with its use.

Postprocedure Considerations: Postprocedure considerations focus on the patient's disease state. The severity of the presenting symptoms may dictate postprocedure recovery. One should not take postprocedure blood pressure in the surgical arm. A bruit or thrill should be present when auscultated with a stethoscope over the surgical site. The absence of a bruit or thrill may signify occlusion of the newly created fistula. Patients may be returned to the dialysis unit, the medical surgical floor, or home once discharge criteria are met.

Nursing Diagnoses: Ineffective breathing pattern secondary to cardiopulmonary response associated with chronic renal failure; alterations in fluid volume; alteration in elimination pattern; potential for skin injury due to the length of the procedure and poor skin condition; potential for dysrhythmia.

Arthroscopy

Description: A local anesthetic may be infiltrated into the joint prior to introduction of the fiberoptic camera source. Once the local anesthetic is injected, a small incision is made in the affected joint area. Additional incisions are made to introduce grabbers, irrigation, and debriding devices.

Indications: Degenerative joint disease, acute injury, loose bodies, arthritis.

Estimated Time: 30 to 60 minutes.

Considerations: The success of this

technique is dependent on the quality of local anesthetic infiltration. Light sedation may suffice for injection of the local anesthetic into the affected joint. A tourniquet is generally applied above the surgical site. Tourniquet pain may become severe during the procedure and is extremely difficult to alleviate. Administration of additional opioids and sedatives may reduce the pain to some degree. The only effective treatment for tourniquet pain (pain at the tourniquet site, hypertension, tachycardia, and agitation) is release and removal of the tourniquet. Release of the tourniquet results in revascularization of the limb with venous return of metabolic byproducts and local anesthetic to the systemic circulation. **Postprocedure Considerations:** Documentation of neurovascular status of the affected extremity is required. Young, healthy patients are treated for acute sports injuries, whereas elderly, debilitated patients may present for debridement or examination of degenerative, arthritic joints. Postprocedure care is dependent on the patient population. Mobility is a concern in the elderly patient. **Nursing Diagnoses:** Alteration in the musculoskeletal system; alteration in comfort; potential for reduced activity.

Automatic Implantable Cardioverter-Defibrillator (AICD) Placement

Description: A nonthoracotomy approach uses a left pectoral subcutaneous patch or transvenous sensing/pacing defibrillating leads. Devices currently on the market include the following:

- CPI Ventak AICD
- Medtronic PCD
- Venitrex Cadence

Additional devices are currently in clinical trials.

Indications: Hemodynamically significant arrhythmias, ventricular fibrillation/ventricular tachycardia. Transvenous, nonthoracotomy implantation may be conducted with local anesthesia and conscious sedation. General anesthesia is required for thoracotomy, median sternotomy, and subcostal approaches. The purpose of the AICD is twofold:

1. It continuously monitors cardiac rhythm
2. It delivers dysrhythmic therapy

Estimated Time: 2 hours.

Considerations: Transvenous endocardial leads and epicardial or subcutaneous patches with abdominal subcutaneous implanted generators may be inserted under conscious sedation in the operating room or cardiac laboratory. One defibrillating electrode or patch is connected to the right atrium or ventricle and one to the cardiac apex. A separate electrode is used to pace and sense. The AICD can then sense ventricular tachycardia or fibrillation and deliver up to four consecutive countershocks of 25 to 30 joules. Low-impedance gel electrodes are routinely placed on the patient's chest and back to allow synchronous cardioversion or defibrillation if needed. AICD devices must be turned off during periods of electrocautery. Electrocautery triggers AICD devices. Intraprocedure care is directed at the hemodynamic profile of the patient. Placement and testing may require frequent intentional electrically induced periods of cardiac arrest. An external defibrillator and advanced cardiac life support (ACLS) medications should be present in the room to effectively deal with cardiac arrest. Patients with AICDs must not be placed in MRI units. AICD patients generally have significant ventricular dysfunction, a high incidence of arrhythmias, and concomitant chronic disease states.

Postprocedure Considerations: One should be prepared to deal with a device that may not function properly. An external defibrillator must be immediately available for use. Some 10% to 20% of transvenous implanted AICDs require conversion to thoracotomy secondary to high DFTs greater than 25 joules. Postprocedure report to recovery personnel includes the status of the AICD (on or off) and the rate-sensing parameters.

Nursing Diagnoses: Hemodynamic instability; impaired cardiac conductance; alteration in cardiovascular system.

Blepharoplasty

Description: Excision of redundant upper or lower eyelid skin and subcutaneous tissue.

Indications: Decreased visual acuity, redundant skin.

Estimated Time: 90 to 120 minutes.

Considerations: Conscious sedation medications administered 3 to 5 minutes before injection of local anesthetic to the upper or lower eyelids increases the patient's tolerance during administration of the local anesthetic. Several minutes is required for the local anesthetic to take effect. It is important for the patient to remain immobile during the procedure. Removal of fat pads from the lower eyelids is uncomfortable for many patients. Additional local anesthesia may be required during excision of lower eyelid subcutaneous tissue. The patient's airway is not readily accessible; therefore it is best to avoid heavy sedation. The administration of oxygen is required under the surgical drapes. It is important to allow oxygen to dissipate into the room by tenting of the surgical drapes when electrosurgical cautery is in use. Reassurance may be conveyed through hand holding and verbal communication.

Postprocedure Considerations: Immediately after the procedure, the patient should be positioned at a 30- to 45-degree head-up angle to avoid bleeding and prevent swelling. Visual inspection of the eye may reveal blood or small clots in the area. This material is generally flushed out in the procedure room. The physician may request the postprocedure staff to irrigate the eye with 20 to 30 ml of normal saline solution. Irrigation is accomplished with the patient's head turned to the side and the saline solution flushed to remove any heme or clot formation. The patient should be informed that bending and heavy lifting may produce bleeding. Pain and swelling may be decreased with the application of iced saline compresses or ice. Triple antibiotic ointment may be prescribed by the physician for direct application onto the incision. Visual acuity, visual assessment, and satisfactory mobility are required prior to discharge.

Nursing Diagnoses: Decreased visual acuity; alteration in mobility; potential for bleeding.

Breast Biopsy

Description: The surgical exploration and removal of breast tissue for definitive diagnosis by frozen section or permanent pathologic determination.

Indications: Breast mass, fibrocystic disease, mammographic abnormalities.

Estimated Time: 30 to 60 minutes.

Considerations: Superficial breast biopsies may be performed under intravenous conscious sedation. However, lesions that lie deep within the breast tissue may require deep sedation techniques or the induction of general anesthesia. Prior to localization of the breast tissue with local anesthesia, a short-acting opioid may be administered 2 to 3 minutes before the injection of the local anesthetic. Some physicians oppose the use of narcotics and rely on the sedative effects of benzodiazepines. The benzodiazepine should be administered 3 to 5 minutes before the planned localization. Benzodiazepines or opioids administered 30 to 45 seconds prior to the localization do not accomplish their full pharmacologic effect or produce an optimal state of sedation for the patient. Patients who experience pain after the administration of a local anesthetic may require supplemental sedation. However, anesthesia of the breast tissue is produced by the infiltration of a local anesthetic administered by the surgeon. No amount of sedative medication short of general anesthesia can atone for poor localization of the breast tissue.

Generally, patients presenting for breast biopsy are extremely anxious. The neuroendocrine response associated with stress and the increased release of catecholamines produce fearful, frightened patients. Verbal reassurance and kindness go a long way with this patient population. At times, the patient's response to the administration of sedative medications may sur-

prise the clinician. Patients may appear extremely anxious and frightened and become very somnolent with the administration of small amounts of medications. Many times these patients have not slept for days prior to the planned procedure and are fearful of the postprocedure diagnosis. One should be careful not to oversedate this patient population.

Postprocedure Considerations: Incisional pain may be minimal. Localization of breast tissue generally provides postoperative analgesia. Patients experiencing pain often respond to acetaminophen or mild oral opioid pain medications prescribed by the physician. The patient should be given specific postprocedure instructions prior to discharge. These instructions should address bathing, diet, activity, medication precautions, and dressing change.

Nursing Diagnoses: Alteration in skin integrity; alteration in neurologic status secondary to the administration of conscious sedation; potential for bleeding.

Bronchoscopy

Description: Flexible bronchoscopy permits direct or indirect visualization of the pharynx, larynx, esophagus, trachea, and bronchi.

Indications: Biopsy, identification of airway anatomy, removal of foreign bodies, mucus plugs, washings, assessment of hemoptysis, or chronic cough.

Estimated Time: 20 to 45 minutes.

Considerations: Topical anesthesia is required prior to initiation of the procedure. Initial localization of the posterior pharynx is critical to the success of the procedure. A variety of methods to localize the posterior pharynx exist. The following popular localization technique yields a profoundly anesthetized oropharynx:

- Atomizer application (4% lidocaine [Xylocaine]): several sprays into the posterior pharynx.
- Application of 5% lidocaine ointment to a tongue blade.

- Place tongue blade into the posterior pharynx.
- Allow the patient to suck on the tongue blade for a period of not less than 5 minutes.
- Remove tongue blade and apply several additional sprays of the 4% lidocaine spray.

NOTE: During localization of the posterior pharynx, do not exceed maximum lidocaine dosage. Death has been reported in cases where excessive amounts of lidocaine have been used.[5]

4% lidocaine = 40 mg/ml

5% lidocaine ointment = 50 mg/ml

With application of the local anesthetic identified above, the patient generally tolerates passage of the bronchoscope with minimal sedation. Procedure time may vary, according to visualization, biopsy, or treatment required. Heavy sedation may lead to airway obstruction or the development of hypoxia. Systemic reactions may occur secondary to the local anesthesia toxicity. Signs and symptoms include hypotension, circumoral numbness, auditory or visual stimuli, convulsions, and cardiac arrest. Emergency resuscitative equipment should be immediately available.

Postprocedure Considerations: Topical application of anesthetic obliterates the gag reflex. Patients must be kept NPO until the gag reflex returns (2 to 8 hours). Once the gag reflex has returned, throat lozenges may be offered to relieve sore throat. Diet may be advanced as tolerated. Subcutaneous emphysema may signify tracheal or bronchial perforation. The patient must be watched for the development of dyspnea or airway obstruction. Edema or laryngospasm requires immediate intervention to restore air flow. Administration of humidifed oxygen decreases edema.

Nursing Diagnoses: Ineffective breathing secondary to procedure; impaired gas exchange; potential for bleeding.

Cardiac Catheterization

Description: The venous and arterial system is cannulated. Contrast material is injected to identify the anatomy of the heart and central vessels.

Indications: Suspicion of coronary artery disease or occlusion.

Estimated Time: 30 to 60 minutes.

Considerations: Cardiac catheterization is indicated in specific situations to define cardiac anatomy, congenital lesions, or valvular dysfunction and to detect coronary artery disease and alterations in cardiac physiology. Cardiac catheterization provides the clinician with data by comparing the pressure and oxygen content of blood in the four heart chambers, pulmonary vasculature, and great vessels. As the data are gathered in stages, measurement of these parameters requires the patient to remain physiologically stable. The administration of conscious sedation gives the patient the ability to remain still and calm while all elements of testing are completed. To assure constant calculations, it is important to maintain oxygenation and ventilation. Nausea may be associated with insertion and withdrawal of the catheter. Procedural complications include nausea, vomiting, hemodynamic compromise, allergic dye reaction, and arrhythmias. Little or no sedation may be required in the hemodynamically compromised patient.

Postprocedure Considerations: Continued hemodynamic monitoring until discharge criteria are met. A girdle device is required for pressure on the vascular insertion point. One should encourage oral fluids and monitor urine output when dye is used. Assessment and documentation of distal pulses.

Nursing Diagnoses: Potential for hemodynamic instability; potential for bleeding; potential for allergic reaction secondary to administration of contrast medium.

Cardioversion

Description: Normal sinus rhythm is dependent on automaticity (spontaneous depolarization) and the dispersion of coordinated electrical activity through the myocardium. The application of external electrical current to the heart is beneficial in converting some dysrhythmias to normal sinus rhythm.

Indications: Supraventricular tachycardia, atrial fibrillation, atrial flutter, ventricular tachycardia with a pulse.

Estimated Time: 5 to 10 minutes.

Considerations: Patients presenting for cardioversion may already be hemodynamically compromised (loss of atrial depolarization). Successful cardioversion occurs when the patient is returned to a normal sinus rhythm. Cardioversion paddles (8 to 12 cm in adults) are placed to the right side of the upper sternum below the clavicle and the remaining paddle in the midaxillary line below the left nipple. Conductive pads or gel is applied to the thoracic area prior to cardioversion. Sedative medications (midazolam, propofol, methohexital) have all been used successfully. Medications should be titrated to effect (nystagmus, slurred speech). Once it is deemed that an adequate state of sedation has been achieved, the paddles are placed and a preselected shock (joules) is delivered to the patient according to the presenting arrhythmia. Use of a bag valve device may be required to deliver an increased FiO$_2$ to the patient. If the initial attempt at cardioversion is unsuccessful, a second attempt is performed by the attending cardiologist. Additional medications may be required if subsequent attempts at cardioversion fail to result in the resumption of normal sinus rhythm.

Postprocedure Considerations: The patient requires continuous postprocedure ECG monitoring. The patient may report mild sternal discomfort. Assessment of hemodynamic parameters and documentation of rhythm changes are required after the procedure. Additional complications include arrhythmias induced by nonsynchronous shock and embolic phenomena.

Nursing Diagnoses: Hemodynamic instability; alteration in level of comfort; potential for respiratory compromise.

Cataract Extraction

Description: A small incision is made around the corneal rim. The lens and nucleus are then removed. Current ultrasound techniques are generally used (phacoemulsification). A replacement lens is deposited into the lens capsule. The incision may be closed with fine nylon sutures.

Indications: Cataract.

Estimated Time: 15 to 120 minutes.

Considerations: The patients presenting for cataract extraction and intraocular lens implant are generally elderly. Chronic disease states (chronic hypertension, history of congestive heart failure, etc.) may make intraprocedural management difficult. The presence of chronic obstructive pulmonary disease or congestive heart failure may make it difficult for the patient to tolerate the supine position for extended periods of time. The eye may be anesthetized by a variety of methods. Retrobulbar block anesthetizes the eye through injection of a local anesthetic into the muscle conus behind the globe of the eye near the ciliary nerve. The orbicularis oculi (motor branch of the facial nerve) is blocked after the retrobulbar injection. Sedation administered before injection of the block increases patient comfort during administration of the local anesthetic. It is surprising that heavy sedation is generally not required for the administration of the retrobulbar block. Small increments of midazolam (0.5 to 1 mg), with or without narcotics, frequently produces adequate sedation and increases the patient's tolerance of the procedure. Complications associated with the administration of retrobulbar block include hemorrhage, optic nerve trauma, increased intraocular pressure, and loss of consciousness. Loss of consciousness and apnea are associated with the infiltration of the local anesthetic along the neural sheath with associated brainstem anesthesia. Apnea may be treated with positive pressure ventilation or intubation if required. The oculocardiac reflex may be elicited during the actual administration of the retrobulbar block. Afferent impulses are mediated by the trigeminal nerve, while efferent impulses are mediated by the vagus nerve. Hypotension, bradycardia, nausea, vomiting, and diaphoresis are common manifestations of the oculocardiac reflex. Administration of oxygen, intravenous fluid, and atropine to relieve pressure on the eye and informing the surgeon are all effective mechanisms to reduce the oculocardiac reflex. Some facilities use topical local anesthesia with tetracaine and minimal sedation. Topical anesthesia is facilitated with several drops of tetracaine and placement of a small pledget along the inner canthus of the eye.

Postprocedure Considerations: At the conclusion of the procedure it is important to orient the patient to time, place, and person. One should assess visual acuity of the nonoperative eye. The patient's head should be positioned at a 30- to 45-degree angle. Recent advances in ophthalmic surgery have led to patients returning from the procedure room without the operative eye patched. It is important to realize that the patient has diminished sight in the operative eye. Mobility and the ability to ambulate must be assessed prior to discharge. Nausea and vomiting must be dealt with effectively to prevent an increase in intraocular pressure.

Nursing Diagnoses: Decreased visual acuity; alterations in mobility secondary to decreased visual acuity; alteration in comfort.

Cervical Cone Biopsy

Description: An area of the cervix is resected by cold knife conization or a loop excision electrocautery procedure (LEEP). Once resected, the area is cauterized and the procedure is completed.

Indications: Abnormal Papanicolaou smear.

Estimated Time: 15 to 30 minutes.

Considerations: Biopsy may be performed with the administration of sedation and local anesthesia. If the addition of local anesthetic with epinephrine is required to assist in hemostasis, tachycardia and hypertension may develop in patients with limited cardiac reserve.

Postprocedure Considerations: Assessment and documentation of postprocedure vaginal bleeding.

Nursing Diagnoses: Alteration in comfort; potential for bleeding; anxiety associated with planned procedure.

Closed Fracture Reduction/Dislocated Joint

Description: Anatomic reduction and maintenance of the fracture site may require a brief period of analgesia and sedation for alignment of the fracture site and casting.

Indications: Fractured bone, dislocated joint.

Estimated Time: 10 to 30 minutes with casting.

Considerations: Many times conscious sedation for fracture reduction, alignment, and casting is provided in the emergency room. These patients may have a full stomach, and deep sedation predisposes to aspiration and the development of respiratory distress. Neurologic or vascular compromise requires immediate reduction. Signs of neurovascular or vascular compromise include pain, discoloration (pale skin), coldness, reduced or absent pulsatile flow, reduced capillary refill, sensation, and swelling.

Postprocedure Considerations: Postprocedure neurovascular assessment should initially be documented every 30 minutes. Components of the assessment include flexion and movement of the fingers or toes. Absence of normal sensation may indicate neural compression and ischemia to the extremity. The pulse oximeter probe may be placed on the affected extremity to assess pulsatile blood flow. This should be noted in postprocedure documentation. The extremity should be elevated and the pulse of the affected extremity compared with that of the unaffected limb. It is important to document and report any signs of pain, weakness, or decreased sensation. These signs may represent the development of compartment syndrome.

Nursing Diagnoses: Alteration in the musculoskeletal system; potential for the development of compartment syndrome; alteration in comfort.

Colonoscopy

Description: A fiberoptic scope is inserted into the rectum and permits visualization of the ascending, transverse, and descending colon.

Indications: Rectal bleeding, anemia, abdominal cramping, diverticulitis, colonic polyps/mass, family history of colon cancer.

Estimated Time: 30 to 60 minutes.

Considerations: Administration of sedation 3 to 5 minutes prior to initiation of the procedure generally decreases the initial discomfort associated with insertion of the colonoscope. Additional sedation may be required during placement of the colonoscope. Patients are generally in the supine or lateral position during the procedure. In the event of respiratory obstruction, access to the patient's airway is reduced in the lateral position. Once the physician has reached the cecum with the scope, patients generally do not require additional sedation during the remainder of the examination or biopsy procedure. Intense pain during insertion of the colonoscope may be decreased not only with the use of sedative medications but also with deep breaths and reassurance from the gastroenterology team members.

Postprocedure Considerations: Patients must be monitored after the procedure for signs of perforation (intense abdominal pain, tense abdomen, fever, etc.). Patients may resume use of oral fluids and solid food when bowel sounds are present. Patients should be reassured that the presence of flatus, abdominal cramping, and small amounts of rectal bleeding are normal in the immediate postprocedure period; however, if they continue for more than 24 hours they should notify their physician.

Nursing Diagnoses: Potential for respiratory compromise; impaired gastrointestinal function; potential for bleeding.

Computed Tomography: The CT Scan

Description: Computed tomography is conducted through cross-sectional image of the area.

Indications: Imaging of the head, thorax, and abdominal area. Diagnoses of bleeding, neoplasms, hydrocephalus, biopsy, and needle aspiration. A motion-free study is required.

Estimated Time: 30 to 40 minutes.

Considerations: A variety of patients will present for CT scanning. Many adults tolerate CT scanning without the use of supplemental sedation. Patients who are anxious, nervous, or claustrophobic may require small doses of sedative medications to provide an anxiolytic effect during the actual scan. Pediatric patients require sedation appropriate to age and physiologic status (see Chapter 7 for medication review and dosage). Sedation may be administered and titrated to achieve anxiolysis. Once the patient is sedate, he or she is placed on the CT scanning device and the scanning begins. Considerations during the actual scan include maintaining a motion-free state with supplemental sedation with reduced accessibility to the patient's airway. Standard monitoring is required to ascertain the first signs of respiratory or hemodynamic distress. Patients may receive intravenous or oral contrast media. Patients required to consume oral contrast media are given full-stomach precautions. Oral contrast media are hypertonic and capable of inducing aspiration pneumonitis and pulmonary edema if aspirated.

Postprocedure Considerations: Patients must be monitored after the procedure until discharge criteria are met. Continued assessment for reaction to contrast material.

Nursing Diagnoses: Alteration in mobility; potential for aspiration; potential for allergic reaction to contrast media.

Cystoscopy

Description: Passage of a rigid or flexible cystoscope through the urethra and into the bladder.

Estimated Time: 10 to 30 minutes.

Considerations: Minor urologic procedures may be performed with conscious sedation and local anesthesia. Lidocaine (Xylocaine) jelly has been used successfully when instilled into the urethra. The administration of opioids and sedative medications increases patient comfort when the cystoscope is inserted. Once inserted, the bladder is filled with an irrigation solution. A distended bladder can lead to vagal response, profound bradycardia, hypotension, and vomiting. Conscious sedation and local anesthesia are not well tolerated for patients who require prolonged bladder distention or urethral dilation.

Postprocedure Considerations: Patients may complain of back pain, bladder fullness, or bladder spasms. Urine output should be documented prior to discharge. Postprocedure teaching should inform the patient that a burning sensation, frequency, and full bladder sensation are common after the procedure. Light pink urine is to be expected for the first several voidings. Bright red blood or clots is not normal and should be reported to the attending physician. Sepsis may manifest as fever, tachycardia, chills, and malaise. Abdominal pain or a tense, rigid abdomen may indicate bladder perforation or internal hemorrhage.

Nursing Diagnoses: Procedure-related urinary retention; alterations in comfort level; alteration in elimination.

Dilatation and Curettage

Description: A weighted speculum is inserted and the cervical os is grasped firmly with the tenaculum. The cervix is progressively dilated with cervical dilators. A curette or vacuum aspirator is used to remove portions of the endometrial lining for biopsy or to remove the products of conception.

Indications: Diagnosis and treatment of disseminated uterine bleeding, incomplete abortion, removal of cervical lesions, or dilation of a stenotic cervix.

Estimated Time: 15 to 30 minutes.

Considerations: Nonpregnant female patients may tolerate conscious sedation for the completion of a dilation and curet-

tage. Patients presenting for removal of retained placental products are generally upset, nervous, and anxious. Reassurance and careful titration of medications are required to accomplish the goals of conscious sedation. After titration of sedative medications, the surgeon administers a paracervical block. The cervix is grasped with the tenaculum, which is gently pulled toward the surgeon. Cervical manipulation may predispose the patient to the onset of bradydysrhythmias. The patient may display signs of discomfort with the application of the tenaculum. Progressive dilation and use of the curette or vacuum aspirator may produce cramping or discomfort. Additional sedative medication may be given in conjunction with gentle surgical manipulation to complete the procedure. At the completion of a dilatation and evacuation for retained products of conception, oxytocin (Pitocin) may be requested by the surgeon.

Postprocedure Considerations: Chronic anemia associated with disseminated uterine bleeding predisposes the patient to hypotension and decreased oxygen-carrying capacity. Continued administration of oxygen into the postprocedure period is strongly advised. Uterine cramping may be relieved with medications ordered by the obstetrician or gynecologist. Postprocedure vaginal blood loss should be documented. In the event of heavy blood loss, additional oxytocin may be ordered. Postprocedure complications include uterine perforation, which must be treated surgically.

Nursing Diagnoses: Hemodynamic instability; alteration in comfort; potential for bleeding.

Electrophysiologic Testing and Radiofrequency Catheter Ablation

Description: Destruction of conduction tissue via
- Current
- Laser
- Surgical interruption

Indications: To define the mechanism, origin, and pathways of cardiac dysrhythmias. Catheters are placed in the heart. These catheters have the capability to
- Pace the heart
- Provide electrical stimulation
- Sense electrical signals

Estimated Time: Several hours.

Considerations: Antiarrhythmic medications are generally discontinued before the electrophysiologic study.

Postprocedure Considerations: Continued monitoring until discharge criteria are met.

Nursing Diagnoses: Potential for hemodynamic compromise; potential for dysrhythmias.

Embolectomy/Thrombectomy

Description: The surgical removal of an embolus from a blood vessel. An embolus is defined as a portion of free-floating foreign matter, which may be composed of clotted blood, air, fat, or other foreign material. A thin catheter (Fogarty) is generally inserted into the vessel with the balloon not inflated. Once the catheter is inserted deeply into the vessel, the balloon is inflated and then removed from the vessel. The embolus is removed, and the vessel and incision are closed.

Indications: Vascular occlusion.

Estimated Time: 30 to 60 minutes.

Considerations: Intravenous sedation is successful when combined with local anesthetic infiltration of the affected area.

Complications associated with embolectomy include inability to remove the embolus and the potential for revascularization procedures. Typically, patients with a variety of chronic illnesses (coronary artery disease, effects of smoking, hypertension, hyperlipidemia) present for embolization procedures. Management of chronic disease states may be more challenging than the conscious sedation required for the procedure. Once the embolus has been removed, flushing of emboli from the vessel may cause significant blood loss and hypotension.

Postprocedure Considerations: Management of the chronic disease state is continued into the postprocedure period.

Assessment of peripheral pulse consists of palpation for pulsation in the peripheral arteries. Dressings and drainage must be documented after the procedure. Dressings should remain dry and intact. The surgeon must be notified in the event of bleeding.

Nursing Diagnoses: Potential for bleeding; alteration in mobility; alteration in circulation.

Endoscopic Retrograde Cholangiopancreatography (ERCP)

Description: Visualization and x-ray study of the biliary system through an endoscope passed through the stomach, duodenum, and into the common bile duct.

Indications: To assess inflammatory conditions and identify the presence of stones in the common bile duct.

Estimated Time: 30 to 60 minutes.

Considerations: Patients presenting for ERCP may be dehydrated as a result of nausea and vomiting. Electrolyte abnormalities may manifest secondary to the condition requiring ERCP diagnostic procedures. The presence of concomitant disease states requires adequate preprocedure evaluation. Prior to insertion of the scope, adequate localization of the oropharynx is required. The scope is inserted into the oropharynx after placement of a bite-block. Use of a bite-block protects both the patient's teeth and the endoscope. Once the endoscope is placed, patients may be turned prone for a portion of the procedure. It is important to titrate medications slowly to the clinical end point of nystagmus and slurred speech. The presence of the endoscope coupled with the patient's prone position presents an additional challenge to the clinician. Access and assessment of the patient's airway present a concern for the nurse monitoring the patient. Rapid assessment and intervention are required in the presence of respiratory depression or obstruction during ERCP procedures.

Postprocedure Considerations: Patients must be assessed for the return of the gag reflex. The patient should not be allowed to drink or eat prior to the return of the gag reflex. Determination of an adequate gag reflex includes demonstration of the patient's ability to swallow and cough. Patients are monitored for procedural complications, which include perforation (severe pain or subcutaneous air), dysphagia, and pancreatitis.

Nursing Diagnoses: Alteration in gastrointestinal function; potential for respiratory compromise; impaired hydration status.

Functional Endoscopic Sinus Surgery (FESS)

Description: Endoscopic sinus surgery is accomplished with a rigid fiberoptic scope to visualize the sinuses. Visualization permits sinus drainage, polyp removal, or mucosal biopsy.

Indications: Chronic sinus infection, nasal polyps, neoplasm.

Estimated Time: 30 minutes to 2 hours.

Considerations: 4% cocaine is applied to the nasal mucosa, followed by injection of a local anesthetic with epinephrine. Patients with coronary artery disease may be predisposed to the development of dysrhythmias. Misdirection of the endoscope could result in injury to the optic nerve or the arterial system or entrance into the brain. Polyp removal and biopsy may be performed with the patient under conscious sedation. However, attempts to perform extensive endoscopic sinus surgery during conscious sedation may predispose the patient to unnecessary risks. Bleeding into the posterior oropharynx may produce decreased oxygen saturation, aspiration, or laryngospasm. Swallowed blood irritates the gastric mucosa and may produce nausea and vomiting.

Postprocedure Considerations: Patients recovering from the sedative effects of conscious sedation and ENT procedures should be positioned with the head elevated 30 degrees. This prevents pooling of blood and secretions, which may accumulate in the posterior pharynx when the patient is in the supine position. Postproce-dure pain may be minimal secondary to the continued effects of the local anesthetic used for the procedure. Patients who are nauseated or vomit should be positioned on their side to promote drainage and allow suctioning of the oropharynx. Antiemetics may be required and should be administered as ordered by the physician.

Nursing Diagnoses: Potential for bleeding; ineffective breathing due to nasal packing; alteration in comfort level.

Hysteroscopy

Description: The cervix is secured with the tenaculum and the hysteroscope is advanced into the uterus. Distention of the uterus is accomplished with a variety of mediums (carbon dioxide or dextran). The uterine mucosa is examined by direct vision or with the attachment of the hysteroscope to an external video system.

Indications: Abnormal uterine bleeding, examination of uterine mucosa, or removal of intrauterine polyps.

Estimated Time: 15 to 60 minutes.

Considerations: Sedative medication is administered prior to dilation of the cervix. During application of the tenaculum and dilation of the uterus, the patient may experience additional discomfort. Additional local anesthetic may be required if bradycardia is evident. The procedure is generally brief.

Postprocedure Considerations: Cramping may be treated with naproxen (Anaprox) or similar medications prescribed by the gynecologist. Postprocedure bleeding should be assessed and documented prior to discharge of the patient.

Nursing Diagnoses: Alteration in comfort; potential for bleeding; anxiety associated with planned procedure.

Inguinal Hernia Repair

Description: Inguinal hernias require repair of weakened areas in the abdominal wall. Abdominal contents will continue to protrude through the weakened area in the abdominal wall unless the hernia is repaired. An incision is made to open the inguinal ring. The hernia sac is ligated, with the surrounding area strengthened with reinforced suture material or Marlex mesh.

Indications: Inguinal hernia.

Estimated Time: 45 to 60 minutes.

Considerations: Inguinal hernia repairs have been performed with the combination of local anesthesia and oral sedatives or intravenous supplementation. When intravenous sedatives are used, opioids or anxiolytics should be administered 3 to 5 minutes prior to localization of the inguinal region. As the surgeon continues the dissection, exploration of the spermatic cord or peritoneal traction produces profound stimulation. These maneuvers enhance vagal activity. The nurse monitoring the patient may observe bradycardia, hypotension, nausea, and vomiting. It is important to notify the surgeon to discontinue peritoneal traction. Surgical pain requires administration of additional local anesthetic. Conscious sedation allows the patient to assist the surgeon during the procedure by coughing and straining to ascertain the strength of the repair.

Postprocedure Considerations: Many surgeons use an ilioinguinal nerve block or wound infiltration with local anesthesia to provide postoperative analgesia. Inability to void after the procedure may delay discharge. The patient should be observed for signs and symptoms of bladder distention. Patients must be instructed in ways to right themselves from the supine position to decrease incisional stress. Coughing and straining require wound reinforcement with the patient's hand to decrease incisional stress and pain associated with this activity.

Nursing Diagnoses: Alterations in mobility; alteration in levels of comfort; urinary retention associated with surgery; potential for vagal response.

Insertion of Peritoneal Dialysis Catheter

Description: Local infiltration may not suffice to achieve adequate anesthesia. Deep sedation or regional anesthesia may be required. Placement of peritoneal dialysis catheters may be extremely difficult with the use of conscious sedation and local anesthesia alone. A small incision is created in the abdominal area (generally in the area of the umbilicus). The subcutaneous tissue, muscle, and fascia are dissected down to the omentum, and the catheter is placed into the peritoneum. Several liters of dialysate is infused once the catheter is placed successfully. The dialysate must drain back into the bags to assure proper placement of the peritoneal catheter. Infusion of the dialysate may also increase intra-abdominal pressure. Patients with limited cardiopulmonary reserve may experience shortness of breath or associated respiratory symptoms during dialysate dwell time.

Indications: Peritoneal dialysis for acute or chronic renal failure.

Estimated Time: 45 to 90 minutes.

Postprocedure Considerations: Dialysate infusion and dwell time should be ordered by the physician. During dwell time the patient should be observed for signs of respiratory compromise. Patients with renal failure may have severe metabolic disruption, fluid imbalance, or both. The patient must be monitored for signs and symptoms of electrolyte disturbance, fluid overload, and acidosis.

Nursing Diagnoses: Alterations in elimination; potential for respiratory compromise; alterations in fluid volume.

Liposuction

Description: Removal of subcutaneous fat with cannulas that loosen and remove fat via a vacuum device connected to the end of the liposuction cannula.

Indications: Excessive fat tissue in an affected area.

Estimated Time: 60 to 120 minutes.

Considerations: There are currently two different types of liposuction, which may be accomplished with conscious sedation or straight local anesthesia. For tumescent liposuction, dilute local anesthetic concentrations are infused into the affected area prior to mechanical manipulation and vacuum evacuation. Dilute local anesthetic solution is infused in liter bags into the affected area. A variety of concentrations are currently used. The volume of local anesthetic and diluent is eventually absorbed into the vascular space. Therefore large volumes of intravenous solution are not required for tumescent liposuction techniques.

The standard liposuction technique performed with conscious sedation and local anesthesia includes infiltration of lidocaine and epinephrine solution into the affected area. The volume of the local anesthetic is more concentrated, and less is used.

Postprocedure Considerations: Large areas of liposuction may require postoperative narcotic analgesia. Postprocedure pain associated with small areas of liposuction may be treated with acetaminophen. Aspirin and nonsteroidal anti-inflammatory agents are avoided to prevent bleeding. Infection and postprocedure bleeding are additional complications associated with liposuction.

Nursing Diagnoses: Potential for bleeding; alteration in comfort; alteration in fluid volume.

Lithotripsy

Description: First introduced into clinical practice in 1984, the lithotripter disintegrates urinary stones in the kidney and upper ureter. Lithotripters use an energy source, a system to focus the shock wave, and a system to visualize and localize the stone in focus (fluoroscopy or ultrasound).

Indications: Urinary tract calculi.

Estimated Time: 60 minutes.

Considerations: Original lithotripters used a water bath in a steel tub. Use of the water bath is associated with physiologic changes on immersion and emersion from the bath. Increased central blood volume and pulmonary artery pressure and decreased tidal volume and functional residual capacity are seen with bath immersion. Patients treated with the original lithotripter are generally cared for by anesthesia personnel.

Newer lithotripters have eliminated the need for the water bath. Second- and third-generation lithotripters allow the patient to be treated on a water mattress or pad. These newer reduced-pain lithotripters allow some patients to be successfully treated with conscious sedation.

It is important to assure patient immobility during the lithotripsy treatment to keep the stone in the shock wave focus area. Cardiac dysrhythmias are avoided with ECG synchronization of the shock wave. To avoid lithotripsy-induced dysrhythmias, avoidance of artifact and bradycardia is advised, since shock waves are triggered on the R wave.

The following are absolute contraindications to lithotripsy:

- Pregnancy
- Untreated bleeding disorders
- Pacemakers placed in the abdominal area

Patients with pacemakers in the pectoral area may be safely treated under the following conditions:

- Pacemaker programmability is established.
- Pacemaker programmability may be switched to a nondemand mode if the lithotripsy shock waves interfere with normal pacemaker function.
- Alternate mechanisms of pacing are available in the event of pacemaker failure.

Postprocedure Considerations: Urine may be tinged with blood as a result of the trauma associated with the shock waves. Patients should be assured that this generally clears within several hours. Redness, bruising, and petechiae may be evident on the treatment area. Ice packs may relieve localized pain associated with the force of the shock waves.

Nursing Diagnoses: Renal colic secondary to stone fragmentation; alterations in comfort; alteration in genitourinary function.

Magnetic Resonance Imaging

Description: Patients are placed in a magnetic field, and radiofrequency pulses are emitted to generate an image. Advantages of MRI imaging include its ability to produce a three-dimensional image, excellent soft tissue contrast, absence of ionizing radiation, and noninvasiveness.

Indication: MRI has capabilities similar to computed tomography for body imaging and scanning.

Estimated Time: 30 to 60 minutes.

Considerations: The magnetic field is so strong that the use of ferromagnetic equipment is prohibited. The magnitude of magnetic force on ferromagnetic materials is dependent on

- Strength of the magnet
- Field configuration
- Magnitude and shape of the field gradient
- Mass and position of the ferromagnetic object

Monitoring equipment constructed of aluminum and nonmagnetic steel must be used in the MRI suite. All patients and personnel must remove ferromagnetic materials before entering the MRI room. Pacemakers, cerebrovascular and surgical clips, and cochlear and stapedial implants are hazardous. Monitoring in the MRI suite is made even more difficult in the presence of incandescent lighting and a copper mesh screen maintained over the observation window. Noise levels can exceed 95 decibels as the magnet rotates. The magnetic field may

- Interfere with the safe and reliable function of monitors
- Render monitors inoperable secondary to distortion by the magnetic field
- Cause looped monitor wires to absorb signal meant for the MRI receiver coil, thereby distorting the image
- Produce heated current in monitor cables, causing burns to the patient

Fatalities have occurred in association with MRI procedures.[6] In 1992 the Safety Committee for Magnetic Resonance Imaging published guidelines and recommendations concerning the monitoring of patients during MRI procedures. Table 9–5 lists these recommendations.[7]

- *ECG:* Continuous ECG monitoring may lead to image degradation and patient burns from looped cables. Several companies have introduced specially developed circuitry and inherent filtration to produce stable, clear ECG waveforms. Fiberoptic technology and conductive plastic ECG lead

TABLE 9–5. *Examples of Patients Who Require Monitoring During MR Procedures*

1. Patients who are physically or mentally unstable
2. Patients who have their normal physiologic function(s) compromised in any way
3. Patients who are unable to communicate
4. Neonatal and pediatric patients
5. Sedated or anesthetized patients
6. Patients undergoing interventional MR procedures
7. Patients undergoing MR procedures using experimental MR systems (e.g., EPI systems, MR systems with static magnetic field strengths that exceed 2 tesla, etc.)
8. Patients who may have a reaction to an MR contrast agent

From Shellock F, Lipczak H, Kanal E. Monitoring patients during MR procedures: a review. *Appl Radiol.* February 1995.

wires minimize the risk of burn from radio frequency current.

- **Blood pressure:** Noninvasive blood pressure may be monitored with long cables and ferrous material located far away from the magnet.
- **Pulse oximetry:** Pulse oximetry may involve problems similar to those of standard ECG monitoring. Pulse oximeters with advanced fiberoptic cable minimize patient injury from radiofrequency current.

Recommendations for prevention of burns associated with the use of physiologic monitoring equipment during MRI procedures are given in Table 9–1.

The following monitoring companies currently provide equipment for monitoring in the MRI suite:

- *Invivo Research, Inc.*, Orlando, Florida
- *Nonin Medical, Inc.*, Plymouth, Minnesota
- *Magnetic Resonance Equipment Corporation*, Bay Shore, New York
- *Biochem International*, Waukesha, Wisconsin

Because of limited access to the patient, patients receiving conscious sedation and monitoring for MRI scanning require reassurance and diligent assessment to assure adequate oxygenation.

Movement by the patient produces significant artifact. The long, narrow scanning device is not conducive to anxious, claustrophobic patients. Newer MRI scanners now feature roomier accommodations for the scan. These larger scanners are ideal for patients with a history of claustrophobia and anxiety disorders.

Oral Surgery/Odontectomy/Dental Caries

Description: The patient's mouth is opened. Impacted teeth are removed or the dental restorative procedure is completed on carious teeth.

Indications: Dental caries, impacted molars, preprosthetic surgery.

Estimated Time: 30 to 90 minutes.

Considerations: Deeply impacted third molars may require general anesthesia in an ambulatory surgery center or hospital. However, removal of partial impactions, restoration of carious teeth, and minor prosthetic surgery may be performed with the patient under conscious sedation. Major complications associated with oral surgery include completion of a procedure within close proximity to the airway. Sponges, pledgets, manipulation of the tongue, blood, and debris in the upper airway predispose the patient to respiratory obstruction, laryngospasm, and aspiration. It is imperative that the oral surgeon or dentist remove all gauze, pledgets, and debris from the airway. Careful suctioning and hemostasis minimize the risk of blood and secretions pooling in the posterior

pharynx. Blood swallowed or drained into the stomach acts as a gastric irritant and may cause vomiting. Metoclopramide, 0.15 mg/kg, stimulates gastric emptying and increases lower esophageal sphincter tone. Metoclopramide also has a central antiemetic effect. A procedural hazard with any oral or dental surgery is working with sedate patients in a "wet" airway. Blood, debris, secretions, and foreign bodies may precipitate rapid oxygen desaturation, laryngospasm, and aspiration.

Postprocedure Considerations: Patients recovering from sedation following oral surgery should be positioned with the head elevated 30 degrees to prevent pooling of blood and secretions that may accumulate in the posterior pharynx in the supine position. Postextraction patients should be instructed to bite down on gauze pads to decrease the incidence of postoperative bleeding and decrease swelling. Postprocedure pain is generally minimal secondary to the continued effects of the local anesthetic used for the procedure. The application of petroleum-based ointments to the lips and corners of the mouth moisturizes and prevents drying of the oral area. Ice applied to the jawline promotes patient comfort. Patients who are nauseated or vomit should lie on their side to promote drainage and allow for suctioning of the orophar-ynx. Antiemetics may be required and should be administered as ordered by the physician.

Nursing Diagnoses: Potential for respiratory compromise; impaired ventilatory exchange; potential for bleeding.

Percutaneous Transluminal Coronary Angioplasty (PTCA)

Description: *Angioplasty:* A catheter with a balloon located at the distal tip is passed percutaneously to the stenotic lesion. The balloon is inflated and deflated to compress the stenotic area and increase the vessel lumen size. A cardiac stent may be used to maintain the diameter of the vessel lumen. *Atherectomy:* A rotary cutting device excises intraluminal obstruction.

Indications: Intraluminal obstruction.

Estimated Time: Varied.

Considerations: Heparin, vasodilators, and calcium channel blockers may be ordered prior to catheter insertion. During inflation of the balloon, hypotension, is-chemia, pain, and ventricular arrhythmias may occur. Ventricular tachycardia generally responds to lidocaine (75 to 100 mg). Intracoronary stents may be used to treat coronary artery closure and the complications associated with vessel collapse. For additional considerations, see section on cardiac catheterization.

Postprocedure Considerations: Continued hemodynamic monitoring for ischemia or pain. Discharge criteria must be met prior to transfer from the cardiology suite.

Nursing Diagnoses: Cardiovascular instability; potential for hemodynamic compromise; potential for bleeding.

Permanent Pacemaker Insertion

Description: Pacemaker leads are inserted transvenously; the pulse generator is implanted in the subcutaneous tissue, generally in the upper anterior thoracic area.

Indications: Complete heart block, sick sinus syndrome, symptomatic bradycardia.

Estimated Time: 30 to 60 minutes.

Considerations: Patients presenting for pacemaker insertion may have a compromised hemodynamic profile. Medications that depress cardiac output or produce negative inotropic effects are contraindicated. Small doses (0.5 mg) of midazolam coupled with adequate local anesthesia work well with this patient population. Adequate local anesthesia in the area of the thoracic pocket eliminates the need for deep sedation or additional sedative for implantation of the generator unit. During insertion of the venous pacing leads, one should beware of the sudden onset of arrhythmias. Ventricular and atrial irritability is common during insertion of the guide wire and pacing leads. The cardiologist or surgeon will be as intent as the nurse in watching the ECG monitor. When the wire is pulled back, arrhythmias generally dissipate. If the attending physician becomes intent on technical aspects of the procedure, he or she should be reminded of the development of new arrhythmias. Once the generator is placed and pacemaker leads are tested and secured to the generator, the incision is closed and the procedure is completed. In the event that defibrillation is required, paddles should not be placed within 12 cm (1 inch = 2.54 cm) of the permanent pacemaker.

Postprocedure Considerations: It is important to note which type of pacemaker was implanted. This information is recorded in the patient's chart by the pacemaker representative or pacemaker identification insert card. Pacemaker modalities are identified as follows:

A = Atrium
V = Ventricle
D = Dual
I = Inhibited
T = Triggered
0 = None
S = Single-chamber atrial or ventricular pacing
R = Rate adaptive generator
M = Multiprogrammable

A five-letter nomenclature identifies pacemaker function:

First letter   = Chamber paced
Second letter = Chamber sensed
Third letter   = Response to pacing
Fourth letter = Programmability and rate responsiveness
Fifth letter   = Antitachycardia response

Example:

VVI The ventricle is paced and sensed, and the mode of response is inhibited.

AAT The atrium is paced and sensed, and the mode of response is triggered.

Additional information that should be recorded on the patient's chart is type of pacemaker, programming, and the effects a magnet or electrocautery may have on it.

Nursing Diagnoses: Alteration in cardiovascular function; alteration in circulation; potential for hemodynamic compromise.

Rhinoplasty/Septoplasty

Description: The nasal cartilage is resected to functionally restore air flow or to reduce the size of the preexisting nasal cartilage. For rhinoplasty, tip reduction, osteotomies, and nasal bone restructuring.

Indications: Cosmetic; restoration of air flow.

Estimated Time: 60 to 90 minutes.

Considerations: The nasal cavity is anesthetized with 4% cocaine and local anesthesia. Epinephrine is generally added to provide hemostasis. Transient hypertension and tachycardia should be avoided in patients with coronary artery disease or limited myocardial reserve.

Postprocedure Considerations: Patients should be positioned in a 30-degree head-up position to prevent pooling of blood and secretions that may accumulate in the posterior oropharynx. Patients who are nauseated or vomit should be positioned on their side to promote drainage and allow for suctioning of the oropharynx. Antiemetics may be required and should be administered as ordered by the physician.

Nursing Diagnoses: Potential for airway compromise; alteration in breathing pattern; potential for bleeding.

Stereotactic Radiotherapy

Description: Powerful radiation beams are used in the treatment of tumors and vascular malformations.

Indications: Intracranial tumors, vascular malformations.

Estimated Time: Varied.

Considerations: A head frame is applied with local anesthesia and sedation. The head frame remains in place throughout the entire procedure. The airway cannot be manipulated once the head frame is in place; therefore deep sedation is contraindicated. CT scan or angiography is performed. The patient is transported to a critical care area while the radiation beam orientation computations are performed. The patient is then taken to the radiology department for completion of treatment. The head frame is removed in the critical care area or radiology suite.

Postprocedure Considerations: Post-procedure monitoring until the patient meets discharge criteria. Specific postprocedure instructions are dependent on the neurologist or neurosurgeon.

Nursing Diagnoses: Potential for airway compromise; alterations in level of consciousness.

Tracheostomy

Description: An incision is made in the trachea with insertion of a tracheostomy tube.

Indications: Prolonged ventilatory assistance, emergency airway support.

Estimated Time: 30 to 60 minutes.

Considerations: Tracheostomy may be performed as either an elective or an emergency procedure. Tracheostomies performed in the operating room generally occur under ideal circumstances. The otolaryngologist or surgeon localizes the tracheal area to be incised. An incision is made through the tracheal cartilage, and the tracheostomy tube is inserted. In the event that the patient is intubated, the surgeon frequently deflates the balloon of the endotracheal tube with the incision into the trachea. Close communication between the surgeon and the nurse is required to coordinate removal of the endotracheal tube and insertion of the tracheostomy tube. Anesthesia personnel are frequently present for tracheostomy in intubated patients. However, nurses engaged in the administration of conscious sedation may be required to coordinate endotracheal tube removal in critical care settings. The surgeon may request suction after initial placement of the tracheostomy tube. Once the patient is suctioned and bilateral breath sounds are confirmed, the patient may be ventilated with a bag valve device if required. The tracheostomy tube must be secured by the surgeon. Tracheostomy tapes in conjunction with suture material may be used. It is imperative that the tracheostomy tube be secure before the patient is transferred from the operating room or before the operating clinician leaves the critical

care setting. It is extremely difficult to replace tracheostomy tubes that dislodge within the first 24 to 48 hours.

Postprocedure Considerations: Patency of the tracheostomy is critical. Initial postprocedure assessment must ascertain and document bilateral breath sounds. As an additional assessment tool, pulse oximetry should be used in patients recovering from tracheostomy. Frequent atraumatic suctioning ensures patency. Steps in tracheostomy suctioning include the following:

- Hyperventilate with 100% oxygen
- Select an appropriately sized sterile suction catheter
- Use a sterile glove or plastic sleeve suction catheter
- Inject 4 to 5 ml of sterile saline solution for viscous secretions
- Insert the catheter 15 to 20 cm (6 to 8 inches) into the new tracheostomy tube site
- During insertion, keep catheter crimped and *do not* apply suction during insertion
- Apply intermittent suction while removing the catheter
- Do not suction for periods > 5 seconds
- Hyperventilate with 100% oxygen when suctioning is completed
- Auscultate breath sounds to ascertain effectiveness of suctioning

Frequent dressing changes may be required because of tracheobronchial secretions and small amounts of blood around the newly created tracheostomy tube site. Complications associated with newly created tracheostomy tubes include inadvertent removal, excessive secretions, and obstruction of the tracheostomy tube. Obstruction of the tracheostomy tube in spite of effective suctioning requires immediate intervention by members of the anesthesia or surgical team. An obturator that is furnished with the tracheostomy tube must be kept at the bedside at all times. The obturator assists in reinsertion of the tracheostomy tube.

Nursing Diagnoses: Impaired gas exchange; potential for bleeding; ineffective airway clearance.

Transesophageal Echocardiography (TEE)

Description: Detection of regional and global ventricular abnormalities, chamber dimensions, valvular anatomy, and the presence of intracardiac air. Views of the heart are obtained from the upper esophagus and the lower esophagus.

Indications: History of poor myocardial or cardiac valvular dysfunction.

Estimated Time: 30 minutes.

Considerations: Advantages of TEE include the following:

- Close proximity to the heart, with separation offered only by the soft tissue of the mediastinum.
- Ability to provide continuous stable views of the heart for prolonged periods of time.
- Excellent image quality.

Absolute contraindications to use include esophageal disease, active upper gastrointestinal bleeding, and severe cervical spine instability. Relative contraindications include recent esophageal surgery, esophageal varices, severe cervical arthritis, and unexplained symptoms of dysphagia. Oropharyngeal anesthesia is achieved with topical anesthesia (see upper endoscopy). The end of the transducer is lubricated with water-soluble gel and introduced orally. A bite-block protects the patient's teeth and the TEE probe. Most basic TEE examinations initially use the three-chamber view, which visualizes the left atrium, ventricle, and left ventricular outflow tract. Once the three-chamber examination is complete, advancement of the probe 1 to 2 cm provides a four-chamber view. The four-chamber view displays the right atrium, tricuspid valve, and the interventricular and interatrial septa. Passage of the probe into the stomach reveals regional wall motion abnormalities.

Postprocedure Considerations: Postprocedure monitoring is conducted until the patient satisfies discharge criteria. Patients must demonstrate an adequate gag reflex and cough prior to the ingestion of liquids. One should not attempt to administer oral fluids or solid food in the absence of a positive gag reflex. The absence of the gag and cough reflex predisposes the patient to aspiration. A sore throat may also be expected when the effects of the local anesthesia dissipate. Patients should be reassured that the sore throat generally resolves within 24 hours. Patients presenting for echocardiography have a variety of symptoms and diseases. Patients should be instructed to advance their diet as prescribed by their physician.

Nursing Diagnoses: Potential for hemodynamic instability; impaired gag reflex; potential for airway compromise.

Upper Endoscopy

Description: Passage of a lighted endoscope via the throat and into the stomach. Direct visualization of the esophagus, stomach, and duodenum is achieved. Cauterization, suction, instillation of air/medications, and biopsy may be performed through the endoscope.

Indications: Esophageal varices, bleeding, ulcer disease, dyspepsia.

Estimated Time: 15 to 30 minutes.

Considerations: Initial localization of the posterior pharynx is critical to the success of the procedure. Various methods to localize the posterior pharynx exist. A popular localization technique yields a profoundly anesthetized oropharynx:

- Atomizer application (4% lidocaine): several sprays into the posterior pharynx.
- Application of 5% lidocaine ointment to a tongue blade.
- Place tongue blade into the posterior pharynx.
- Allow the patient to suck on the tongue blade for a period of not less than 5 minutes.
- Remove tongue blade and apply several additional sprays of the 4% lidocaine spray.

NOTE: During localization of the posterior pharynx, do not exceed maximum lidocaine dosage. Death has been reported in cases where excessive amounts of lidocaine have been used.[5]

4% lidocaine = 40 mg/ml
5% lidocaine ointment = 50 mg/ml

Through application of the local anesthetic identified above, the patient generally tolerates passage of the endoscope with minimal sedation. Procedure time may vary with visualization, biopsy, or treatment required. Heavy sedation may lead to airway obstruction or the development of hypoxia. Attempts at verbal or physical stimulation precede the need to remove the endoscope. In the event that the patient does not respond to verbal, physical stimulation or in the presence of apnea and decreasing oxygen saturation, the physician should remove the endoscope to provide positive pressure ventilation or placement of a nasal/oropharyngeal airway. Conscious sedation procedures that entail instrumentation of the oropharynx require increased vigilance. It is important to rapidly assess, diagnose, and intervene in the event of airway obstruction. Preparation and intervention to reestablish air flow are imperative. Cardiac stimulation with instrumentation of the lower esophagus may lead to dysrhythmias. If dysrhythmias occur, the physician should be informed immediately. Repositioning of the scope away from the lower esophagus relieves the anterior displacement of the scope on the heart. Additional complications include esophageal perforation, which is evidenced by severe pain. Severe bleeding associated with esophageal varices may require intubation to prevent aspiration of blood and secure the airway.

Postprocedure Considerations: Patients must demonstrate an adequate gag reflex and cough prior to the ingestion of liquids. One should not attempt to administer oral fluids or solid food in the absence of a positive gag reflex. The absence of the gag and cough reflex predisposes the patient to aspiration. A sore throat may also be expected when the effects of the local anesthesia dissipate. Patients should be reassured that the sore throat generally resolves within 24 hours. Patients presenting for endoscopy have a variety of symptoms and diseases. The patient should be instructed to advance the diet as prescribed by the physician.

Nursing Diagnoses: Potential for bleeding; alteration in comfort level; alteration in gastrointestinal function.

Vascular Access

Description: The subclavian vein is identified with a small-gauge finder needle. Once identified, a wire is threaded through the subclavian vein into the superior vena cava. The infusion port and catheter are secured with sutures. *Catheter types:* Hickmann, Groshong, Mediport, Broviac, and Portacath.

Indications: Vascular access for chemotherapy, total parenteral nutrition, short-term dialysis, antibiotic therapy.

Estimated Time: 15 to 60 minutes.

Considerations: Patients presenting for vascular access are chronically ill. Sepsis, cancer, or long-term home care may require permanent venous access. Placement of the catheter depends on the patient's anatomy, the surgeon's skill, and the specific type of device to be implanted. During threading of the wire through the subclavian vein and into the heart, dysrhythmias may occur. Ventricular dysrhythmias are common and require close communication between the nurse and the physician. Ventricular dysrhythmias generally cease once the wire is pulled back slightly. Patients who are chronically ill or end-stage carcinoma patients may require larger doses of opioids and sedatives. Titration to the clinical end point of conscious sedation (nystagmus and slurred speech) and adequate local anesthesia create a working environment conducive for successful placement of the vascular access.

Postprocedure Considerations: Postprocedure considerations focus on the patient's presenting symptoms and the rationale for vascular access. Sterile dressings should be applied to catheter sites. The IV team should be notified for inpatients and home health care for outpatients to arrange for postprocedure patient instruction. Postprocedure chest x-ray should be obtained to verify catheter tip location and rule out pneumo/hemothorax.

Nursing Diagnoses: Alteration in fluid volume status; alteration of skin integrity; potential for infection.

REFERENCES

1. Fitzpatrick K, Duey M. Anesthesia outside the operating room. In: Duke J, Rosenberg SG. *Anesthesia Secrets.* Philadelphia: Mosby; 1996:421.
2. Messick J, MacKenzie R, Southorn P. Anesthesia at remote locations. In: Miller RD, ed. *Anesthesia.* 4th ed. New York: Churchill Livingstone; 1994.
3. Practice Guidelines for Sedation and Analgesia by Non-Anesthesiologists. A Report by the American Task Force on Sedation and Analgesia by Non-Anesthesiologists. *Anesthesiology.* 1996;84(2).
4. Association of Operating Room Nurses. Position statement on the role of the RN in management of patients receiving IV conscious sedation for short term therapeutic, diagnostic, or surgical procedures. *AORN J.* 1992;55:207.
5. Briley J. Death of a healthy college student volunteer in a research study. Clinical Trials Advisor; Special Report. Naples, Fla: Global Success Corporation; 1996.
6. Shellock F, Lipczak H, Kanal E. Monitoring patients during MR procedures: a review. *Appl Radiol.* 1995;11.
7. Kanal E, Shellock FG. Policies, guidelines and recommendations for MR imaging safety and patient management. *J Magn Reson Imag.* 1992;2:247.

*Postprocedure Care
of the Patient*

PART III

Postprocedure Monitoring and Discharge Criteria

CHAPTER 10

AORN RECOMMENDED PRACTICE VII

Patients who receive intravenous conscious sedation/analgesia should be monitored postprocedure, receive verbal and written discharge instructions, and meet specified criteria before discharge.

JCAHO:TX 2.2.4

The patient's postprocedure status is assessed on admission to the postanesthesia recovery area and before discharge from the postanesthesia recovery area or setting.

Postprocedure recovery and monitoring after the administration of intravenous conscious sedation depends on a number of variables:

- Diagnostic or surgical procedure performed
- Length of procedure
- Preprocedure physiologic condition
- Presence of intraprocedure complications
- Medication administered
- Quantity of medication administered

The purpose of postprocedure monitoring is to assure the return of physiologic function prior to discharge or return to the inpatient setting. The postprocedure period provides a time to assess, diagnose, and treat complications associated with the administration of conscious sedation. It also provides a time period for the patient to meet institutionally approved discharge criteria. Postprocedure monitoring and discharge policies are required by accrediting bodies and recommended by professional practice organizations.[1-3]

The success of a conscious sedation program depends not only on providing preprocedure evaluation and the administration of intravenous sedation, it must also embrace adequate postprocedure monitoring and proper discharge planning. To avoid allegations of premature patient discharge, mechanisms must be in place to assess home readiness. Documentation of discharge based on adherence to specific objective clinical parameters is also required. The American Society of Perianesthesia Care Nurses identifies characteristics unique to perianesthesia nursing practice.[4] These characteristics are identified in Table 10–1. Nurses engaged in the postprocedure management of patients receiving conscious sedation participate in postanesthesia phase II as defined by the American Society of Perianesthesia Care Nurses. However, depending on the level of sedation or in the event of an adverse reaction, the nurse must be capable of providing acute emergent care.

TABLE 10–1. *Characteristics Unique to Perianesthesia Nursing Practice*

Preanesthesia phase	Patient preparation (physical and emotional)
	Data collection, assessment, planning for postprocedure disposition
Phase I	Implementation of nursing care to provide a safe transition from the fully anesthetized state to a physiologic state requiring less acute care.
Phase II	Implementation of nursing care to prepare the patient for self-care or to be cared for by another.

Postprocedure monitoring may be provided in a variety of settings. Patients may remain monitored in the treatment area or be transferred to a designated postprocedure recovery area. The recovery area should be physically conducive to meet the needs of the patient and the caregiver. Postprocedure recovery areas must be well lighted and located in a central area with appropriate monitoring and emergency resuscitative equipment available. Recommended equipment for PACU phase I and phase II are identified in Table 10–2. If the registered nurse

TABLE 10–2. *Recommended Postprocedure Equipment and Supplies*

1. Mechanism to deliver O_2 to each patient
2. Suction and suctioning equipment
3. Monitoring equipment
   - ECG
   - Blood pressure
   - SaO_2
4. Oxygen-delivery devices and equipment
   - Bag valve mask/appropriate size masks
   - Face mask extension and connectors
   - Oropharyngeal airway
   - Nasal airway
   - Endotracheal tubes (age appropriate)
   - Nonrebreather mask
   - Wall oxygen/backup cylinders
   - Yankauer suction tip
   - Laryngoscope/blades
   - Stylets
   - Magill forceps
   - Nasal cannula
5. Defibrillator (cardioversion/transthoracic pacing capability, readily available)
6. Emergency medication resuscitation cart (adult/pediatric)
   - Adenosine
   - Bretylium
   - Diltiazem
   - Flumazenil
   - Methylprednisolone
   - Procainamide
   - Verapamil
   - Aminophylline
   - Calcium
   - Dopamine
   - Furosemide
   - Naloxone
   - Propranolol
   - Atropine
   - 50% dextrose
   - Epinephrine
   - Lidocaine
   - Norepinephrine
   - Sodium bicarbonate
7. Intravenous supplies
   - Age-appropriate IV catheters
   - Macro/microdrip tubing
   - IV solutions
   - Dextrose
   - Normal saline solution
   - Lactated Ringer's solution
   - Gloves
   - Alcohol swabs
   - Betadine
   - 4 × 4 inch gauze pads
   - Tape
   - Central vein catherization set

TABLE 10–3.   *Components of Postprocedure Report*

• Patient's name	• Response/reaction to medications
• Age	• Adverse response/reaction
• Diagnostic or surgical procedure	– ECG, blood pressure, SaO_2, respira-
• Past medical history	tions
• Routine medications	– Complications
• Allergies	– Treatment
• Preoperative and procedural vital signs	• Fluid balance
• Level of consciousness	– Site and size of IV catheters
• Airway	– IV solution infused and amount
• Conscious sedation medications admin-	– Blood loss
istered	• Postprocedure concerns
– Total dose administered	– Review of medical orders
– Antagonist administered (time)	• Location of responsible physician

participating in the administration and procedural care of the patient does not monitor the patient after the procedure, the patient must be safely transported to a postprocedure recovery area. Before transport, the patient should have a stable, patent airway. Oxygen equipment should be available for transport to the postprocedure area. The patient is accompanied by the registered nurse participating in the procedure who is knowledgeable about the patient's condition. Prior to the transfer of care to another provider, a verbal report must be given to the registered nurse assuming care of the patient. Components of the postprocedure report are outlined in Table 10–3. Documentation of the transfer of care should be recorded in the initial assessment area of the postprocedure record. Facilities that provide postprocedure care in the same unit where conscious sedation was administered may use the conscious sedation flow sheet for postprocedure documentation. To clearly delineate this separate and distinct period of care, various postprocedure documentation forms have been developed. Postprocedure documentation should include the following:

- Initial assessment area
- Postprocedure recovery scoring
- Graphic vital signs recording area

These components are summarized in a concise format on page 212.

POSTPROCEDURE RECORD

A postprocedure recovery scoring mechanism was introduced into clinical practice in 1970 by Aldrete and Kroulik.[5] Modifications of the Aldrete Scoring System have been used since its original inception. The Aldrete system assigns a predetermined score to objective criteria, which include the following:

- Activity
- Respiration
- Circulation
- Consciousness
- Oxygenation

Postprocedure Intravenous Conscious Sedation Record

Procedure: _____

Attending
Physician:_____

Name

ID #

Unit

Date

ECG
SaO2
220
200
180
160
140
120
100
80
60
40
20
Resp
0

	Time	Comments
Activity		
Sitting		
Up in chair		
Ambulates		
Tolerates PO fluid		
Voids		

Nurses Notes:

Aldrete Scoring System

Activity	Able to move four extremities voluntarily on command	2
	Able to move two extremities voluntarily on command	1
	Unable to move	0
Respiration	Able to deep breathe and cough freely	2
	Dyspnea or limited breathing	1
	Apneic	0
Circulation	B/P & H/R +/- 20% of preanesthetic level	2
	B/P & H/R +/- 20-50% of preanesthetic level	1
	B/P & H/R +/- 50% of preanesthetic level	0
Consciousness	Fully awake (Able to answer questions)	2
	Arousable on calling (arousable only on calling)	1
	Unresponsive	0
Oxygenation	Able to maintain O2 saturation > 92% on room air	2
	Needs O2 inhalation to maintain saturation> 90%	1
	O2 saturation < 90% even with O2 supplement	0

Postprocedure Follow-Up:

Telephone # (   ) _____ - _____

Date: _____/_____/_____

Contacted: _____

[ ] Postprocedure teaching completed
[ ] No complications noted
[ ] Complications:

Actions taken: _____

Attending physician notified

Date: _____ Time: _____

Discharge Care:

[ ] Postprocedure teaching completed, questions answered.

[ ] Postoperative/medication instructions given.

[ ] Responsible adult verbalized understanding.

[ ] Discharge criteria met.

[ ] Discharged in care of:

_____

Via _____

Time:_____

RN:_____

TABLE 10–4. *Aldrete Scoring System*

ACTIVITY	
Able to move four extremities voluntarily on command	2
Able to move two extremities voluntarily on command	1
Unable to move	0
RESPIRATION	
Able to deep breathe and cough freely	2
Dyspnea or limited breathing	1
Apneic	0
CIRCULATION	
BP and HR ± 20% of preanesthetic level	2
BP and HR ± 20% to 50% of preanesthetic level	1
BP and HR ± 50% of preanesthetic level	0
CONSCIOUSNESS	
Fully awake (able to answer questions)	2
Arousable on calling (arousable *only* to calling)	1
Unresponsive	0
OXYGENATION	
Able to maintain O_2 saturation > 92% on room air	2
Needs O_2 inhalation to maintain saturation > 90%	1
O_2 saturation < 90%, even with O_2 supplement	0

Reprinted by permission of the publisher from Aldrete A. Postanesthesia recovery score revisited. J Clin Anesthesiol 7:84. Copyright 1995 by Elsevier Science Inc. Elsevier Science Inc., 655 Avenue of the Americas, New York, NY 10010.

The complete Aldrete Scoring System is summarized in Table 10–4. Use of the variables identified provides objective clinical parameters for postprocedure assessment. Through the evolution of anesthesia and surgery, variations of the Aldrete Scoring System have evolved.[6,7] A postprocedure scoring system must be clearly understood by the nursing staff to provide accurate documentation and assure the safe discharge of the patient when all discharge criteria have been met. Use of a scoring system provides objective parameters related to the patient's postprocedure recovery and readiness for discharge. Criteria-based recovery parameters provide a mechanism to objectively assess the needs of the patient. Discharge criteria specific to intravenous conscious sedation are highlighted in Table 10–5. These criteria provide objective assessment parameters to ascertain the degree of recovery from sedative medications administered.

ACTIVITY

Patients who will be discharged to home after the procedure may prepare to ambulate once a postprocedure score greater than or equal to 8 has been achieved. Patients recovered on a gurney or recliner should be placed in a 30- to 40-degree head-up position. Dizziness or light-headedness is assessed, and the patient's activity level is advanced accordingly. If the patient tolerates the head-up position, sitting or dangling the legs for 5-minute increments precedes sitting in a chair and

TABLE 10–5.   *IV Conscious Sedation Discharge Criteria*

- Respiratory assessment
  - The patient retains the ability to maintain and protect the airway
  - The patient displays no signs of respiratory distress (snoring, stridor, suprasternal retraction, decreased O_2 saturation, or respiratory rate)
  - Demonstrates the ability to cough, tolerates liquids/light nourishment
  - A minimum of 30 minutes after the administration of the last dose of narcotic
  - Patients treated with reversal agents (flumazenil/naloxone) are monitored for a minimum of 120 minutes after the administration of the reversal agent
- Consciousness
  - Fully oriented to time, person, and place or return to baseline mentation
  - Absence of vomiting; patients who have been treated for vomiting must retain oral fluids and demonstrate the ability to swallow and cough
  - Dizziness or lightheadedness (if present) does not interfere with mobility
  - Able to void on instruction; contact physician if has not voided within 8 hours
- Circulation
  - Stable vital signs for a minimum of 30 minutes
- Activity
  - The patient performs age-appropriate ambulation (walk, sit, stand)
  - The patient demonstrates controlled, coordinated movements
  - Presence of a responsible adult for discharge and home environment
- Oxygenation and color
  - The patient maintains oxygen saturation > 95% on room air or attains preprocedure oxygen saturation value
  - Skin color is pink
- Procedure site
  - No bleeding on the dressing, dressing dry and intact
- Pain
  - The patient shall have minimal or no pain prior to discharge

© 1996, Specialty Health Consultants

ambulation. Absence of diaphoresis, bradycardia, hypotension, nausea, or vomiting is required prior to ambulation of the patient. Assisted ambulation is recommended to assess steadiness of gait. Patients may appear alert and prepared to ambulate, only to discover that they are not quite sure-footed enough to enter the bathroom or dressing area. An assisted ambulation method may prevent unexpected falls by patients who overextend their capabilities at any given time.

Patients who have received intravenous conscious sedation generally retain the ability to tolerate oral fluids without incident. The encouragement of oral fluids is contraindicated in patients who have received oropharyngeal topical anesthetics. Prior to oral fluid intake, the presence of a gag reflex and the ability to cough must be documented. Small amounts of oral fluid may then be encouraged prior to discharge or removal of the intravenous catheter. Oral fluids should not be forced in the presence of nausea and vomiting. Patients with nausea or vomiting may benefit from the administration of additional intravenous fluids in anticipation of discharge. For protracted nausea and vomiting, medications identified in Table 10–6 have been used in postoperative patients with some success. Pa-

TABLE 10–6. *Postprocedure Complications*

COMPLICATION	ETIOLOGY	TREATMENT OPTIONS
Pain	Postprocedure pain Pain associated with chronic conditions (arthritis, etc.)	1. Acetaminophen 2. NSAIDs 3. Prescribed opiates

Nausea/
  vomiting
	Increased vagal tone
	Hypotension
	Pain
	Opiate administration
	Hypovolemia
	Hypoglycemia associated
	  with NPO status
		1. IV droperidol 25 µg/kg
		2. Metoclopramide 0.15 mg/kg
		3. Ondansetron 0.05–0.1 mg/kg
		4. Liberal IV fluid replacement
		5. Suctioning

Airway
  obstruction
	Tongue against posterior
	  pharynx
	Secretions
	Vomit
	Blood
		1. Verbal/physical stimulation
		2. Head tilt
		3. Chin lift
		4. Jaw thrust
		5. Oral/nasal airway
		6. Intubation

Hypoventilation
  ($Paco_2 > 45$
  mm Hg)
	Residual sedative effects
	Preexisting pulmonary
	  disease
	Inadequate reversal
	Overdose
		1. Verbal/physical stimulation
		2. Continue administration of oxygen
		3. Encourage deep breathing
		4. Administration of additional rever-
		  sal agent
		5. Assisted/controlled ventilation
		6. Endotracheal intubation in the
		  event of unresponsive respiratory
		  depression

Hypotension	Enhanced vagal tone
	Left ventricular dysfunc-
	  tion
	Hypovolemia
	Pain
	Hemorrhage
	Spinal anesthesia
		1. Reduce factors that enhance vagal
		  tone (pain, anxiety, agitation, etc.)
		2. Correct factors that impair left ven-
		  tricular performance (myocardial
		  ischemia, fluid overload, etc.)
		3. Liberal IV fluids
		4. Pain relief
		5. Ephedrine, Trendelenburg position

Hypertension	Neuroendocrine response
	  to procedural pain
	Bladder distention
	Hypoxemia
	Hypercapnia
	Preexisting history of
	  hypertension
		1. Administration of mechanisms to
		  relieve pain
		2. Relieve noxious stimuli (full
		  bladder)
		3. Correct respiratory obstruction
		  < Sao_2, ventilatory depression
		4. Administration of beta/alpha
		  blockers

Conscious Sedation Medication
Discharge Instructions

Patient: _____   Date: __/__/__

Procedure Performed: _____

Medication discharge instructions:

You received the conscious sedation medications indicated below.

☐   Midazolam   ☐   Diazepam

☐   Fentanyl   ☐   Alfentanil   ☐   Remifentanil

☐   Hydromorphone ☐   Morphine   ☐   Meperidine

☐   Pentothal   ☐   Methohexital ☐   Propofol

Common side effects associated with these medications include:

- Drowsiness, dizziness, euphoria, sleepiness or confusion
- Impaired memory recall
- Unsteady gait, loss of fine muscle control and delayed reaction time.
- Visual disturbances: difficulty focusing, blurred vision

You may experience some of these side effects or you may not be cognizant of subtle changes in your behavior or reaction time. **Because you received these medications, we are giving you the following instructions.**

- Do not drive for 24 hours

- Do not operate equipment for 24 hours
  - ~ Lawnmowers, power tools etc.
  - ~ Kitchen accessories: stove, etc.

- Do not consume **any** alcoholic beverages for a minimum of 24 hours.

- Do not make important personal, legal or business decisions for 24 hours

- Move slowly and carefully, do not make sudden position changes. Be alert for dizziness or lightheadedness and move accordingly. Have responsible assist you.

© 1996, Specialty Health Consultants

tients with severe protracted nausea and vomiting require additional observation and should not be discharged.

The requirement to have a patient void after the procedure is not universally accepted. Patients receiving intravenous conscious sedation may not have the normal urinary retention experienced by postoperative surgical patients, and voiding is generally not a problem. However, in the presence of intravenous narcotics, patients may experience some urinary retention with altered bladder tone. Patients

Conscious Sedation Medication
Discharge Instructions *Continued*

- Drink liberal amounts of fluid today. Advance your diet as tolerated (unless you have received specific instructions from your doctor). If you feel nauseated, advance your diet as tolerated. Notify your physician if you have not voided within 8 hours postprocedure.

- Do not take any of the following medications unless prescribed by your physician.

    ~ Muscle relaxants
    ~ Sedatives
    ~ Hypnotics
    ~ Mood altering medications
    ~ Narcotics

Contact your physician or this facility if you have any questions or concerns regarding your postprocedure care.

Contact person: _____ Telephone #: _____

☐ Discharge instructions received
☐ Instructions given to responsible adult:_____
☐ Verbalized understanding

If you report to an emergency room, doctor's office or hospital within 24 hours postprocedure, BRING THIS SHEET WITH YOU and give it to the physician or nurse attending to you.

Date:_____ Time: _____

Responsible Adult:_____ _____
                        Signature   Printed

Instructions given by: _____ _____
                          Signature   Printed

© 1996, Specialty Health Consultants

who have not voided must be instructed when to return to the treatment facility in the event of bladder distention or the prolonged inability to void.

POSTPROCEDURE TEACHING AND INSTRUCTION

Postprocedure teaching should be conducted in the presence of the responsible adult assuming care of the patient on discharge or the registered nurse accepting care of the patient immediately after the procedure. Written discharge instructions addressing medications, diet, and procedure specific information must be reviewed with each patient and responsible adult. The postprocedure discharge teaching should take place in an unhurried atmosphere, much like the preprocedure assessment process. Use of written discharge instructions (procedure and medication) serves both the patient and the facility. The medication discharge form shown on pages 216–217 identifies medication used, side effects, and specific postprocedure guidelines to protect the patient. Instructions should also address diet, activity, and postprocedure expectations and should identify personnel to contact in the event of an emergency.

In addition to conscious sedation medication instructions, postprocedure specific discharge instructions should be reviewed and given to the patient. Postprocedure discharge instructions (below) address specific requirements associated

Postprocedure Discharge Instructions

☐ Rest today. If you feel up to it, you may move about but do not overdo it or engage in any strenuous activity.

☐ You may/may not shower or bathe today. If bathing/showering prohibited today, you may shower or bathe _____ hours postprocedure. A sponge bath today is permitted.

☐ Notify your physician if you have not voided within 8 hours of the procedure.

☐ Advance your diet as tolerated; refer to conscious sedation medication discharge instructions.

☐ Postprocedure medication:
Unless otherwise directed by your physician
- You may resume your regularly scheduled medications when you arrive home.
- Take prescribed pain medication as directed by your physician (or acetaminophen tablets every 3–4 hours for minor discomfort).

☐ Contact your physician's office, ( ) _____ - _____ for a follow-up appointment.

☐ You may return to work in _____ hours/days.

☐ Procedural site:
○ There should be no/minimal bleeding.
○ Minimal discomfort may be treated with pain medication prescribed. If severe pain occurs, contact your physician.
○ You may remove the dressing within _____ hours.
○ Replace dressing with _____.
○ If any signs of redness, fever, pus, swelling, or bleeding occur, contact your physician.

Additional Considerations:

_____

_____

_____

_____

If you have persistent nausea or vomiting, contact your physician. If you are experiencing complications and cannot contact your physician, report to the hospital emergency room. Please bring your discharge instructions with you.

RN: _____   Responsible adult: _____

Date: _____

with diagnostic or surgical procedures. They also address activity and diet as well as specific instructions related to the procedure.

POSTPROCEDURE FOLLOW-UP

A mechanism to ascertain postprocedure patient status is recommended for patients discharged on the day of the procedure. Inpatient information may be gathered by the conscious sedation practitioner or the physician following the procedure. Methods of gathering data include the following:

- Patient questionnaire
- Telephone interview
- Satisfaction survey

The purpose of postprocedure assessment is to evaluate the following:

- Incidence of complications related to the administration of conscious sedation
- Delayed recovery
- Procedural complication rate
- Return to function

Follow-up telephone conversations give the nurse the ability to receive direct feedback from the patient. Postprocedure follow-up featured on page 212 identifies complications and documents completion of the teaching process. Consistent postprocedure assessment is an accurate method to identify complications and assure the delivery of quality conscious sedation services.

SUMMARY

Use of discharge criteria and the postprocedure recovery period provides time to assess and verify the patient's return to preprocedure physiologic status. Use of scoring mechanisms, assessment of activity level, postprocedure teaching, and the provision of discharge instructions prepare the patient to return to the primary care setting or home.

REFERENCES

1. Practice Guidelines for Sedation and Analgesia by Non-Anesthesiologists. A Report by the American Society of Anesthesiologists Task Force on Sedation and Analgesia by Non-Anesthesiologists. *Anesthesiology.* 1996;84(2).
2. Joint Commission on Accreditation of Healthcare Organizations. *1997 JCAHO Manual.* Oakbrook Terrace, Ill: JCAHO; 1997.
3. Association of Operating Room Nurses. Recommended Practices for Managing the Patient Receiving Conscious Sedation/Analgesia. *AORN J.* 1997;••:149–154.
4. The American Society of Post Anesthesia Nurses. *Standards of Perianesthesia Nursing Practice.* New Jersey: ASPAN; 1995.
5. Aldrete J, Kroulik D. A postanesthetic recovery score. *Anesth Analg.* 1970;49:924.
6. Chung F. Are discharge criteria changing? *J Clin Anesth.* 1992;5:64S.
7. Aldrete A. Postanesthesia recovery score revisited. *J Clin Anesth.* 1995;71.

CHAPTER 11

Effective Risk-Management Strategies and Implementation of a Conscious Sedation Educational Program

DEVELOPMENT OF A RISK-MANAGEMENT STRATEGY

Quality has been broadly defined as the comprehensive positive outcome of a product.[1] Achievement of excellence in healthcare requires quality care and service evaluation. The quality of conscious sedation services is based on compliance with prescribed standards and recommended practice. Implementation of a successful conscious sedation program is based on the delivery of the high-quality technical aspects of care combined with positive outcomes. The delivery of quality conscious sedation services is also dependent on the patient's perception of care rendered. Today consumers are more cognizant than ever of the care they receive. The environment of managed care attempts to create the perception of acceptable value in return for the cost of healthcare.[2] The Joint Commission on Accreditation of Healthcare Organizations (JCAHO) states that *quality* is the "degree to which patient care services increase the probability of undesired outcomes, given the current state of knowledge."[3] To assure the delivery of high-quality care and reduce patient injury, strategic risk-management programs are designed. As emphasized throughout this text, the delivery of conscious sedation requires vigilance, clinical competence, proficient monitoring, and assessment skills. Adherence to state statutes, accrediting body regulations, and promulgated standards of care provides the clinician with parameters and guidelines to provide safe, high-quality conscious sedation services. However, unexpected events and complications may occur as a result of human error, periods of reduced observation, environmental factors (reduced lighting, limited patient access), poor communication, haste, and lack of preparation. When undesirable events occur, they must be rapidly diagnosed with appropriate intervention to restore body homeostasis. To prevent or reduce the development of adverse events, a risk-reduction strategy should be implemented for all units and personnel engaged in the administration of conscious sedation.

Individual injury prevention strategies include the following:

1. Development of a complete conscious sedation plan (Chapter 1).
2. Preprocedure preparation and patient assessment (Chapter 2).
3. Application and use of required monitoring equipment (Chapter 6).

4. Selection of appropriate pharmacologic medications and techniques (Appendix D, Chapters 3 and 5).
5. Preparation and presence of emergency resuscitative equipment and personnel (Chapter 4).
6. Preparation for specific procedures and locations (Chapter 9).
7. Postprocedure monitoring and discharge planning (Chapter 10).

Ideally, through implementation of individual risk-reduction strategies, prevention of injury precedes the occurrence of an adverse incident or event.

Application of a risk-management program on a departmental/institution basis requires development and implementation of mechanisms aimed at risk identification, analysis, and control. As depicted in Figure 11–1, creation of a conscious sedation database program is essential. A coordinator (nurse manager, department chairman) guides input into the conscious sedation database. Once the database has been instituted, strategies to implement change are used.

INSTITUTION/OFFICE POLICY AND PROCEDURE

The development of policies and procedures related to the administration of conscious sedation is a multidisciplinary process. Comprehensive policy development requires consultation with members of the administrative, nursing, medical, and anesthesia staff. As outlined throughout this manual, policy and procedure development must include components from regulations and guidelines promulgated by the following:

- JCAHO
- State statutes
- Professional organizations
- Recommended practice guidelines

JCAHO policy and guidelines are presented in Appendix A. State board of nursing position statements or nurse practice acts must be readily available for review. Professional organizations that have addressed recommended practice guidelines or promulgated position statements for clinical care of the conscious sedation patient are listed in Table 11–1. Policy and procedure development must encompass the following issues:

Nursing Care
- Professional standards
- Credentials and qualifications
- Medication administration
- Monitoring
- Patient selection
- Postprocedure care and discharge instruction

Patient Care
- Assessment, diagnosis, and intervention
- Protocols

- Discharge criteria and postprocedure care
- Management of complications

Institution Administrative Issues
- Standards and policies
- JCAHO, state practice issues
- Personnel requirements
- Scheduling practices

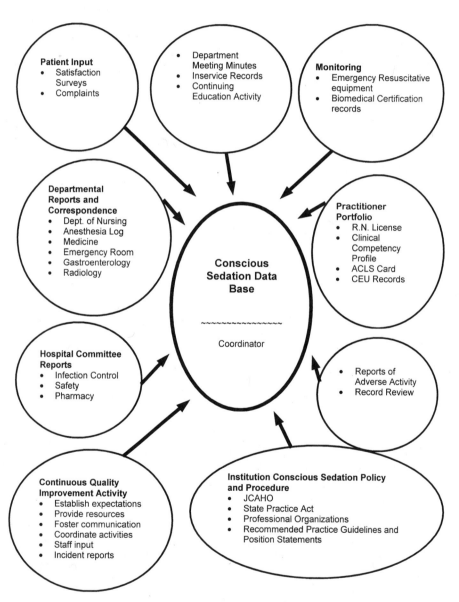

Patient Input
- Satisfaction Surveys
- Complaints

- Department Meeting Minutes
- Inservice Records
- Continuing Education Activity

Monitoring
- Emergency Resuscitative equipment
- Biomedical Certification records

Departmental Reports and Correspondence
- Dept. of Nursing
- Anesthesia Log
- Medicine
- Emergency Room
- Gastroenterology
- Radiology

Conscious Sedation Data Base

~~~~~~~~~~~~~~~

Coordinator

Practitioner Portfolio
- R.N. License
- Clinical Competency Profile
- ACLS Card
- CEU Records

Hospital Committee Reports
- Infection Control
- Safety
- Pharmacy

- Reports of Adverse Activity
- Record Review

Continuous Quality Improvement Activity
- Establish expectations
- Provide resources
- Foster communication
- Coordinate activities
- Staff input
- Incident reports

Institution Conscious Sedation Policy and Procedure
- JCAHO
- State Practice Act
- Professional Organizations
- Recommended Practice Guidelines and Position Statements

FIGURE 11–1.   Conscious sedation database program. (© 1996, Specialty Health Consultants.)

TABLE 11–1. *Professional Organizations Conscious Sedation Position Statements*

AMERICAN NURSES ASSOCIATION
Position Statement on the Role of the Registered Nurse in the Management of Patients
  Receiving Intravenous Conscious Sedation
—Endorsed by 23 Professional Nursing Organizations

ASSOCIATION OF OPERATING ROOM NURSES
Recommended Practices for Managing the Patient Receiving Conscious
  Sedation/Analgesia

AMERICAN SOCIETY OF ANESTHESIOLOGISTS
Practice Guidelines for Sedation and Analgesia by Non-Anesthesiologists
A Report by the American Society of Anesthesiologists Task Force on Sedation and
  Analgesia by Non-Anesthesiologists

AMERICAN ASSOCIATION OF NURSE ANESTHETISTS
Position Statement
Qualified Providers of Conscious Sedation

AMERICAN ACADEMY OF PEDIATRICS
Committee on Drugs
Guidelines for Monitoring and Management of Pediatric Patients During and After Seda-
  tion for Diagnostic and Therapeutic Procedures

- Equipment and supplies
- Emergency preparedness

Appropriate policy development must address:

1. A statement of purpose
2. Policy development
3. Procedure implementation

The JCAHO intravenous conscious sedation sample policy is outlined in Appendix A.

PRACTITIONER PORTFOLIO

A clinical portfolio should be maintained on all personnel engaged in the administration of intravenous conscious sedation. Components of this portfolio include the following:

- Registered nursing license
- Advanced cardiac life support/basic cardiac life support (ACLS/BCLS) status
- Clinical competence profile
- Educational inservice records
- Clinical privilege/position description

The granting of clinical privileges begins by defining the clinical position and role. See Table 11–2 for a conscious sedation nurse position description. Prior

TABLE 11–2. *Conscious Sedation Nurse Position Description*

Job Description: Conscious Sedation Nurse

Supervisor: _____

The registered nurse participating in the administration of intravenous conscious sedation is accountable for the preprocedure, intraprocedure, and postprocedure nursing care as prescribed by the policies, procedures, philosophies, and objectives of this institution. The registered nurse engaged in the administration of conscious sedation works under the direct supervision of the attending physician.

QUALIFICATIONS
- Graduation from an accredited school of nursing
- BCLS/ACLS recognition/completion of a dysrhythmia course
- Licensure as a professional registered nurse in the Commonwealth of
  _____
- Completion of intravenous conscious sedation educational modules as prescribed by this institution
- Hands-on practicum: Airway management, monitoring modalities, emergency resuscitative procedures

DIRECT PATIENT CARE
- Practices within the guidelines of the state nurse practice act
- Participates in preprocedure patient assessment
- Implements all aspects of clinical and technical care in accordance with established institution policy and procedure
- Uses universal precautions in all aspects of patient care
- Provides direct 1:1 patient care
- Provides a safe practice environment for patient care
- Uses infection-control practices to decrease the spread of nosocomial infection
- Acts as a patient advocate
- Respects the dignity and confidentiality of all patients
- Provides comprehensive transfer and discharge summary of patient care
- Provides patient education: before, during, and after the procedure

CLINICAL COMPETENCE
Displays clinical competence to:
- Assess the preprocedure, intraprocedure, and postprocedure needs of the patient
- Understand the goals and objectives of conscious sedation/analgesia
- Monitor the patient with no other responsibility that would require the nurse to leave the patient unattended or compromise continuous patient monitoring during the procedure
- Demonstrate function, interpretation, and use of resuscitative medications and monitoring equipment
- Monitors for adverse reactions and physiologic and psychologic changes associated with the administration of sedative/analgesic medications
- Document patient care where conscious sedation is administered
- Provide postprocedure care and assessment of discharge criteria
- Request physician consultation when indicated
- Participate in the quality-improvement process
- Teach patients using adult learning theories

TABLE 11–2. *Conscious Sedation Nurse Position Description* Continued

LEADERSHIP
Functions as a role model in:
- Patient care
- Patient education
- Communication
- Attendance

PROFESSIONAL GROWTH
Maintains a current knowledge base and professional development via:
- Participation in required educational inservice programs
- Attendance at department meetings
- Participation in professional organizations
- Participation in the personal evaluation process
- Maintains ACLS/BCLS certification
- Shares educational information gathered at seminars with staff members
- Identifies professional and educational needs
- Contributes to organizational goals
- Supports the philosophy, objectives, and goals of the institution
- Participation in patient care, conferences, staff meetings, annual review, revision of goals and objectives, and identification of measures for cost containment

© 1996, Specialty Health Consultants

clinical experience, educational preparation and training, and the clinical privileges outlined on pages 226–227 may be granted with or without restriction. Maintenance of a clinical competence profile ascertains the skill level of newly assigned personnel and provides annual renewal of intravenous conscious sedation privileges. A complete clinical competency list is presented in Appendix G.

MONITORING/EMERGENCY RESUSCITATIVE EQUIPMENT, BIOMEDICAL CERTIFICATION RECORDS

Biomedical certification of medical equipment is recommended on a biannual basis.[4] Preventive maintenance and biomedical certification are used on monitoring and resuscitative equipment to inspect, clean, lubricate, adjust, and replace worn and damaged parts. The purpose of biomedical certification is also to assure proper functioning of routine monitors and diagnostic and emergency resuscitative equipment. The following equipment requires routine inspection and certification:

- ECG monitors
- Noninvasive blood pressure monitor
- Pulse oximeters
- Defibrillators
- Diagnostic equipment
- Electrosurgical units

Application for Clinical Privileges
Intravenous Conscious Sedation

Category: **Administration of Intravenous Conscious Sedation**

Personal Background Information

Name:_____
           (Last)   (First)   (Middle Initial)

Home Address:_____

City:_____ State:_____ Zip Code:_____

Date of Birth:_____/_____/_____   Sex: Male   Female

Education:

Nursing Education: School of Nursing: _____

                       Date of Graduation:_____/_____/_____ Degree:_____

Additional Education: University:_____

                       Address:_____

                       City:_____ State:_____

Professional Clinical Experience:

Licensure: State_____ RN License #_____ Expires:_____

             BCLS Expiration Date: _____/_____/_____ **ACLS** Expiration Date: _____/_____/_____

Employment:

     Institution Name & Address: _____

                                  _____

         Phone Number:_____Supervisor:_____

         Dates of Employment: _____to_____Reason for Leaving:_____

     Institution Name & Address: _____

                                    _____

         Phone Number:_____Supervisor:_____

         Dates of Employment: _____to_____Reason for Leaving:_____

     Institution Name & Address: _____

                                    _____

         Phone Number:_____Supervisor:_____

         Dates of Employment: _____to_____Reason for Leaving:_____

Application for Clinical Privileges *Continued*
Intravenous Conscious Sedation

References (3): _____
(Name and Address)

_____
(Name and Address)

_____
(Name and Address)

Professional Organization Memberships:

1)_____

2)_____

3)_____

<u>Clinical Privilege Delineation</u>

Type of Request   ☐   **Initial**   ☐   **Annual Renewal**

Name:_____

Please check all clinical procedures for which you are applying:

☐ **Preprocedure assessment**
☐ **Intravenous access**
☐ **Administration of conscious sedation medications listed below:**

- _____
- _____
- _____
- _____

Intraprocedure Monitoring   **Administration of oxygen via:**
  ☐ EKG   ☐ Nasal cannula
  ☐ NIBP   ☐ Face mask
  ☐ Pulse Oximetry   ☐ Humidified mask
  ☐ Capnography   ☐ Bag valve mask
Postprocedure Management:
  ☐ Postprocedure monitoring
  ☐ Discharge assessment
  ☐ Postprocedure instructions (Procedure and Conscious Sedation)

Management of Complications:
  ☐ Cardiopulmonary resuscitative management
  ☐ Respiratory resuscitation

☐ Approved	☐ With Restriction	☐ Denied
_____ Clinical Manager	_____ Supervisor	
Practitioner notified: _____/_____/_____		
**Above clinical privileges are granted for a period of one year.		

© 1996, Specialty Health Consultants

Documentation and Record Keeping

It is important to maintain a separate file within the conscious sedation database for preventive maintenance, service, and biomedical certification records. Documentation provides a written record of service performed on specific monitoring and resuscitative equipment. Information that should be recorded on the biomedical service sheet includes the following:

- Date of purchase
- Serial number
- Description of device
- Instructions for servicing
- Name, address, and telephone number of manufacturer
- Name, address, and telephone number of biomedical service company

Routine (biannual) maintenance should be documented, including service performed, parts replaced, and the name of the person servicing the equipment. Core components of a biomedical certification evaluation are identified on page 229. Service or instruction manuals for all monitoring equipment should be readily available for the clinician's use. Storage of service manuals in the purchasing department or manager's office or removal from the immediate vicinity is not recommended.

DEPARTMENT/UNIT-RELATED ACTIVITY

Business and education activity related to the department or unit must also be documented and stored in the database. Department meeting minutes, inservices, or continuing educational activities should be readily available for staff members who are not able to attend. Continuing education activity reports should be completed by staff members returning from seminars, inservices, or national meetings. This information is then disseminated at an upcoming staff meeting or available in written form for individual review. An example of a continuing education activity report is featured on page 230. Through implementation of a brief summary report, unit personnel benefit from a variety of educational seminars and activities attended by clinicians throughout the year.

Effective department meeting strategy includes completion of old business and introduction of new business combined with a mechanism to introduce educational activities. Case reports, journal articles, and professional organization updates are easily coordinated into staff development. Management modalities to assist practitioner development include the assignment of several staff members to briefly review medical journals, articles, and professional organization guidelines on a monthly basis. A condensed summary and clinical pertinence report (professional development summary) is presented at each staff meeting. Three or four professional journals pertinent to the unit's activity are reviewed monthly, with selection of appropriate topics for presentation. A professional development summary report is highlighted on page 231. Implementation of this type of program reduces time and energy expenditure while providing high-quality educational presentations. Documentation of educational activities and minutes of de-

Biomedical Certification Form
AC Line-Powered Equipment

Completed by: _____   Date of Inspection:___/___/___

Equipment Description:_____

Tag No._____Location:_____

Next Inspection Date: _____

		OK	Service Required	Service Completed	Date	Initials
1.	General Condition					
2.	Line Cord, Strain Reliefs					
3.	Attachment Plug					
4.	Grounding Check_____OHMS_____					
5.	AC Chassis Leakage Properly Grounded On _____ Off_____					
	Ungrounded, Correct Polarity: On_____ Off_____					
	Ungrounded, Reversed Polarity On_____ Off_____					

Additional Information: _____

_____

_____

_____

_____

partment meetings are added to the conscious sedation database by the coordinator or designated representative. A sample of department meeting minutes is given on page 232.

PATIENT INPUT

Results of patient satisfaction surveys or questionnaires should be summarized and entered into the database. Areas consistently addressed by patients require further evaluation. Patient care issues require action to avoid potential in-

Continuing Education Activity Report

Name: _____

Conference Attended: _____

Dates of Attendance: _____

Date of Report: _____

Speaker: _____

Speakers:

    A._____

    B._____

    C._____

Presentation Content:

Relevance to Clinical Practice

Recommendations

☐   See Attached Enclosures

☐   See Educational Articles Enclosed

---

jury and improve quality of care. Intangible complaints offered by patients may be difficult to address (parking, elevators, etc.). To reduce patient anxiety and enhance communication with patients, these areas are addressed in subtle ways. Preprocedure preparation strategy includes clear communication and patient instruction. Patients must be given clear (preferably written) instructions for planned activities. These instructions include the following:

Professional Development Summary Report

Title of Article: _____ **Author:** _____

Journal: _____ **Pages:** _____ **Date:** _____

SUMMARY:

CLINICAL SIGNIFICANCE:

RECOMMENDATIONS:

ACTIONS TAKEN:

Submitted by: _____ **Date:** _____/_____/_____

- Where to report (building/floor)
- What paperwork or insurance information is required
- Where to park
- What time to report

A user-friendly facility with adequate signs may reduce patient anxiety and complaints. Use of good communication skills and assessment of consistent patient suggestions are required to enhance patient care.

Department Meeting Summary Report

Date: ____/____/____

Department:____/____/____

Recorder/Secretary: _____

Members Present:

Members Excused:

Meeting called to order _____ **AM/PM By:**_____

Old Business:

   Actions taken:

New Business

   Actions Taken

Professional Development Summary Reports:

**Presented
by:**_____

(See attached reports)

Meeting Adjourned: _____ **AM/PM By:**_____

Respectfully submitted,

DEPARTMENTAL REPORTS AND CORRESPONDENCE

Interdisciplinary reports and memos should be readily available for staff review. Nursing, anesthesia, emergency room, gastroenterology, radiology, and all applicable departments interacting with the conscious sedation unit should be posted in an accessible area. Memos, minutes, and reports are initialed by staff members. A mechanism to assure that all information has been disseminated to the appropriate personnel is presented below.

Staff Memo Confirmation

Date of Memo: _____/_____/_____

Memo Number:_____

Written By:_____

Regarding:_____

I have read and understand the contents of Memo #:_____

Staff Members:

1) (Name)	Date:	Initials
2)		
3)		
4)		
5)		
6)		
7)		
8)		
9)		
10)		
11)		
12)		
13)		
14)		
15)		
16)		
17)		
18)		
19)		
20)		

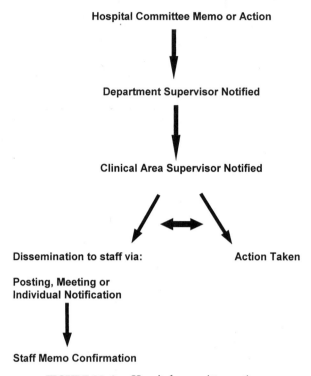

Hospital Committee Memo or Action

Department Supervisor Notified

Clinical Area Supervisor Notified

Dissemination to staff via: **Action Taken**

**Posting, Meeting or
Individual Notification**

Staff Memo Confirmation

FIGURE 11–2.   Hospital committee action.

HOSPITAL COMMITTEE REPORTS

Reports and actions of the institution's committee structure must also be disseminated to appropriate unit personnel. A system of communication outlined in Figure 11–2 facilitates the communication process within the unit.

CONTINUOUS PERFORMANCE IMPROVEMENT

Continuous performance improvement attempts to provide a systematic approach to detection and correction while at the same time improving efficiency in the care that is rendered to patients by healthcare providers. Continuous performance improvement attempts to address all facets of the organization that affect patient outcomes.[5] Continuous performance improvement is a continuous process committed to long-term improvement in patient outcome. JCAHO requires the use of outcome indicators as a basis for quality monitoring. Use of individual specialty indicators attempts to identify deviations in quality of care. An example of continuous quality indicators used in conscious sedation follows:

- Presedation status documentation
  - Preprocedure patient assessment
  - NPO status

TABLE 11–3. *Examples of Accepting Less Than 100% Quality*

If you settle for 99.9% quality, you get
- One hour per month of unsafe drinking water.
- 16,000 pieces of mail lost per hour.
- 20,000 wrong presciptions per year.
- 500 incorrect surgical operations per week.
- 50 newborns dropped by the doctor per day.
- 22,000 checks deducted from the wrong account per hour.
- Two unsafe landings per day at O'Hare International Airport.
- 3200 missed heartbeats per person per year.

From INS (Intravenous Nurses Society). *Intravenous Therapy: Clinical Principles and Practice.* Philadelphia: WB Saunders; 1995:52.

- – Allergies
- – Medications
- Physician documentation for conscious sedation medications
- Physician discharge orders
  - – Evidence of postprocedure monitoring
  - – Satisfaction of discharge criteria
- Evidence of continuous monitoring
  - – Intraprocedure
  - – Postprocedure
- Documentation of adverse reactions or events

See page 236 for an example of a conscious sedation clinical indicator form. The ultimate goal of continuous quality improvement is to achieve 100% quality. Examples of the effects of accepting less than 100% quality are listed in Table 11–3. The conscious sedation database is an integral component of the continuous quality improvement process. Through total staff involvement and commitment, employees are empowered to participate in key components of the quality improvement process.

IMPLEMENTATION OF A CONSCIOUS SEDATION EDUCATIONAL PROGRAM

The administration of conscious sedation is both challenging and rewarding. However, the development of a quality-conscious sedation program and the education of clinicians engaged in the administration of conscious sedation involve policy, educational, and operational issues.

POLICY DEVELOPMENT

As outlined in Chapter 1, policy development is required in any setting in which conscious sedation is administered. Prior to inception, any good business sets forth a mission statement to outline the goals and objectives of the organization. A conscious sedation educational program should clearly delineate its goals,

Conscious Sedation: Clinical Indicator Form

Patient Identification #_____   Age:_____   Date of Service:____/____/____

Attending Physician: _____   Procedure:_____

CS Nurse: _____   Location:_____

MONITORING INDICATORS

A. Continuous ECG monitoring?   ☐ Yes   ☐ No

B. Continuous respiratory monitoring?   ☐ Yes   ☐ No

C. Continuous blood pressure monitoring?   ☐ Yes   ☐ No

D. Continuous pulse oximetry monitoring?   ☐ Yes   ☐ No

E. Continuous level of consciousness monitoring?   ☐ Yes   ☐ No

F. Continuous patient monitoring by nurse?   ☐ Yes   ☐ No

PREPROCEDURE INDICATORS

☐ Preprocedure assessment complete

☐ Incomplete informed consent/no signature

☐ Incomplete patient chart

☐ Incomplete labwork

☐ Medical consult required

☐ Noncompliance: NPO status

☐ Noncompliance: preprocedure medication instructions

PROCEDURE INDICATORS

☐ Respiratory depression

☐ Respiratory complication: stridor/laryngospasm/arrest

☐ Cardiovascular complications: cardiac arrest/ischemia/CHF/pulmonary edema

☐ Cardiovascular complications: hypotension/hypertension/dysrhythmias

☐ Level of consciousness: unresponsive/obtunded reflexes/agitation

☐ Medication: allergic reaction/wrong medication administered

☐ All medications administered as per facility policy

☐ Reversal agents administered (Flumazenil/Naloxone)

POSTPROCEDURE INDICATORS

☐ Prolonged somnolence

☐ Unexpected admission secondary to sedation

☐ Additional reversal agents administered (Flumazenil/Naloxone)

☐ Nausea/Vomiting: _____times post discharge, current status:_____

☐ Evidence of postprocedure monitoring

☐ Documentation of discharge criteria

☐ Evidence of patient/family dissatisfaction

☐ Postprocedure follow-up complete

---

objectives, and expectations (see p 237). Once a mission statement has been established, the scope of services must be delineated. A conscious sedation program scope of services is outlined in Table 11–4.

    Conscious sedation policies and procedures, the mission statement, and the scope of services must be readily available in all patient care areas. As outlined in Chapter 1, policy and procedure development must address the following:

Mission Statement

The mission of the conscious sedation program at _____ and
the clinicians in the administration of conscious sedation in this facility is to provide the
highest quality medical care. We will continually attempt to improve the level of care which
we provide through clinical service and education. We will develop a system in which the
administration of intravenous conscious sedation services are provided in a stable and supportive environment. Intravenous conscious sedation will be administered in accordance
with regulatory agency guidelines, state practice statutes, and professional organization
recommended practices.

Conscious Sedation Continuing Education Goals, Objectives, and Expectations

I. Purpose
The purpose of the continuing education program is to provide a mechanism for clinical case conference, research, and new product information dissemination to all staff
involved in the procedural care of patients receiving intravenous conscious sedation.

II. Learning Objectives
At the conclusion of the program, participants will:
- Demonstrate an awareness of available literature pertinent to the subject of con-
scious sedation.
- Discuss current trends and changes in the administration of conscious sedation
and care of patients receiving conscious sedation services.
- Demonstrate clear evaluation and review of current literature.
- Discuss scientific principles related to a variety of clinical case scenarios.
- Discuss challenging questions and relate them to the role of continuous quality im-
provement and risk reduction strategy.
- Present a concise, accurate report and lead a group discussion when applicable.

III. Teaching Methods
Teaching methods include:
- Lecture
- Discussion
- Slides
- Handouts
- Authorized reprints
- Clinical case management synopsis

- Preprocedure assessment
- Patient selection criteria
- Monitoring requirements and clinician responsibility
- Methods of recording patient data
- Frequency of patient documentation
- Medications that may be administered by the registered nurse
- Treatment of complications

TABLE 11–4.   *Scope of Service: Clinical Departments*

Department: Intravenous Conscious Sedation Unit

☐ GI Laboratory   ☐ Radiology   ☐ Emergency Room
☐ Operating Room   ☐ Physician's Office   ☐ Other

Services Provided: The _____ unit is engaged in the administration of intravenous conscious sedation to provide a reduced state of anxiety for minor surgical or diagnostic procedures.

1. Types and ages of patients served (ages, patient groups, frequent diagnostic categories, etc.).
Intravenous conscious sedation services will be afforded to all patients within this facility with the exception of [*applicable exceptions*]. Clinical services are available for all minor surgical or diagnostic procedures with the exception of [*applicable exceptions*].

2. Methods used to assess and meet patients' care needs (How are patient care or service needs identified and how are they met?):
Methods used to assess and meet patient needs include:
- Preprocedure assessment
- Intraprocedural monitoring
- Selection of appropriate pharmacologic medications based on patient assessment
- Provision of postprocedure monitoring, discharge information, and follow-up

3. Scope and complexity of patients' care needs (diagnosis, conditions, etc.):
The scope of care is dependent on preprocedure patient assessment, diagnostic or surgical procedure, patient reaction to pharmacologic medications, and recovery from the residual effects of sedatives.

4. Appropriateness, clinical necessity, and timeliness of service provided.
The appropriateness, clinical necessity, and timeliness of services are provided through periodic review. Mechanisms of review include:
- Medical chart review
- Participation in continuous quality-improvement process
- Management of a risk-management database coordinated by [*individual's name*]

5. Availability of necessary staff (staffing model/assignment methodology, hours of operation, needs related to credentials, age-specific competence, continuing education, etc.):
Conscious sedation services are provided on a 1:1 basis. Patients will be continuously monitored during the procedure and in the postprocedure period.
Hours of operation: _____ to _____
On call services are available.
The following competencies will be evaluated on an annual basis:
- Knowledge of the goals and objectives of conscious sedation
- ACLS certification
- ECG rhythm interpretation
- Airway evaluation and resuscitation
- Mechanism of actions; treatment of adverse reactions associated with the administration of sedatives, hypnotics, and narcotics
- Intravenous insertion skills
- Conscious sedation annual education module examination

© 1996, Specialty Health Consultants

TABLE 11–4. *Scope of Service: Clinical Departments* **Continued**

Continuing education and clinical competency records outlined above are maintained in an individual practitioner portfolio. Continuing education inservices are based on patient population, staff needs, technologic advances, and performance appraisals. *Annual competency validation.*

6. *Extent to which the level of service or care provided meets the patient's needs (treatments, procedures and/or activities provided, patient satisfaction):*
The conscious sedation unit (Department of _____) is a _____ bed unit which provides conscious sedation for short diagnostic and minor surgical procedures. Patients are provided the highest quality of medical care as promulgated by regulatory agencies, state statutes, and professional organization recommendations. Patient satisfaction is assessed via a discharge patient satisfaction survey reviewed by management.

Department Goals for Patient Care
- Continue to provide the highest medical care to the patient population
- Enhance patient teaching
- Implement programs to improve patient satisfaction

Written: _____/_____/_____
Revised: _____/_____/_____

© 1996, Specialty Health Consultants

- Discharge criteria
- Postprocedure instructions

Policy and procedures must clearly delineate lines of responsibility and accountability. The interdisciplinary development of conscious sedation policy should attempt to reduce risk factors, provide the highest-quality patient care, and *assure the same level of care throughout the institution.*

EDUCATION

Once the goals and objectives of a conscious sedation program have been outlined, implementation of the service is accomplished through education. Identification of problems that obstruct these goals may include the following:

- ACLS training
- Interpretation of ECGs and completion of a dysrhythmia course
- Pharmacologic education
- Provision of monitoring and resuscitative equipment

Problem areas must be addressed and rectified to the satisfaction of regulatory agencies and state law. Use of a multidisciplinary approach includes education related to the following:

- Pharmacology (Chapter 3)
- Drug dosages (Appendix D)
- Administration techniques (Chapter 5)

- Adherence to policy and procedures (Chapter 1)
- Preprocedure patient assessment (Chapter 2)
- Monitoring requirements (Chapter 6)
- Airway management (Chapter 4)
- Postprocedure monitoring (Chapter 10)
- Continuous performance improvement (Chapter 11)

As emphasized throughout this text, identification of variables that affect conscious sedation services, staff education, and patient care issues must be addressed as core components of a conscious sedation program. Policy development, which addresses preprocedure patient assessment, monitoring, pharmacologic education, postprocedure monitoring, and patient education coupled with assessment of discharge criteria, enhances quality patient care. Credentialing of clinical competencies provides clinicians with the confidence to rapidly assess, diagnose, and intervene when providing conscious sedation services. Through proper clinical training and education, the clinician remains confident in his or her ability to effectively stabilize the patient and provide resuscitative care until additional assistance becomes available.

References

1. Graham N. *Quality Assurance in Hospitals: Strategies for Assessment and Implementation.* Rockville, Md: Aspen; 1990.
2. Gillen TR. Deming's 14 points and hospital quality: responding to the consumer's demand for the best value health care. *J Nurs Qual Assur.* 1988;2:70–78.
3. Joint Commission on Accreditation of Healthcare Organizations (JCAHO). *1997 Accreditation Manual for Hospitals.* Oak Terrace, Ill: JCAHO; 1997.
4. Dorsch J. *Understanding Anesthesia Equipment.* 2nd ed. Baltimore: Williams & Wilkins; 1994.
5. Koch MW, Fairley TM. *Integrated Quality Management.* St. Louis: Mosby; 1993.

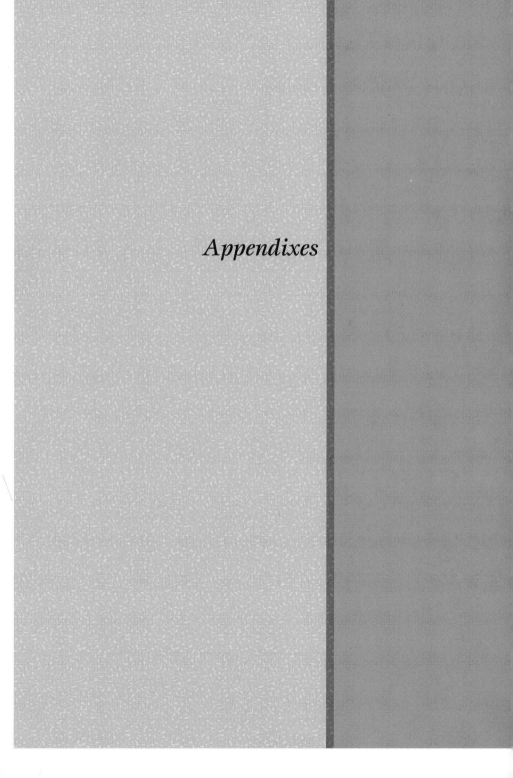

Appendixes

Joint Commission on Accreditation of Healthcare Organizations

APPENDIX A

SAMPLE POLICY AND PROCEDURE FOR INTRAVENOUS CONSCIOUS SEDATION

Intravenous Conscious Sedation Policies and Procedures

SAMPLE POLICY AND PROCEDURE FOR INTRAVENOUS CONSCIOUS SEDATION— INTRODUCTION TO TX.2. The following sample policy and procedure illustrates one organization's approach to developing definitions and protocols of care for patients undergoing procedures using intravenous conscious sedation.

ADMINISTRATIVE MANUAL

POLICY. Our organization provides guidelines for monitoring intravenous conscious sedation administered to patients undergoing invasive, manipulative, or constraining procedures.

DEFINITION. IV conscious sedation is the proper administration of drugs to obtund, dull, or reduce the intensity of pain and awareness without loss of defensive reflexes. Conscious sedation of the patient is generally achieved when there is slurred speech but the patient is arousable and is able to respond. This policy does not apply to IV conscious sedation used for therapeutic management of pain control or seizures. It also does not apply to IV conscious sedation used in the operating room or family birthing unit.

This policy is applicable to

- patients from 18 to 60 years old who receive intravenously > 5 mg of Versed or > 20 mg of Valium or any dosage of narcotic;
- patients 60 years of age and older who receive intravenously > 3.5 mg of Versed or > 10 mg of Valium or any dosage of narcotic;
- all pediatric patients; and
- patients receiving any combination of drugs.

At the discretion of the physician, this policy can be initiated for patients receiving dosages of drugs less than those listed above.

From *Comprehensive Accreditation Manual for Hospitals: The Official Handbook.* Copyright by Joint Commission on Accreditation of Healthcare Organizations, Oakbrook Terrace, IL: 1997, pages TX-76 to TX-80. Reprinted with permission.

LOCATION. IV conscious sedation is practiced in various departments within the organization, for example, endoscopy lab, radiology.

PROCEDURE. Intravenous conscious sedation practices throughout the organization shall be monitored and evaluated by the Department of Anesthesia, according to the policy outlined and performed to assure optimal patient outcome.

All patients must have an intravenous access secured prior to administering conscious sedation.

The medical director of each department administering intravenous conscious sedation will be responsible for ensuring that policies and procedures exist in that department and are applicable to that department's practice.

All IV conscious sedation will be ordered and supervised by the physician credentialed for the specific procedure and administration of anesthetics. The licensed professional nurse (RN) responsible for managing the care of the patients receiving IV conscious sedation will complete and maintain competency in the skill.

All patients requiring IV conscious sedation will have a preprocedure assessment, a minimal preanesthetic assessment including, but not limited to:

- History and physical performed by a physician (this should include age, review of systems specific to cardiopulmonary disease) and current medications and a history of any adverse or allergic drug reactions with anesthesia or sedation;
- Vital signs: heart rate, blood pressure, respiratory rate, and oxygen saturation;
- Level of consciousness;
- NPO status;
- Proper consents signed; and
- Pregnancy.

Emergency equipment must be immediately accessible to every location where IV conscious sedation is administered, and includes at least the following: defibrillator, suction device, oxygen, airways, emergency drugs (Narcan, Romazicon), intubation equipment, and ECG monitor.

Monitoring of the patient is to be continuous throughout the procedure and will include documentation of

- vital signs, including blood pressure, pulse rate, percentage of oxygen saturation, and respirations taken and recorded on the chart prior to initiation of sedation and at the end of the procedure;
- pulse rate, respirations, and oxygen saturation must be documented at regular intervals during the procedure, at a minimum of every 15 minutes. Blood pressure shall be taken as needed during the procedure or as ordered by physician;
- continuous pulse oximetry with both digital and auditory displays;
- level of consciousness documented every 15 minutes;
- hypersensitivity reactions; and

- postprocedure documentation of patient's tolerance, level of consciousness, vital signs including oxygen saturation maintenance on room air, and unit and name of person receiving the patient.

NOTE: Prior to discontinuing the postprocedure monitoring, patient's vital signs must be stable compared to baseline (preprocedure readings).

Intravenous Conscious Sedation Human Resources

QUALIFICATIONS FOR ADMINISTERING AND MONITORING IV CONSCIOUS SEDATION. All persons are responsible for maintaining proficient skills necessary to provide quality patient care, prior to administering and monitoring IV conscious sedation. The person administering or monitoring IV conscious sedation patients are required to

- be familiar with proper dosages, administration, adverse reactions, and interventions for adverse reactions and overdoses;
- know how to recognize an airway obstruction and demonstrate skills in basic life support;
- assess total patient care requirements or parameters, including but not limited to respiratory rate, oxygen saturation, blood pressure, cardiac rate, and level of consciousness; and
- have the knowledge and skills to intervene in the event of complications.

Administration and/or monitoring IV conscious sedation may be performed by a qualified physician or a registered nurse trained in administering or monitoring IV conscious sedation.

Only a physician is qualified to prescribe, order, or select the medication(s) to be used to achieve IV conscious sedation.

Upon discharge, the outpatient or the responsible person will be provided verbal and written instructions regarding diet, medications, activities, and signs and symptoms of complications with course of action to take if any complication develops.

DEFINITIONS

Examples of Definitions Developed by Two Organizations and Supported by Several Professional Nursing Organizations

DIFFERENCES BETWEEN CONSCIOUS SEDATION AND DEEP SEDATION TECHNIQUES

Conscious Sedation	Deep (Unconscious) Sedation
Mood altered	Patient unconscious
Patient cooperative	Patient unable to cooperate
Protective reflexes intact	Protective reflexes obtunded
Vital signs stable	Vital signs labile
Local anesthesia provides analgesia	Pain eliminated centrally
Amnesia may be present	Amnesia always present
Short recovery room stay	Occasional prolonged recovery room stay or overnight admission required

Conscious Sedation	*Deep (Unconscious) Sedation*
Perioperative complications infrequent	Perioperative complications reported in 25% to 75% of cases
Uncooperative or mentally handicapped patient cannot always be managed	Useful in managing difficult or mentally handicapped patients

1. The various degrees of sedation defined in the following paragraphs occur on a continuum. The patient may progress from one degree to another, based on the medications administered, route, and dosages. The determination of patient monitoring and staffing requirements should be based on the patient's acuity and the potential response of the patient to the procedure.

    light sedation   The administration of oral medications for the reduction of anxiety. In this stage the following should be present:
    1. Normal respirations;
    2. Normal eye movements; and
    3. Intact protective reflexes.

    Amnesia may or may not be present. The patient is technically awake, but under the influence of the drug administered. Groups of drugs that may be used for this purpose include
    - sedative-hypnotics;
    - antianxiety;
    - benzodiazepines;
    - antihistamines; and
    - narcotics.

    conscious sedation   A medically controlled state of depressed consciousness that
    1. allows protective reflexes to be maintained;
    2. retains the patient's ability to maintain a patent airway independently and continuously; and
    3. permits appropriate response by the patient to physical stimulation or verbal command, for example, "open your eyes."

    deep sedation   A medically controlled state of depressed consciousness or unconsciousness from which the patient is not easily aroused. It may be accompanied by a partial or complete loss of protective reflexes, and includes the inability to maintain a patent airway independently and respond purposefully to physical stimulation or verbal command.

2. Because the administration of sedative agents intravenously (for example, Versed, Valium, Demerol, morphine, fentanyl, Propofol, Brevital, Nubain, Stadol) could result in a risk of loss of protective reflexes, an ambulatory care organization defined its protocol for the use of sedation.

    According to the protocol, the physician responsible for managing the patient receiving conscious sedation must be competent in the use of anesthesia techniqes and able to provide a level of monitoring that includes respiratory rate, oxygen saturation, blood pressure, cardiac rate and rhythm, and determining the patient's level of consciousness. The physician must also be able to manage complications that may occur related to the administration of conscious sedation. The physician is to be trained in basic life support, and training in advanced life support is recommended.

The protocol stresses that, in addition to the physician, an additional qualified practitioner is included whose responsibilities cover continuous uninterrupted monitoring of the patient's physiological parameters and to assist in supportive or resuscitation measures, if necessary.

3. General competency for the qualified individual managing the care of a patient receiving conscious sedation includes the ability to
   a. demonstrate the acquired knowledge of anatomy, physiology, pharmacology, cardiac arrhythmia recognition, and complications related to conscious sedation and medications;
   b. assess total patient care requirements during conscious sedation and recovery. Physiological measurements should include, but are not limited to, respiratory rate, oxygen saturation, blood pressure, cardiac rate and rhythm, and the patient's level of consciousness;
   c. understand the principles of oxygen delivery, respiratory physiology, oxygen transport and oxygen uptake, and demonstrate the ability to use oxygen delivery devices;
   d. anticipate and recognize potential complications of conscious sedation in relation to the type of medication being administered;
   e. possess the requisite knowledge and skills to assess, diagnose, and intervene in the event of complications or undesired outcomes, and to institute interventions in compliance with orders (including standing orders) or institutional protocols or guidelines; and
   f. demonstrate skill in airway management and resuscitation.

Specific criteria for the registered nurse managing the care of a patient receiving conscious sedation include the following:
1. Advanced cardiopulmonary support (ACLS) is recommended.
2. Basic life support (BLS) annual recertification is required.
3. Training is required in the recognition of the cardiovascular and respiratory side effects of sedatives, as well as the variability of patient response.
4. Training in airway management is required.
5. Recertification of the above criteria is required annually.
6. Successful completion of a basic "Dysrhythmia Class" is mandatory.
7. The person administering the medications knows the pharmacology of the medications administered.

4. In developing its protocols, an ambulatory surgery center identified the following requirements for managing patients across the continuum of sedation:
   I. Definition:
   Except when "light sedation" is administered orally as a premedication, staffing during "conscious sedation" and "deep sedation" should always include a minimum of
   • one qualified practitioner to monitor patient and
   • one physician.

Staffing

II. Staffing:

Additional staffing is based on the patient's acuity, procedure, and the potential response to the medications administered.

Staffing during "light sedation" should include one nurse or qualified practitioner to observe the patient's response to the medication(s). The nurse does not have to be in the continuous presence of the patient.

Equipment

III. Equipment list:
- Emergency cart with a defibrillator
- Suction at bedside
- Positive pressure breathing device
- Oxygen and delivery devices (nasal cannula, mask)
- Appropriate oral and nasal airways (Pediatric and Adult as appropriate)
- Cardiac monitor
- Pulse oximeter
- Ambu bag
- Intubation tray
- Reversal agents (Narcan and Mazicon)
- IV supplies

Self-Directed

IV. Self-directed Learning Module on Patient Monitoring
- Literature review
- QI data

Charting

V. Minimum Required Chart Documentation
- Allergies
- Level of consciousness
- Monitoring devices or equipment used, serial numbers
- Physiologal data from continuous monitoring, documented at 5- to 15-minute intervals and at any significant event
- Dosage, route, time, and effects of sedative medications
- Any interventions, such as oxygen or intravenous therapy, and the patient's response
- Any untoward or significant reactions and resolutions

QI Tool

VI. Use of Required Process and Patient Outcome Measurement Tool
   1. Continuous ECG monitoring   yes ( )   no ( )
      Respiratory rate   yes ( )   no ( )
      Blood pressure   yes ( )   no ( )
      Pulse oximeter   yes ( )   no ( )
      Level of consciousness   yes ( )   no ( )
      Continuous visual monitoring by RN   yes ( )   no ( )
   2. Medications administered according to   yes ( )   no ( )
      policy and procedure?

3. Identify undesirable effects from the administration of IV conscious sedation medications:
( ) None
( ) Unarousable or stuporous
( ) Absent blink reflex
( ) Loss of ability to maintain airway
( ) Respiratory depression
( ) Respiratory arrest
( ) Hypotension
( ) Severely slurred speech
( ) Combativeness or agitation
Describe treatment
rendered _____
Describe patient
outcome _____

Association of Operating Room Nurses

RECOMMENDED PRACTICES FOR MANAGING THE PATIENT RECEIVING CONSCIOUS SEDATION/ANALGESIA

The following recommended practices were developed by the AORN Recommended Practices Committee and have been approved by the AORN Board of Directors. They were published as proposed recommended practices through the AORN fax-on-demand system for comments by members and others. They are effective January 1, 1997.

These recommended practices are intended as achievable recommendations representing what is believed to be an optimal level of practice. Policies and procedures will reflect variations in practice settings and/or clinical situations that determine the degree to which the recommended practices can be implemented.

AORN recognizes the numerous types of settings in which perioperative nurses practice. These recommended practices are intended as guidelines adaptable to various practice settings. These practice settings include traditional ORs, ambulatory surgery units, physicians' offices, cardiac catheterization suites, endoscopy suites, radiology departments, and all other areas where operative and other invasive procedures may be performed.

PURPOSE

"Sedation and analgesia describes a state which allows patients to tolerate unpleasant procedures while maintaining adequate cardiorespiratory function and the ability to respond purposefully to verbal command and/or tactile stimulation. Patients whose only response is reflex withdrawal from a painful stimulus are sedated to a greater degree than encompassed by sedation/analgesia."[1]

These recommended practices provide guidelines for RNs managing patients receiving conscious sedation/analgesia. Patient selection for conscious sedation/analgesia should be based on established criteria developed through interdisciplinary collaboration of health care professionals. The type of monitoring used with patients who receive conscious sedation/analgesia, the medications selected, and the interventions taken must be within the defined scope of perioperative nursing practice.

Certain patients are not candidates for conscious sedation/analgesia with monitoring by RNs. These patients may require more extensive monitoring and sedation, as provided by anesthesia care providers, and should be identified in consultation with anesthesiologists, surgeons, and other physicians. It is not the intent of these recommended practices to address situations that require the services of anesthesia care providers.

The patient care and monitoring guidelines in these recommended practices may be exceeded at any time. Their intent is to encourage quality patient care; however, implementation of these recommended practices cannot guarantee specific patient outcomes. These recommended practices are subject to revision as warranted by advances in nursing practice and technology.

RECOMMENDED PRACTICE I

Registered nurses should understand the goals and objectives of conscious sedation/analgesia.

INTERPRETIVE STATEMENT 1. The primary goal of conscious sedation/analgesia is to reduce the patient's anxiety and discomfort so as to facilitate cooperation between the patient and the caregivers. Conscious sedation/analgesia can be used as an adjunct to local anesthesia during the procedure.

RATIONALE. Adequate preoperative preparation and verbal reassurances from RNs facilitate the desired effects of conscious sedation/analgesia and may allow for a decrease of the dosages of opioids, benzodiazepines, and sedatives used.[2]

INTERPRETIVE STATEMENT 2. Objectives for the patient receiving conscious sedation/analgesia include

- alteration of mood;
- maintenance of consciousness;
- enhanced cooperation;
- elevation of the pain threshold;
- minimal variation of vital signs;
- some degree of amnesia; and
- a rapid, safe return to activities of daily living.

RATIONALE. Conscious sedation/analgesia produces a condition in which the patient exhibits a depressed level of consciousness but retains the ability to independently respond appropriately to verbal commands or physical stimulation. Misunderstanding the objectives of conscious sedation/analgesia may jeopardize the quality of patient care.[3]

RECOMMENDED PRACTICE II

The RN monitoring the patient who receives conscious sedation/analgesia should have no other responsibilities that would require the nurse to leave the patient unattended or compromise continuous patient monitoring during the procedure.

INTERPRETIVE STATEMENT 1. The RN should provide continuous monitoring of the patient who receives conscious sedation/analgesia. The RN must be able to immediately recognize and respond to adverse physiologic and psychological changes during the procedure.

RATIONALE. It is unrealistic to assume that one RN can perform circulating duties and also provide continuous monitoring, physical care, and emotional support for the patient who receives conscious sedation/analgesia.[4]

RECOMMENDED PRACTICE III

The RN monitoring the patient's care should be clinically competent in the function and in the use of resuscitation medications and monitoring equipment and be able to interpret the data obtained from the patient.

INTERPRETIVE STATEMENT 1. The RN who is monitoring the patient should understand how to operate monitoring equipment used during conscious sedation/analgesia.

RATIONALE. Knowledge of the function and proper use of monitoring equipment is essential for providing safe patient care.[5]

INTERPRETIVE STATEMENT 2. The nurse who is monitoring the patient should demonstrate knowledge of

- anatomy and physiology;
- pharmacology of medications used for conscious sedation/analgesia;
- cardiac arrhythmia interpretation;
- possible complications related to the use of conscious sedation/analgesia; and
- respiratory functions (ie, oxygen delivery, transport, uptake).

RATIONALE. Medications used for conscious sedation/analgesia may cause rapid, adverse physiologic responses in the patient. Early detection of such responses allows for rapid intervention and treatment.[6]

INTERPRETIVE STATEMENT 3. The RN who is monitoring the patient should be competent in the use of oxygen delivery devices and airway management.

RATIONALE. Rapid intervention is necessary in the event of complications from the undesired effects of conscious sedation/analgesia.[7]

DISCUSSION. The airway management skill level of the RN who is monitoring the patient receiving conscious sedation/analgesia should be defined by the health care facility's policies and procedures. Basic cardiac life support, which includes maintenance of the patient's airway by use of the head-tilt or chin-lift maneuver, is considered a basic competency for all RNs. The use of oxygen delivery devices (eg, respirator bag, face mask device) may be included as part of the orientation and continuing education process for RNs who monitor patients receiving conscious sedation/analgesia. Advanced cardiac life support (ACLS) certification may be required in some health care facilities. Health care professionals with

ACLS skills (eg, ACLS team members, anesthesia care providers) should be readily available to every location in which conscious sedation/analgesia is being administered.

INTERPRETIVE STATEMENT 4. Health care facilities should provide competency-based education programs for all RNs who manage patients undergoing conscious sedation/analgesia. These programs should offer a variety of learning opportunities based on learners' needs.

RATIONALE. The facility should have an education/competency validation mechanism in place that includes a process for evaluating and documenting RNs' demonstration of knowledge, skills, and abilities related to the management of patients receiving conscious sedation/analgesia. Evaluation and documentation of competence should occur on a periodic basis according to the health care facility's policies and procedures.[8]

RECOMMENDED PRACTICE IV

Each patient who will receive conscious sedation/analgesia should be assessed physiologically and psychologically before the procedure. The assessment should be documented in the patient's record.

INTERPRETIVE STATEMENT 1. A preprocedure patient assessment should include a review of:

- physical examination findings;
- current medications;
- drug allergies/sensitivities;
- current medical problems (eg, hypertension, diabetes, cardiopulmonary disease, liver disease, renal disease);
- tobacco smoking and substance abuse history;
- chief complaint;
- baseline vital signs, including height, weight, and age;
- level of consciousness;
- emotional state;
- communication ability; and
- perceptions regarding the procedure and conscious sedation/analgesia.

RATIONALE. A preprocedure assessment provides health care professionals baseline data and identifies the patient's risk factors.[9]

RECOMMENDED PRACTICE V

Each patient who receives conscious sedation/analgesia should be monitored for adverse reactions to medications and for physiologic and psychological changes.

INTERPRETIVE STATEMENT 1. The RN who administers medications for conscious sedation/analgesia should be responsible for understanding the medications'

- indications and dosages,
- contraindications,
- adverse reactions and emergency management techniques,
- interactions with other medications,
- onset and duration of action, and
- desired effects.

RATIONALE. Patient anxiety and medications used for conscious sedation/ analgesia may cause rapid, adverse physiologic and psychological changes in the patient.[10]

INTERPRETIVE STATEMENT 2. The RN who monitors the patient receiving conscious sedation/analgesia should be knowledgeable of the desirable and undesirable medication effects of conscious sedation/analgesia.

RATIONALE. Observation of the patient for desired therapeutic medication effects, prevention of avoidable medication reactions, early detection and management of unexplained adverse reactions, and accurate documentation of the patient's response are integral components of the monitoring process.[11]

DISCUSSION. Desirable effects of conscious sedation/analgesia include

- intact protective reflexes,
- relaxation,
- comfort,
- cooperation,
- diminished verbal communication,
- patent airway with adequate ventilatory exchange, and
- easy arousal from sleep.

Potential complications of conscious sedation/analgesia include

- aspiration,
- severely slurred speech,
- unarousable sleep,
- hypotension,
- agitation,
- combativeness,
- hypoventilation,
- respiratory depression,
- airway obstruction, and
- apnea.

INTERPRETIVE STATEMENT 3. Before conscious sedation is administered, an oxygen delivery device should be in place or immediately available, an IV access line should be established, and appropriate monitoring devices should be in place.

RATIONALE. Sedatives and benzodiazepines used for conscious sedation/analgesia may case somnolence, confusion, coma, diminished reflexes, and depressed respiratory and cardiovascular functions. Opioids used for conscious sedation/

analgesia may cause respiratory depression, hypotension, nausea, and vomiting. Overdosage and adverse reactions may occur any time during the procedure and may be reversible.[12]

DISCUSSION. The following equipment should be present and ready for use in the room in which conscious sedation/analgesia is administered:

- oxygen,
- suction apparatus,
- oxygen delivery devices,
- noninvasive blood pressure device,
- electrocardiograph, and
- pulse oximeter.

Monitoring parameters should include

- respiratory rate,
- oxygen saturation,
- blood pressure,
- cardiac rate and rhythm,
- level of consciousness, and
- skin condition.

Undesirable changes in patient condition should be reported immediately to the physician.

INTERPRETIVE STATEMENT 4. Each patient who receives conscious sedation/analgesia intravenously should have continuous IV access. If medications are not administered intravenously, the need for IV access should be determined on a case-by-case basis. In all instances, an individual with the skills to establish IV access should be immediately available.

RATIONALE. Continuous IV access provides a means for administering medications used for conscious sedation/analgesia and for implementing emergency medications and fluids to counteract adverse medication effects.[13]

DISCUSSION. Continuous IV access may be obtained using an IV access device or by infusing IV fluids through an access port. The type of continuous IV access chosen will vary depending on health care facilities' policies and procedures and physicians' preferences.

INTERPRETIVE STATEMENT 5. An emergency cart with appropriate resuscitative medications, including narcotic and sedative reversal medications, and equipment (eg, defibrillator) should be immediately available to every location in which conscious sedation/analgesia is being administered.

RATIONALE. Medication overdoses or adverse reactions may cause respiratory depression, hypotension, or impaired cardiovascular function requiring immediate intervention and/or cardiopulmonary resuscitation (CPR).[14] Equipment for CPR or emergency medication reversals should be available for immediate use because diminished reflexes, depressed respiratory function, and impaired cardiovascular function may occur within seconds or minutes after the administration of medications used for conscious sedation/analgesia.[15]

RECOMMENDED PRACTICE VI

Documentation of patient care during conscious sedation/analgesia should be consistent with the AORN "Recommended practices for documentation of perioperative nursing care" wherever conscious sedation/analgesia is administered.

INTERPRETIVE STATEMENT 1. Nursing diagnoses applicable to patients receiving conscious sedation/analgesia may include the potential for

- anxiety related to the unfamiliar environment and procedure,
- ineffective breathing patterns or impaired gas exchange related to altered level of consciousness or airway obstruction,
- knowledge deficit related to poor recall secondary to medication effects,
- cardiac output changes related to medication effects on the myocardium, and
- injury related to altered level of consciousness.

RATIONALE. Use of nursing diagnoses for planning the care of patients who receive conscious sedation/analgesia provides for patient care that focuses on patients' responses to the procedures and/or nursing interventions. Nursing interventions are directed toward positive patient outcomes.[16]

INTERPRETIVE STATEMENT 2. Documentation should include:

- preprocedure assessment;
- dosage, route, time, and effects of all medications and fluids used;
- type and amount of fluids administered, including blood and blood products, monitoring devices, and equipment used;
- physiologic data from continuous monitoring at 5- to 15-minute intervals and upon significant events;
- level of consciousness;
- nursing interventions taken and the patient's responses; and
- untoward significant patient reactions and their resolution.

RATIONALE. Documentation of nursing interventions promotes continuity of patient care and improves communication among health care team members. Documentation also provides a mechanism for comparing actual versus expected patient outcomes.[17]

RECOMMENDED PRACTICE VII

Patients who receive conscious sedation/analgesia should be monitored postprocedure, receive verbal and written discharge instructions, and meet specified criteria before discharge.

DISCUSSION. Postprocedure patient care, monitoring, and discharge criteria should be consistent for all patients. Patients and their family members or caregivers should receive verbal and written discharge instructions and verbalize an understanding of the instructions to the nurse. Preprocedure and postprocedure instructions, as well as verbalization of understanding, is encouraged because medications used for conscious sedation/analgesia may cause significant patient amnesia that directly affects recall ability.[18]

Discharge guidelines provide specific criteria for assessing and evaluating the patient's readiness for discharge and home care. Discharge criteria should reflect indications that the patient has returned to a safe physiologic level. These indicators should include

- adequate respiratory function;
- stability of vital signs, including temperature;
- preprocedure level of consciousness;
- intact protective reflexes;
- return of motor/sensory control;
- absence of protracted nausea;
- skin color and condition;
- satisfactory surgical site and dressing condition when present; and
- absence of significant pain.[19]

The presence of a responsible adult escort is necessary for discharge. Discharge criteria should be developed by representatives from the medical staff, anesthesia, nursing, and other departments as appropriate.

RECOMMENDED PRACTICE VIII

Policies and procedures for managing patients who receive conscious sedation/analgesia should be written, reviewed periodically, and readily available within the practice setting.

DISCUSSION. Policies and procedures for managing patients receiving conscious sedation/analgesia should include

- patient selection criteria,
- extent of and responsibility for monitoring,
- method of recording patient data,
- data to be documented,
- frequency of the patient's physiologic data documentation,
- medications that may be administered by the RN, and
- discharge criteria.

Policies and procedures are operational guidelines that are used to minimize patient risk factors, standardize practice, assist staff members, and establish guidelines for continuous quality improvement activities by establishing authority, responsibility, and accountability.

GLOSSARY

Benzodiazepines: A pharmacologic family of central nervous system depressants possessing anxiolytic, hypnotic, and skeletal muscle-relaxant properties. These medications are used to allay anxiety and fear and produce varying amnesic effects during conscious sedation/analgesia. Diazepam and midazolam are two benzodiazepines commonly used for conscious sedation/analgesia.

Conscious sedation/analgesia: A minimally depressed level of consciousness that allows a surgical patient to retain the ability to independently and continuously maintain a patent airway and respond appropriately to verbal commands and physical stimulation.

Managing the patient: The use of the nursing process to deliver and direct comprehensive nursing care during a procedure in a practice setting.

Monitoring: Clinical observation that is individualized to patient needs based on data obtained from preprocedure patient assessments. The objective of monitoring patients who receive conscious sedation/analgesia is to improve patient outcomes. Monitoring includes the use of mechanical devices and direct observation.

Opioid: Natural or synthetic pharmacologic agents that produce varying degrees of analgesia and sedation and relieve pain. Fentanyl and meperidine hydrochloride are two opioid analgesic medications that may be used for conscious sedation/analgesia.

Sedatives: Pharmacologic agents that reduce anxiety and may induce some degree of short-term amnesia.

NOTES

1. American Society of Anesthesiologists, *Guidelines for Sedation and Analgesia by Non-Anesthesiologists,* (American Society of Anesthesiologists: Park Ridge, Ill, 1995).
2. D S Watson, D S James, "Intravenous conscious sedation: Implications of monitoring patients receiving local anesthesia," *AORN Journal* 51 (June 1990) 1513–1522.
3. *Ibid;* "Position statement on the role of the RN in the management of patients receiving IV conscious sedation for short-term therapeutic, diagnostic, or surgical procedures," *AORN Journal* 55 (January 1992) 207–208; Watson, James, "Intravenous conscious sedation: Implications of monitoring patients receiving local anesthesia," 1513.
4. "Position statement on the role of the RN in the management of patients receiving IV conscious sedation for short-term therapeutic, diagnostic, or surgical procedures," 207–208; Watson, James, "Intravenous conscious sedation: Implications of monitoring patients receiving local anesthesia," 1520.
5. Watson, James, "Intravenous conscious sedation: Implications of monitoring patients receiving local anesthesia," 1522.
6. *Ibid,* 1520.
7. *Ibid,* 1512.
8. "Position statement on the role of the RN in the management of patients receiving IV conscious sedation for short-term therapeutic, diagnostic, or surgical procedures," 207–208.
9. J A Kidwell, "Nursing care for the patient receiving conscious sedation during gastrointestinal endoscopic procedures," *Gastroenterology Nursing* 13 (Winter 1991)

136–137; Watson, James, "Intravenous conscious sedation: Implications of monitoring patients receiving local anesthesia," 1514.

10. Watson, James, "Intravenous conscious sedation: Implications of monitoring patients receiving local anesthesia," 1520.

11. *Ibid,* 1514; Kidwell, "Nursing care for the patient receiving conscious sedation during gastrointestinal endoscopic procedures," 137–138.

12. Watson, James, "Intravenous conscious sedation: Implications of monitoring patients receiving local anesthesia," 1514, 1517.

13. Kidwell, "Nursing care for the patient receiving conscious sedation during gastrointestinal endoscopic procedures," 137.

14. Watson, James, "Intravenous conscious sedation: Implications of monitoring patients receiving local anesthesia," 1516, 1520.

15. P L Bailey et al, "Frequent hypoxemia and apnea after sedation with midazolam and fentanyl," *Anesthesiology* 73 (November 1990) 826–830; "Position statement on the role of the RN in the management of patients receiving IV conscious sedation for short-term therapeutic, diagnostic, or surgical procedures," 208.

16. S V M Kleinbeck, "Introduction to the nursing process," in *Perioperative Nursing Care Planning,* ed J C Rothrock (St. Louis: The C V Mosby Co, 1990) 8.

17. "Recommended practices for documentation of perioperative nursing care," in *AORN Standards and Recommended Practices* (Denver: Association of Operating Room Nurses, Inc, 1996) 151–153.

18. Watson, James, "Intravenous conscious sedation: Implications of monitoring patients receiving local anesthesia," 1513.

19. *Standards of Perianesthesia Nursing Practice: 1996* (Thorofare, NJ: American Society of Post Anesthesia Nurses, 1995) 45.

SUGGESTED READING

American Association of Nurse Anesthetists. *American Association of Nurse Anesthetists Guidelines for Practice of the Certified Registered Nurse Anesthetist.* Park Ridge Ill: American Association of Nurse Anesthetists, 1983.

Originally published April 1993, *AORN Journal,* as "Recommended practices for monitoring the patient receiving intravenous conscious sedation." Revised November 1996; to be published January 1997, *AORN Journal.*

APPENDIX C

American Association of Nurse Anesthetists Latex Allergy Protocol

This latex allergy protocol was developed by the AANA Infection/Environmental Control Task Force and was approved by the AANA Board of Directors in April 1993.

INTRODUCTION

In the past four to five years, latex allergy has been recognized as a significant problem for specific patients (e.g., patients with spina bifida requiring multiple surgeries) and healthcare workers.[1]

Approximately 0.8% of the population is latex sensitive. However, patients and/or healthcare workers who have frequent exposure to latex devices such as gloves, catheters, and drains may be sensitized.[2] It has been reported that 6–7% of surgical personnel and 18–40% of spina bifida patients are latex sensitive.[3] It is estimated that 7.5% of surgeons and 5.6% of nurses are sensitive to latex or the chemicals used in processing latex.[2] Latex, the sap of the rubber tree *Hevea Brasiliensis,* contains low molecular weight soluble proteins which are the likely allergy cause. New rubber products, especially very soft ("dipped") products contain the greatest proportion of these soluble proteins.[3]

Immediate hypersensitivity reactions to latex vary from contact urticaria to systemic anaphylaxis that requires lifesaving intervention.

Anaphylactic reactions have complicated a variety of common medical procedures including surgery (particularly of the genitourinary tract) and anesthesia, barium enemas, as well as oral, vaginal, and rectal examinations utilizing latex gloves. In most cases, there has been contact between latex products and mucous membranes. However, in some exquisitely sensitive individuals, exposure through inhalation of aerosolized latex or through intravenous administration has led to severe reactions. The type of reactions is similar to immediate drug reactions or stinging insect venom and may be associated with rapidly progressive anaphylaxis and death.[1]

The most reliable screening test for predicting an anaphylaxic reaction to latex is a medical history, as sensitive and specific reagents for testing for latex allergy are not commercially available at this time.[1]

POPULATION CONSIDERED HIGH RISK FOR DEVELOPING LATEX ALLERGY

Individuals considered high risk for developing latex allergy should be labeled *latex risk,* and those that have known or suspected allergy to latex should be labeled *latex allergy.*

Patients (particularly of the pediatric age group) who are considered *high risk* include:

- Those with neural tube defects—
  Myelomeningocele/meningocele
  Spina bifida
  Lipomyelomeningocele
- Patients requiring chronic bladder catheterizations—
  Spinal cord trauma
  Exstrophy of the bladder
  Neurogenic bladder
- Patients that have multiple operations
- Those with a history of atopy and multiple allergies, including food allergies
- Patient with occupational exposure to latex—
  Workers in latex industry
  Healthcare workers
- Those with a history of allergic reaction after touching balloons, rubber gloves or powder from rubber gloves, dental dams, latex consumer products, and medical devices; especially atopic patients
- Those with a history of having experienced anaphylactic reaction during surgery, urinary catheterization, rectal or vaginal examination, and/or bladder stimulation
- Healthcare personnel and others who wear latex gloves, due to the generalized usage of universal precautions, may become sensitized.
- Healthcare providers or other workers who give a history of mild latex glove eczema rarely have anaphylactic events. However, a history of severe or worsening latex glove induced eczema, urticaria, or work-related conjunctivitis, rhinitis, asthma, or urticaria may indicate allergic sensitization and increase the risk for more severe reactions in the future.

LATEX AVOIDANCE PRECAUTIONS

By touching any latex object, the healthcare worker can transmit the allergen by hand to the patient. Caution should be taken to keep the powder from the gloves away from the patient because the powder will act as a carrier for the latex protein. Therefore, in order to reduce the possibility of the latex protein becoming airborne, care must be taken not to snap gloves on and off.

Patients should be identified as being *latex sensitive.* The room needs to be labeled *latex free* to avoid personnel from bringing rubber products (wrist bands, chart labels, bed, room signs, etc.) into the room.

A readily available master list of *latex-free* devices and products should be developed.*

Establish a latex consultant in your institution; an allergist is recommended.

Develop programs to educate healthcare workers in the care of *latex-sensitive* patients.

Develop educational programs for patients and their families in the care and precautions that should be taken to prevent latex exposure. This should encompass a first-aid protocol in the event a severe reaction should arise.

Encourage *latex-sensitive* patients to obtain and carry with them, at all times, some type of identification such as a medical alert bracelet.

RECOMMENDATIONS FOR PATIENT CARE— PATIENTS WITH LATEX ALLERGY OR LATEX RISK[1,4,5]

Schedule *latex-allergy* and/or *latex-risk* patients as the first case(s) in the morning. This will allow latex dust (from the previous day) to be removed overnight.

The Operating Room

- Remove all latex products from the operating room.
- Bring a *latex-free* cart (if available) into the room.
- Use a *latex-free* reservoir bag.
- Use a *non-latex* circuit with plastic mask and bag.
- Ventilator bellows must be a *non-latex* bellows.
- Place all monitoring devices, cords/tubes (oximeter, blood pressure, ECG wires) in stockinet and secure with tape.

Intravenous Line Preparation

- Use intravenous (IV) tubing without latex ports.
- If unable to obtain IV tubing without latex ports, cover latex ports with tape.
- Cover all rubber injection ports on IV bags with tape and label in the following way: *Do not inject or withdraw fluid through the latex port.*

Operating Room Patient Care

- Use *non-latex* gloves. *(Use caution when selecting non-latex gloves. Not all substitutes are equally impermeable to bloodborne pathogens; care and investigation should be taken in the selection of substitute gloves.)*
- Use *non-latex* tourniquets/may use *non-latex* examination glove or polyvinyl chloride tubing.
- Draw medication directly from opened multidose vials (remove stoppers) if medications are not available in ampoules.

---

*A sample letter to manufacturers requesting latex information and resource articles regarding latex allergy are available in a *Latex Packet* from the Practice Department, American Association of Nurse Anesthetists, 222 South Prospect Avenue, Park Ridge, IL 60068-4001. Phone: (708) 692-7050, ext. 305.

- Draw up medications just prior to the beginning of the case. The rubber allergen could leach out of the plunger of the syringe causing a reaction.
- Glass syringes are another alternative.
- Use stopcocks to inject drugs rather than latex ports.
- Minimize mixing/agitating lyophilized drugs in multidose vials with rubber stoppers.
- Notify Pharmacy and Central Supply that the patient you are caring for is latex sensitive so that these departments can use the appropriate procedure when preparing preparations for the patient.

SIGNS AND SYMPTOMS OF ALLERGIC REACTIONS TO LATEX[6]

Symptoms usually occur within 30 minutes from anesthesia induction. However, the time of onset can range from 10–290 minutes.

Awake Patient	Anesthetized Patient
Itchy eyes	Tachycardia
Generalized pruritis	Hypotension
Shortness of breath	Wheezing
Feeling of faintness	Bronchospasm
Feeling of impending doom	Cardiorespiratory arrest
Nausea	Flushing
Vomiting	Facial edema
Abdominal cramping	Laryngeal edema
Diarrhea	Urticaria
Wheezing	

MANAGEMENT

All the following should be done to manage a latex allergic reaction:

- Remove latex agents, if possible. **Do not delay immediate emergency therapy.**
- Stop treatment/procedure.
- Support airway—administer 100% oxygen.*
- Start intravascular volume expansion with **Ringer's lactate*** or **normal saline.***
- Administer **epinephrine*** 0.5–1.0 µg/kg bolus (10 µg/mL dilution). May need to repeat dose or give subcutaneously or by continuous infusion.

Secondary Treatment

- **Diphenhydramine*** 1 mg/kg IV (maximum dose 50 mg).
- **Methylprednisolone*** 2 mg/kg IV (maximum dose 125 mg).
- **Ranitidine*** 0.5 mg/kg IV every 6 hours for 2–4 doses (maximum dose 50 mg).

---

*These drugs and fluids should be readily available for timely administration.

RECOMMENDED PREMEDICATION PRIOR TO PROCEDURE[5,6]

The use of preoperative prophylaxis may not change the rate of anaphylaxis but may lessen the severity of a reaction. All of the following are recommended:

Outpatient

- **Prednisone:** 1 mg/kg by mouth every 6 hours (maximum dose 40 mg/dose) for 12–24 hours prior to the patient arriving at the hospital and 1 hour prior to the induction of anesthesia
- **Hydroxyzine:** 0.7 mg/kg by mouth every 6 hours (maximum dose 50 mg/dose) for 12–24 hours prior to the patient arriving at the hospital and 1 hour prior to the induction of anesthesia

Inpatient

- **Methylprednisolone:** 1 mg/kg IV every 6 hours for 2–4 doses (maximum dose 125 mg)
- **Diphenhydramine:** 1 mg/kg IV every 6 hours for 2–4 doses (maximum dose 50 mg)
- **Ranitidine:** 0.5 mg/kg IV every 6 hours for 2–4 doses (maximum dose 50 mg)

Medication may be discontinued postoperatively if there is no evidence of an allergic reaction intraoperatively or postoperatively.

Inpatients with known *latex allergy* should be continued on the inpatient protocol for 24 hours postoperatively.

COMMON LATEX MEDICAL DEVICES USED IN THE HOSPITAL[4-6]

- Mattresses found on stretchers
- Rubber gloves
- Adhesive tape
- Urinary catheters
- Electrode pads
- Wound drains
- Stomach and intestinal tubes
- Condom urinary collection devices
- Protective sheets
- Enema tubing kits
- Dental cofferdams
- Rubber pads
- Fluid circulating warming blankets
- Hemodialysis equipment
- Ambu bags
- Bulb syringes
- Elastic bandages, Ace™ wraps

- Medication vial stoppers
- Stethoscope tubing
- Band-Aids™ and other similar products
- Gloves—examination and sterile
- Patient controlled analgesia syringes
- Tourniquets

ANESTHESIA EQUIPMENT CONTAINING LATEX

- Rubber masks
- Electrode pads, e.g., electrocardiogram, peripheral nerve stimulator
- Head straps
- Rubber tourniquets
- Rubber nasal-pharyngeal airways
- Rubber oral-pharyngeal airways
- Teeth protectors
- Bite blocks
- Blood pressure cuffs (inner bladder and tubing)
- Rubber breathing circuits
- Reservoir breathing bags
- Rubber ventilator hoses
- Rubber ventilator bellows
- Rubber endotracheal tubes
- Latex cuffs on plastic tracheal tubes
- Latex injection ports on intravenous tubing
- Certain epidural catheter injection adapters
- Multidose vial stoppers
- Patient controlled analgesia syringes
- Rubber suction catheters
- Injection ports on intravenous bags

REFERENCES

1. *Interim Recommendations to Health Professionals and Organizations Regarding Latex Allergy Precautions.* Palatine, Illinois: American College of Allergy and Immunology. March 1992.
2. Latex Allergies: Anesthesia Concerns. *AANA NewsBulletin/Anesthesia Quality Plus.* 1992;46(9)(suppl):3.
3. U.S. Food and Drug Administration. Allergic reactions to latex-containing medical devices. *FDA Medical Bulletin.* 1991;21:2.
4. Holzman R. *Latex-Free Environment Precautions for Patients with a Latex Allergy/Patients at High Risk for Latex Allergy.* Boston, Massachusetts: Boston Children's Hospital (Departmental Policy). 1992.
5. Pasquariello CA, Lowe DA. *Protocol for the Management of Patients with Allergy and Risk for Allergy to Latex Products.* Department of Anesthesia and Critical Care, St. Christopher's Hospital for Children, Philadelphia, Pennsylvania. 1992.
6. Roy CA, Barton CR. Intraoperative latex anaphylaxis compounded by atracurium sensitivity: A case report. *AANA Journal.* 1991;59:399–404.

APPENDIX D

Conscious Sedation Medications Pharmacologic Profile

Alfentanil Hydrochloride
(Alfenta)

Classification: Opioid agonist

Schedule: Alfentanil is subject to Schedule II control under the Controlled Substances Act of 1970.

Clinical Pharmacology: Alfentanil is an opioid analgesic with rapid onset of action. Alfentanil is $\frac{1}{5}$ to $\frac{1}{10}$ as potent as fentanyl and has $\frac{1}{3}$ the duration of action of fentanyl. Lower doses provide analgesia while higher doses promote hypnosis and attenuate catecholamine response. Opioids bind to opiate receptors located throughout the CNS. Opioid receptors that have been identified include mu, kappa, delta, and sigma. The pharmacodynamic properties of each opioid are dependent on which specific opioid receptor is occupied.

Onset: *IV:* 1 to 2 minutes

Peak Effect: *IV:* 1 to 2 minutes

Duration: *IV:* 10 to 15 minutes

Indications: For use as an adjunct in the maintenance of anesthesia, continuous infusion, as a primary anesthetic agent, and as the analgesic component for monitored anesthesia care

Contraindications: Known hypersensitivity to alfentanil. Depressed ventilatory function, increased intracranial pressure.

Protein Binding: 92%

Half-Life: 98 minutes

Considerations: Individualize dose. Titrate medication to effect. Reduce dosage in elderly and debilitated patients.

Drug Interactions: Pronounced synergism and respiratory depression occurs when used in conjunction with CNS depressants (barbiturates, benzodiazepines).

Respiratory Effects: Apnea, respiratory depression, hypoxia, and bronchospasm, as well as diminished respiratory reserve. Extreme caution must be used in patients with pulmonary disease, decreased respiratory reserve, or compromised respiratory status. Dose-related muscle rigidity (particularly truncal rigidity) may occur. Facilities must be fully equipped to monitor and treat respiratory depression.

CV Effects: Arrhythmias, bradycardia, tachycardia, hypotension. Bradycardia may be treated with atropine.

CNS Effects: The magnitude and duration of CNS effects are enhanced when alfentanil is used with other CNS-depressant drugs. Dosages of alfentanil and other CNS-depressant drugs should be reduced when used in combination. Caution should be excercised in patients with increased intracranial pressure or head injury. Increased intracranial pressure is associated with the development of hypercapnia and the respiratory depressant effects associated with opioid use. Additional neurologic effects include confusion or euphoria.

Metabolism: Alfentanil is metabolized to inactive metabolites by hepatic mechanisms. Erythromycin can inhibit alfentanil metabolism.

Elimination: Excretion via urine.

Overdose: Signs and symptoms of narcotic overdose include decreased respiratory rate and volume, extreme somnolence, cold clammy skin, bradycardia, and hypotension. In the event of an overdose, maintenance of a patent airway, coupled with cardiac and respiratory support, is required. Ventilation and oxygenation must be maintained until the respiratory depressant effects have dissipated.

Reversal: Naloxone (Narcan) is a narcotic antagonist that will reverse the respiratory and cardiovascular depressant effects associated with alfentanil overdose. Naloxone may also reverse side effects associated with narcotic administration. These side effects include urinary retention, pruritus, respiratory depres-

sion, nausea, and vomiting. Careful titration is required to avoid full reversal of analgesia.

Patients treated with naloxone must remain adequately monitored and reassessed after the procedure to avoid the development of renarcotization and respiratory depression.

Dosage: Should be individualized and reduced in the elderly or debilitated, patients with renal/hepatic disease, or patients with hypothyroidism. Titration to individual patient response is required. If used for conscious sedation, slow IV injection is required.

Supplied: 500 µg/ml (in 2 ml, 5 ml, 10 ml, and 20 ml)

Atropine Sulfate

Classification: Anticholinergic
Clinical Pharmacology: Atropine is a white crystalline alkaloid. Atropine antagonizes the action of acetylcholine at the muscarinic receptor. Atropine decreases salivary, respiratory, and gastrointestinal secretions. Bronchial and lower esophageal sphincter muscle tone is relaxed. As a parasympatholytic medication, atropine increases sinus node automaticity and atrioventricular conduction through a direct vagolytic mechanism of action.
Onset: *IV:* 45 to 60 seconds; *IM:* 5 to 40 minutes; *intratracheal:* 10 to 20 seconds; *oral:* 30 minutes to 2 hours; *inhalation:* 3 to 5 minutes
Peak Effect: *IV:* 2 minutes; *inhalation:* 1 to 2 hours
Duration: *IV/IM* (vagal blockade): 1 to 2 hours
Indications: To decrease salivary, bronchial, and gastric secretions; treatment of sinus bradycardia, vagal episodes, and incorporation within the ACLS algorithm
Contraindications: Extreme care must be used in patients with tachyarrthymias, CHF, acute MI, myocardial ischemia, and myocardial infarction. Use with caution in patients with atrioventricular block at the

His Purkinje level (type II AV block and new third-degree blocks with wide QRS complexes).
Considerations: Large doses may produce mental disturbances, confusion, delirium, flushed, hot skin, and blurred vision. Obstructive uropathy and obstructive diseases of the GI tract. Transient decreases in heart rate have been associated with the administration of low dosages (< 0.5 mg) due to weak peripheral muscarinic effects.
Respiratory Effects: Respiratory depression in excessively large doses may be due to paralysis of the medullary center.
CV Effects: Tachycardia is associated with high dosages; bradycardia is associated with low dosages; palpitations.
CNS Effects: Confusion, hallucinations, drowsiness, excitement, and agitation
Metabolism: Enzymatic hydrolysis
Elimination: 13% to 50% of the drug is excreted unchanged in the urine.
Overdose: If marked excitement is present, a short-acting barbiturate or benzodiazepine may be used for sedation. Ice bags and alcohol sponges help to reduce fever in the presence of hot, flushed skin or febrile states, particularly in children.

Dosage: *Adult:* IV, IM: 0.5 to 1 mg. May be repeated every 3 to 5 minutes. A total of 40 µg/kg is a fully vagolytic dose in most patients.

Pediatrics: IV, IM: 10 to 20 µg/kg (minimum 0.1 mg)
Supplied: 0.3 mg/1 ml, 0.5 mg/ml, 0.8 mg/ml, 1 mg/ml, 0.4 mg/0.5 ml

Diazepam
(Valium)

Classification: Benzodiazepine agonist
Schedule: Diazepam is subject to Schedule IV control under the Controlled Substances Act of 1970.
Clinical Pharmacology: Diazepam is a benzodiazepine, which depresses the central nervous system to produce amnesia, anxiolysis, and a calming effect. The pharmacologic effect of benzodiazepines is primarily exerted via facilitated action of the inhibitory neurotransmitter gamma-aminobutyric acid (GABA). This GABA interaction enhances the inhibitory effects of various neurotransmitters. Benzodiazepines affect the limbic system, thalamus, and hypothalamus, producing a calm, sedate state. The effects of diazepam on the central nervous system are based on
- Dose administered
- Route of administration
- Presence of other premedicants
- Concurrent medications administered (opioids)

Diazepam is the benzodiazepine to which all other benzodiazepines are compared. It possesses a long half-life, active metabolites, and a propylene glycol suspension that causes pain on injection.
Onset: *IV:* 5 minutes; *oral:* 15 to 60 minutes
Peak Effect: *IV:* 3 to 5 minutes; *oral:* 30 to 90 minutes
Duration: *IV:* 15 to 60 minutes; *oral:* 3 to 8 hours
Indications: Anxiety, acute alcohol withdrawal, skeletal muscle spasm, sedation, conscious sedation procedures, preoperative sedation, status epilepticus, severe recurrent seizures
Contraindications: Known hypersensitivity to diazepam. Acute narrow-angle

glaucoma, untreated open-angle glaucoma, shock, coma, acute alcohol intoxication, and children under 6 months of age
Protein Binding: 98%
Half-Life: 21 to 37 hours
Considerations: When given intravenously, diazepam must be injected slowly (1 minute for each 5 mg). A large vein must be used to prevent venous irritation and possible thrombophlebitis. Use of hand and wrist veins may result in increased incidence of venous irritation. Extreme caution must be used to avoid extravasation or intra-arterial administration.
Drug Interactions: Drug effect is accentuated (synergism) by concomitant use of sedatives, hypnotics, or narcotic analgesics. Drug dosage should be decreased according to the type, amount, and time of administration of adjunct medications.

Complications associated with IV diazepam include venous thrombosis, phlebitis, local irritation, swelling, and vascular impairment. It is recommended not to mix or dilute the medication once it is withdrawn into the syringe. Administration via an intravenous Soluset should use the injection site closest to the IV catheter.
Respiratory Effects: Intravenous diazepam may cause respiratory depression and apnea. Extreme caution should be used in patients with decreased respiratory reserve. Coughing and laryngospasm have been reported with the administration of diazepam during endoscopic procedures.
CV Effects: Decreased systemic vascular resistance and cardiac output. Extreme caution should be used in critically ill or hypovolemic patients.
CNS Effects: Drowsiness, confusion, depression, dysarthria, headache, hypoactiv-

ity, slurred speech, syncope, vertigo, tremor, ataxia, restlessness, anterograde amnesia, venous irritation, blurred vision, diplopia, rash, urticaria, hiccoughs. May also cause increased CNS depression with concomitant administration of other CNS-depressant medications.

Physical and psychologic dependence has been reported as well as acute withdrawal after sudden discontinuation in addicted patients.

Metabolism: Hepatic metabolism yields metabolite (desmethyldiazepam) with active pharmacologic effect.

Elimination: Urine

Overdose: In the event of an overdose (respiratory depression, apnea, cardiovascular collapse), maintenance of a patent airway and respiratory and cardiovascular support are required. Reversal with flumazenil, which is a specific benzodiazepine antagonist, generally restores the patient to a clear-headed state. Patients must be continuously monitored after the procedure to assess for

- Resedation
- Respiratory depression
- Residual depressant effects of benzodiazepines

A complete pharmacologic profile of flumazenil and dosage guidelines are listed in this appendix.

Dosage: Individualized and titrated to effect. Prior to the planned procedure, 1 to 2 mg of intravenous diazepam titrated over 2 minutes may be administered. Additional 1 mg increments administered over several minutes provide sedation for the planned procedure. Additional time must be allowed to evaluate pharmacologic effect in geriatric or debilitated patients or patients with decreased cardiac output. Do not administer by rapid or single bolus injection. Titration to effect includes administration of drug until somnolence, slurring of speech, or nystagmus occurs. Extreme care must be exercised when administering diazepam in the presence of concurrent opioid administration.

Supplied: *Injection:* 5 mg/ml; *emulsion:* 5 mg/ml; *tablets:* 2, 5, and 10 mg; *extended release capsules:* 15 mg; *oral solution:* 5 mg/5 ml or 5 mg/ml

Ephedrine

Classification: Nonselective, noncatecholamine adrenergic *stimulant*

Clinical Pharmacology: Ephedrine causes endogenous catecholamine release via indirect mechanism of action and stimulation of adrenergic receptors via a direct effect. Through these combined effects (alpha and beta stimulation), blood pressure, heart rate, contractility, and cardiac output increase. Ephedrine is also a bronchodilator via stimulation of $beta_2$ stimulation. Ephedrine is not as potent as epinephrine and has a longer duration of action.

Onset: *IV:* 30 to 45 seconds (immediate); *IM:* < 5 minutes

Peak Effect: *IV:* 2 to 5 minutes; *IM:* < 10 minutes

Duration: 10 to 60 minutes

Indications: Intraoperative treatment of hypotension, emergency treatment of hypotension of unknown origin

Contraindications: Cautious use in patients with hypertension, tachycardia, or unstable cardiovascular profile

Considerations: Tachyphylaxis occurs with repeated doses. However, temporary cessation of the drug restores its original effectiveness.

Drug Interactions: Decreased responsiveness has been observed in patients treated with beta-blockers. Unpredictable effects in patients with depleted catecholamine stores. Hypertensive crisis may occur in patients treated with MAO or tricyclic antidepressants.

Respiratory Effects: Pulmonary edema

CV Effects: Hypertension, tachycardia, arrhythmias

CNS Effects: Agitation, anxiety, insomnia, tremors
Metabolism: Hepatic
Elimination: Renal
Overdose: Signs and symptoms associated with an overdose (tachycardia, arrhythmias, hypertension, agitation) generally dissipate within several minutes. Symptoms associated with an exaggerated pharmacologic response may be treated with alpha- or beta-blockade.
Dosage: *Adults:* IV: 2.5 to 10 mg increments titrated to effect (0.1 to 0.2 µg/kg); IM: 25 to 50 mg; supplemental doses may be increased to prevent the development of tachyphylaxis.
   Children: 0.1 mg/kg titrated to effect.
Supplied: 50 mg/1 ml ampule

Epinephrine Hydrochloride
(Adrenalin)

Classification: Adrenergic agonist; sympathomimetic
Clinical Pharmacology: Epinephrine is a naturally occurring catecholamine, which is secreted from the adrenal medulla. It has both alpha (peripheral vasoconstriction) and beta (increase in heart rate, bronchodilation) activity. However, its most prominent actions are on the beta-receptors of the heart, vascular, and other smooth muscle. When given intravenously, it produces a rapid rise in blood pressure and direct stimulation of cardiac muscle (positive chronotropic and inotropic effects), which increases the strength of ventricular contraction and cardiac output.
Onset: *IV:* 30 to 60 seconds; *subcutaneous:* 6 to 15 minutes; *inhalation:* 3 to 5 minutes; *intratracheal:* 5 to 15 seconds
Peak Effect: 2 to 3 minutes
Duration: *IV:* 5 to 10 minutes; *intratracheal:* 15 to 25 minutes; *inhalational/subcutaneous:* 1 to 3 hours
Indications: Treatment of cardiac arrest, ventricular fibrillation, and asystole; conditions that require increased inotropy, bronchodilation, treatment of allergic reactions, and prolongation of local anesthetic activity
Contraindications: Cardiac dilation, coronary insufficiency, cardiovascular disorders, thyroid toxicosis, diabetes mellitus, and organic brain damage
Considerations: Caution in patients with hypertension, cardiovascular disease, diabetes, and hyperthyroidism. Contraindicated for intravenous regional anesthesia and local anesthesia to end organs (digits, ears, nose).
Drug Interactions: The cardiovascular effects of epinephrine may be potentiated by tricyclic antidepressants and antihistamines (diphenhydramine). Use with caution in patients taking MAO inhibitors. Vasodilators (alpha-blocking agents) may counteract the pressor effects of epinephrine.
Respiratory Effects: Pulmonary edema
CV Effects: Hypertension, tachycardia, chest pain
CNS Effects: Anxiety, headache, hemorrhage
Metabolism: Enzymatic degradation (hepatic, renal, and GI tract)
Elimination: Kidneys
Overdose: Excessive doses of epinephrine may result in precordial distress, vomiting, headache, dyspnea, and hypertension. Alpha- or beta-blockers may be required to counteract excessive dosage of epinephrine.
Dosage: *Cardiac arrest:* 1 mg or 0.02 mg/kg of 100 µg/ml solution. May be administered every 3 to 5 minutes per ACLS protocol.
   Inotropic support: 2 to 20 µg/minute or 0.1 to 1 µg/kg/minute.
   Anaphylactic reaction (epinephrine 1 mg/ml solution): adults: 0.1 to 0.5 mg SC/IM; pediatric: 0.01 mg/kg SC/IM, not to exceed 0.5 mg
Supplied: 0.01 mg/ml (10 µg/ml), 0.1 mg/ml (100 µg/ml), 0.5 mg/ml (500 µg/ml), 1 mg/ml (1000 µg/ml)

Fentanyl Citrate
(Sublimaze)

Classification: Opioid agonist

Schedule: Fentanyl is subject to Schedule II control under the Controlled Substances Act of 1970.

Clinical Pharmacology: Fentanyl is a phenylpiperidine derivative, which is a potent opioid agonist. The analgesic activity of 100 µg (2 ml) of fentanyl is equivalent to 10 mg of morphine or 75 mg of meperidine. It is approximately 75 to 125 times more potent than morphine. It has a rapid onset of action and a relatively short duration of action. Opioids bind to opiate receptors located throughout the CNS. Opioid receptors that have been identified include mu, kappa, delta, and sigma. The pharmacodynamic properties of each opioid are dependent on which specific opioid receptor is occupied. Fentanyl's principal actions are analgesia and sedation.

Onset: *IV:* 1 to 2 minutes; *IM:* 5 to 8 minutes; *transmucosal:* 5 to 15 minutes

Peak Effect: *IV:* 5 to 15 minutes; *IM:* 15 to 20 minutes; *transmucosal:* 1 to 2 hours

Duration: *IV:* 30 to 60 minutes; *IM:* 1 to 2 hours; *transmucosal:* 1 to 2 hours

Indications: Analgesic action of short duration during anesthetic periods, premedication, induction and maintenance of anesthesia. As a narcotic analgesic supplement in general or regional anesthesia.

Contraindications: Known hypersensitivity to fentanyl, depressed ventilatory function, increased intracranial pressure

Protein Binding: 80% protein bound

Half-Life: 1.5 to 6 hours

Considerations: Titration to effect is required. Dosage reduction and extreme caution must be used when administering to elderly, debilitated patients and patients susceptible to respiratory depression. Chest wall rigidity may result in inability to ventilate the patient.

Drug Interactions: Circulatory and respiratory depression. Profound synergism occurs when used with sedatives and CNS depressants.

Respiratory Effects: Respiratory depression may last longer than analgesic effects. As the dose of narcotic is increased, the degree of pulmonary exchange is decreased. Apnea, respiratory depression, and chest wall rigidity may occur. Extreme caution must be exercised when administered to patients with COPD, decreased respiratory reserve, and compromised respiratory status. Facilities must be fully equipped to monitor and treat respiratory depression.

CV Effects: Tachycardia, bradycardia, shock, cardiac arrest, palpitations, syncope, hypotension

CNS Effects: Euphoria, dysphoria, weakness, sedation, agitation, tremor. Extreme caution should be exercised with patients who have intracranial hypertension. Addition of CNS-depressant drugs produces a synergistic effect and potentiates the effects of CNS-depressant drugs.

Metabolism: Hepatic biotransformation

Elimination: Renal excretion. Caution should be exercised in elderly patients because of decreased clearance rates and those with liver and kidney disease.

Overdose: Signs and symptoms of narcotic overdose include decreased respiratory rate and volume, extreme somnolence, cold clammy skin, bradycardia, and hypotension. In the event of an overdose, maintenance of a patent airway, coupled with cardiac and respiratory support, is required. Ventilation and oxygenation must be maintained until the respiratory depressant effects have dissipated.

Reversal: Naloxone (Narcan) is a narcotic antagonist that will reverse the respiratory and cardiovascular depressant effects associated with fentanyl overdose. Naloxone may also reverse side effects associated with narcotic administration. These side effects include urinary retention, pruritus, respiratory depression, nausea, and vomiting. Careful titration is required to avoid full reversal of analgesia.

Patients treated with naloxone must remain adequately monitored and reassessed after the procedure to avoid the development of renarcotization and respiratory depression.

Dosage: 0.75 to 2 µg/kg titrated in 25 µg increments over several minutes.

Should be individualized and reduced in the elderly, debilitated, patients with renal/hepatic disease, or patients with hypothyroidism. Titration to individual patient response is required. If used for conscious sedation, slow IV injection is required.

Supplied: 50 µg/ml (in ampule of 2, 5, 10, 20, 30, or 50 ml)

Flumazenil
(Romazicon)

Classification: Benzodiazepine receptor antagonist

Clinical Pharmacology: Flumazenil is used for complete or partial reversal of benzodiazepine sedation. It competitively inhibits the activity of the benzodiazepine receptor sites on the GABA–benzodiazepine receptor complex. Flumazenil has been shown to antagonize sedation and psychomotor impairment. The duration and degree of reversal of benzodiazepine effects are related to total dose administered and plasma benzodiazepine concentrations.

Onset: *IV:* 1 to 2 minutes. An 80% response will be achieved within 3 minutes of administration.

Peak Effect: 6 to 10 minutes

Duration: 45 to 90 minutes. Duration of effect is dependent on the total benzodiazepine plasma concentration.

Indications: Complete or partial reversal of the sedative effects of benzodiazepines; management of benzodiazepine overdose

Contraindications: Known hypersensitivity to flumazenil or benzodiazepines. Patients on long-term benzodiazepine therapy for control of life-threatening conditions (status epilepticus) or in patients who show signs of serious cyclic antidepressant overdose.

Half-Life: 41 to 79 minutes

Considerations: Individualized dosage is required. The manufacturer does not recommend the administration of flumazenil to patients under the age of 18. The safety, efficacy, risks, and benefits have not been

established in this age group. Serious adverse effects of flumazenil are related to the reversal of benzodiazepine effects.

Use of more than the minimally effective doses is tolerated by most patients but may complicate the management of patients who are physically dependent on benzodiazepines. Flumazenil has been associated with seizures. Flumazenil-induced seizures have been reported in patients treated with benzodiazepines to control seizures and patients with chronic physical dependence on benzodiazepines. Patients who have responded to flumazenil should be carefully monitored (up to 120 minutes) for resedation. To avoid pain and inflammation at the site of injection, administration of flumazenil via a large vein is recommended.

Drug Interactions: Flumazenil is not recommended in cases of tricyclic antidepressant overdosage.

Respiratory Effects: Respiratory depression is related to the duration of effect of the benzodiazepine administered, which has exceeded the therapeutic effects of flumazenil.

CV Effects: Cutaneous vasodilatation, sweating, and flushing; arrythmias (atrial, nodal, ventricular extrasystole, bradycardia, tachycardia), and hypertension

CNS Effects: Dizziness, headache, abnormal or blurred vision, confusion, and convulsions

Other Adverse Effects: Fatigue, pain at the injection site, thrombophlebitis, or rash

Metabolism: Hepatic metabolism is dependent on hepatic blood flow.
Elimination: Inactive metabolites are excreted via the urine
Overdose: In the presence of benzodiazepine agonists, excessive doses of flumazenil result in anxiety, agitation, increased muscle tone, and possibly convulsions.
Dosage: Individualized dosage is required on the basis of patient response:

IV bolus: 0.2 mg over 1 minute (4 to 20 µg/kg). May repeat at 20-minute intervals. Maximum single dose = 1 mg. Not to exceed 3 mg in any 1-hour period.
Infusion: 30 to 60 µg/minute (0.5 to 1 µg/kg/minute). Total dose not to exceed 3 mg per hour.
Supplied: 0.1 mg/ml in 5 ml vials, 0.1 mg/ml in 10 ml vials

Hydromorphone Hydrochloride
(Dilaudid)

Classification: Opioid agonist
Schedule: Hydromorphone is subject to Schedule II control under the Controlled Substances Act of 1970.
Clinical Pharmacology: Hydromorphone is a semisynthetic opioid agonist (derivative of morphine). It is eight times as potent as morphine, with a shorter duration of action and a more rapid onset. It produces more sedation and less euphoria than morphine.
Onset: *IV:* 1 minute; *subcutaneous/IM:* 15 to 30 minutes; *oral:* 30 minutes
Peak Effect: *IV:* 15 to 30 minutes; *IM:* 30 to 60 minutes; *subcutaneous:* 30 to 90 minutes; *oral:* 1.5 to 3 hours
Duration: *IV:* 2 to 3 hours; *IM:* 4 to 5 hours; *subcutaneous/oral:* 4 hours
Indications: Analgesic agonist for the relief of moderate to severe pain
Contraindications: Known hypersensitivity to hydromorphone; increased intracranial pressure, depressed ventilatory function.
Protein Binding: < 30%
Half-Life: 2 to 3 hours
Considerations: Respiratory depression is dose related. Hydromorphone must be given slowly when used for IV administration (over 3 minutes). Rapid administration of hydromorphone increases narcotic-related side effects.
Drug Interactions: Hypotension, bradycardia, urinary retention, dysphoria, constipation, nausea, pruritus, urticaria. Pa-

tients taking other CNS depressants may have synergistic effects when hydromorphone is used. Decreased doses of hydromorphone are required when used in the presence of other CNS-depressant drugs.
Respiratory Effects: Respiratory depression, decreased respiratory rate, and tidal volume with resultant cyanosis and hypoxemia. Facilities must be fully equipped to monitor and treat respiratory depression.
CV Effects: Orthostatic hypotension, syncope, circulatory depression, bradycardia, hypotension
CNS Effects: Sedation, drowsiness, lethargy, mental/physical impairment, anxiety, fear, dysphoria, dizziness, mood alterations, psychologic dependence
Metabolism: Conjugation in the liver
Elimination: Excreted as glucuronidated conjugate via the kidney
Overdose: Signs and symptoms of narcotic overdose include decreased respiratory rate and volume, extreme somnolence, cold clammy skin, bradycardia, and hypotension. In the event of an overdose, maintenance of a patent airway, coupled with cardiac and respiratory support, is required. Ventilation and oxygenation must be maintained until the respiratory depressant effects have dissipated.
Reversal: Naloxone (Narcan) is a narcotic antagonist that will reverse the respiratory and cardiovascular depressant effects associated with hydromorphone overdose. Naloxone may also reverse side

effects associated with narcotic administration. These side effects include urinary retention, pruritus, respiratory depression, nausea, and vomiting. Careful titration is required to avoid full reversal of analgesia.

Patients treated with naloxone must remain adequately monitored and reassessed after the procedure to avoid the development of renarcotization and respiratory depression.

Dosage: Analgesia: *Slow intravenous administration:* 0.5 to 2 mg; *IM:* 2 to 4 mg (0.04 to 0.08 mg/kg).

Should be individualized and reduced in the elderly, debilitated, patient with renal/hepatic disease, or patients with hypothyroidism. Titration to individual patient response is required. If used for conscious sedation, slow IV injection is required.

Supplied: *Injection:* 1, 2, 3, and 4 mg/ml; *tablets:* 1, 2, 3, 4, and 8 mg; *oral solution:* 1 mg/ml; *suppositories:* 3 mg; *cough syrup:* 1 mg/5 ml with guaifenesin, 100 mg/5 ml; *HPJ:* 10 mg/ml *(only for postdilution use)*

Hydroxyzine Hydrochloride
(Vistaril)

Classification: Ataractic/antihistamine
Clinical Pharmacology: Hydroxyzine is a piperazine ataractic, which is effective in the management of neurosis and emotional disturbances (anxiety, tension, agitation, apprehension, and confusion). Pharmacologic activity may be related to reduced activity in subcortical areas of the central nervous system. Vistaril is often used in conjunction with narcotic premedication to produce a calming, anxiolytic effect.
Onset: *IM:* < 5 minutes
Peak Effect: 5 minutes
Duration: 4 to 6 hours
Indications: For the management of anxiety, tension, agitation during emotional stress conditions
Contraindications: Known hypersensitivity to hydroxyzine
Half-Life: *Adults:* 3 hours; *children:* 7 hours; *geriatrics:* 29 hours
Considerations: Hydroxyzine greatly potentiates CNS effects of depressant drugs, narcotics, and barbiturates. A reduction in dosage of these drugs by 50% is required when hydroxyzine is used.

Thrombosis, gangrene, and local irritation occur with extravasation of hydroxyzine. It should be given only in its oral (PO) or intramuscular (IM) form. For IM injection in adults the upper, outer quadrant of the buttocks or midlateral thigh is indicated.

Drug Interactions: Additive, synergistic actions occur when used with opiates, analgesics, sedatives, and barbiturates.
Respiratory Effects: Respiratory depression, hypoxia, and hypercarbia secondary to resultant synergism when combined with opiates and CNS-depressant medications
CV Effects: Mild antiarrhythmic activity, which is of minimal clinical significance
CNS Effects: Drowsiness, decreased anxiety, slurred speech, and dry mouth. Drowsiness generally dissipates with continued therapy.
Other Adverse Effects: Tremor, convulsions, and involuntary motor activity have been reported.
Metabolism: Liver
Elimination: Urine, feces via biliary elimination
Overdose: Treatment of hydroxyzine overdose is symptomatic and supportive. PO overdose is treated with induced emesis or gastric lavage. A secure airway and cardiovascular and respiratory support are required in the event of an overdose.
Dosage: As a preoperative adjunct: *adults IM:* 25 to 100 mg; *children IM:* 1 mg/kg
Supplied: *Tablets:* 10, 25, 50, and 100 mg; *capsules:* 25 mg and 50 mg; *oral syrup:* 10 mg/5 ml; *oral suspension:* 25 mg/5 ml; *injection:* 25 and 50 mg/ml

Ketamine

Classification: Dissociative anesthetic

Clinical Pharmacology: A phencyclidine derivative that produces rapid dissociative anesthesia, which causes the patient to appear conscious (eyes open, swallowing, enhanced laryngeal-pharyngeal reflexes, muscle contractures, respiratory stimulation). However, the patient loses the ability to process or respond to sensory input. The primary site of action appears to be the thalamoneocortical projection system. Through selective disorganization of nonspecific pathways in the midbrain and thalamic areas, it produces analgesia, amnesia, and unconsciousness. Central sympathetic stimulation occurs with systemic, pulmonary arterial pressure and heart rate and cardiac output increases. Ketamine also produces significant bronchodilation.

Onset: *IV:* <15 seconds; *IM/rectal:* 3 to 4 minutes

Peak Effect: *IV:* 1 minute; *IM/rectal:* 5 to 20 minutes

Duration: *IV:* 5 to 15 minutes; *IM/rectal:* 12 to 25 minutes

Indications: IV, IM anesthetic induction agent. Sedation/analgesia to supplement local and regional anesthesia.

Contraindications: Patients with increased intracranial pressure, open eye injury, or patients with psychiatric illness. Caution must be exercised in patients with ischemic heart disease.

Protein Binding: 12%

Half-Life: 3 hours

Considerations: Because of ketamine's ability to produce hypertension and tachy-

cardia, increased myocardial oxygen consumption occurs. Psychologic reactions (illusions, dreams, fear, anxiety, excitement, and out-of-body experiences), termed *emergence delirium,* occur in 40% of patients. Emergence reactions generally manifest within the first several hours of recovery and are diminished with the administration of small doses of benzodiazepines.

Drug Interactions: A combination of theophylline and ketamine may produce seizures. Diazepam and lithium prolong the elimination half-life of ketamine.

Respiratory Effects: Minimal decrease in ventilatory drive. Potent bronchodilator. Increased upper airway secretions are exhibited, particularly in children.

CV Effects: Hypertension, tachycardia, increased cardiac output

CNS Effects: Euphoria, unconsciousness, disassociation, and production of a cataleptic state; increase in intracranial pressure, cerebral oxygen consumption, and cerebral blood flow

Metabolism: Biotransformation to active and inactive metabolites

Elimination: Excretion via the kidney

Overdose: In the event of overdose, maintenance of a patent airway and respiratory and cardiovascular support are required.

Dosage: Sedation and analgesia: *IV:* 0.5 to 1 mg/kg; *IM/rectal:* 2.5 to 5 mg/kg; *oral:* 5 to 6 mg/kg diluted in 5 to 10 ml of solution

Supplied: 10 mg/ml (20, 25, and 50 ml vials), 50 mg/ml (10 ml vials), 100 mg/ml (5 ml vials)

Lidocaine Hydrochloride
(Xylocaine)

Classification: Antiarrhythmic

Clinical Pharmacology: Lidocaine is a sterile aqueous solution. It suppresses ventricular arrhythmias by decreasing automaticity and excitability via attenuation of

phase IV diastolic depolarization. Lidocaine raises the ventricular fibrillation threshold. It has been shown to cause little or no decrease in ventricular contractility, cardiac output, arterial pressure, or heart rate. Lidocaine readily crosses the placenta and blood/brain barriers.

Onset: *IV:* 45 to 90 seconds

Peak Effect: 1 to 2 minutes

Duration: 10 to 20 minutes

Indications: Treatment of ventricular arrhythmia

Contraindications: Known hypersensitivity to amide local anesthetics. Contraindicated in Stokes-Adams syndrome and Wolff-Parkinson-White syndrome. Severe degrees of SA, AV, or intraventricular block in the absence of an artificial pacemaker.

Protein Binding: 55%

Half-Life: 1.5 to 2 hours; may be increased two to three times for patients with liver dysfunction

Considerations: Dosage should be reduced in children and debilitated and elderly patients. Accumulation may occur in the presence of liver or kidney disease. Caution should be exercised when using lidocaine in the presence of hypovolemia, severe CHF, shock, and heart block.

In patients with sinus bradycardia or incomplete heart block, the IV administration of lidocaine for the elimination of ventricular ectopy may result in more frequent and serious ventricular arrhythmia or complete heart block.

Drug Interactions: Lidocaine should be used with caution in patients with digitalis toxicity. Clearance is reduced with concomitant use of beta-blockers and cimetidine.

Respiratory Effects: Respiratory depression, arrest

CV Effects: Hypotension, bradycardia, arrhythmias, and heart block

CNS Effects: Excitatory phenomena include light-headedness, nervousness, dizziness, apprehension, euphoria, confusion, drowsiness, tinnitus, blurred or double vision, vomiting, sensation of heat, cold, or numbness, twitching, tremors, convulsions, or unconsciousness.

Metabolism: Lidocaine is rapidly metabolized by the liver.

Elimination: 10% of the administered dose is excreted unchanged in the urine.

Overdose: Generally results in CNS or CV toxic manifestations. In the presence of convulsions, respiratory depression, or cardiac arrest, requires intubation and cardiovascular support. Use of benzodiazepines or barbiturates is effective in the treatment of convulsions.

Dosage: *Slow IV bolus:* 1 mg/kg (1% to 2% solution) or 50 to 100 mg at a rate of 25 to 50 mg/minute followed by 0.5 mg/kg every 2 to 5 minutes to a maximum of 3 mg/kg per hour. *Infusion:* 0.1% to 0.4% solution 1 to 4 mg/minute with use of a precision volume control IV pump for continuous IV infusion.

Supplied: 10 mg/ml in 5 ml vial/ampule, 10 mg/ml in 10 ml vial/ampule, 20 mg/ml in 5 ml ampule

Meperidine Hydrochloride
(Demerol)

Classification: Opioid agonist

Schedule: Meperidine is subject to Schedule II control under the Controlled Substances Act of 1970.

Clinical Pharmacology: Meperidine is a narcotic analgesic similar to morphine. Its principal therapeutic actions are analgesia and sedation. May cause less spasm of smooth muscle, constipation, and suppression of the cough reflex than morphine. Meperidine, 60 to 80 mg given parenter-

ally, is equipotent in analgesic effect to 10 mg of morphine. Opioids bind to opioid receptors located throughout the CNS. Opioid receptors that have been identified include mu, kappa, delta, and sigma. The pharmacodynamic properties of each opioid are dependent on which specific opioid receptor is occupied.

Onset: *IV:* 1 minute; *IM:* 10 to 15 minutes; *oral:* 15 to 45 minutes

Peak Effect: *IV:* 5 to 7 minutes; *IM:* 30 to 50 minutes; *oral:* 60 to 90 minutes

Duration: 2 to 4 hours

Indications: Meperidine is indicated for the short-term relief of moderate to severe pain.

Contraindications: Known hypersensitivity to meperidine. Depressed ventilatory function, increased intracranial pressure. Although the exact mechanism of action is unclear, it has been reported that patients treated with MAO inhibitors have had severe to fatal reactions. Reactions include severe respiratory depression, cyanosis, hypotension, hyperexcitability, convulsions, tachycardia, and hypertension. When narcotics are required in this patient population, meperidine is contraindicated. Monitoring and follow-up are required if narcotics are used in the presence of MAO inhibitors.

Protein Binding: 60% to 80%

Half-Life: 3 to 5 hours

Considerations: The administration of intravenous meperidine must be titrated to effect and injected slowly. Rapid injection increases the incidence of adverse reactions, which include severe respiratory depression, apnea, hypotension, circulatory collapse, and cardiac arrest. Pharmacologic breakdown results in toxic metabolite (normeperidine); therefore long-term use is not recommended in the elderly.

Drug Interactions: Dry mouth, constipation, spasm of the sphincter of Oddi (biliary spasm), flushing, urinary retention, pruritus, urticaria, rash, skin wheals, local irritation at the injection site, and antidiuretic effect

Respiratory Effects: Severe respiratory depression and arrest may occur with the IV administration of meperidine. Extreme caution should be exercised in patients with asthma, COPD, cor pulmonale, decreased respiratory reserve, hypoxia, or hypercapnia. Facilities must be fully equipped to monitor and treat respiratory depression.

CV Effects: Tachycardia, bradycardia, shock, cardiac arrest, palpitations, syncope, orthostatic hypotension. Hypotension may be severe in hypovolemic, critically ill patients.

CNS Effects: Euphoria, dysphoria, weakness, headache, sedation, convulsions, agitation, tremor, uncoordinated muscle movements, transient hallucinations, disorientation, and visual disturbances. Extreme caution should be exercised with use of any narcotic in patients with increased intracranial pressure or head injury. Increased intracranial pressure is associated with the development of hypercapnia and the respiratory depressant effects of opioids.

Metabolism: Meperidine undergoes extensive metabolism in the liver.

Elimination: Urinary excretion is pH dependent.

Overdose: Signs and symptoms of narcotic overdose include decreased respiratory rate and volume, extreme somnolence, cold clammy skin, bradycardia, and hypotension. In the event of an overdose, maintenance of a patent airway coupled with cardiac and respiratory support is required. Ventilation and oxygenation must be maintained until the respiratory depressant effects have dissipated.

Reversal: Naloxone (Narcan) is a narcotic antagonist that will reverse the respiratory and cardiovascular depressant effects associated with meperidine overdose. Naloxone may also reverse side effects associated with narcotic administration. These side effects include urinary retention, pruritus, respiratory depression, nausea, and vomiting. Careful titration is required to avoid full reversal of analgesia.

Patients treated with naloxone must remain adequately monitored and reassessed after the procedure to avoid the development of renarcotization and respiratory depression.

Dosage: Should be individualized and reduced in the elderly, debilitated, patients with renal/hepatic disease, or patients with hypothyroidism. Titration to individual patient response is required. If given intravenously for conscious sedation, slow IV injection is required.

IM: 0.5 to 1 mg/kg; *IV:* 0.5 to 1 mg/kg slowly titrated in 25 mg increments

Supplied: *Ampules:* 50 and 100 mg/ml; *vials:* 50 and 100 mg/ml; *oral tablets:* 50 and 100 mg; *syrup:* 50 mg/5 ml. Carpujects and Tubex dispensers also available.

Methohexital Sodium
(Brevital)

Classification: Barbiturate

Schedule: Methohexital sodium is subject to Schedule IV control under the Controlled Substances Act of 1970.

Clinical Pharmacology: Methohexital sodium is an ultra-short-acting barbiturate, which is twice as potent as thiopental. The duration of action is approximately 50% shorter than that of thiopental with fewer cumulative effects. Its primary mechanism of action is via its effect on the reticular activating center and interaction with the gamma-aminobutyric acid receptor complex. Methohexital is a methylated barbiturate, which depresses the sensory cortex, decreases motor activity, and produces dose-dependent degrees of drowsiness, hypnosis, and sedation. It is not an analgesic agent.

Onset: *IV:* 30 seconds; *rectal:* < 5 minutes

Peak Effect: *IV:* 45 seconds; *rectal:* 5 to 10 minutes

Duration: *IV:* 5 to 10 minutes; *rectal:* 30 to 90 minutes

Indications: Induction of general anesthesia. As an adjunct to inhalational anesthesia during short procedures. As an IV anesthetic adjunct for short diagnostic and therapeutic procedures.

Contraindications: Known hypersensitivity to barbiturates. Dosage reduction is required in the presence of shock, coma, porphyria, or acute alcohol intoxication. Caution must be exerted when administered to patient with concomitant disease states.

Half-Life: 6 to 8 hours

Considerations: Methohexital sodium should be administered by qualified personnel specially trained in the administration of anesthesia and in the management of the airway and cardiovascular system.

In the presence of extravascular or intra-arterial injection, necrosis and gangrene occur. Use of local or intra-arterial injection with an alpha-blocker (phentolamine, 2.5 to 5 mg in 10 ml) produces vasodilatation in the affected extremity.

Respiratory Effects: Respiratory depression, hypoxia, laryngospasm, apnea, hiccoughs, cardiorespiratory arrest, bronchospasm, dyspnea

CV Effects: Circulatory depression, thrombophlebitis, vascular collapse, hypotension, cardiorespiratory arrest, tachycardia, and local irritation and pain at the injection site

CNS Effects: May have additive effects with other CNS depressants. Tonic/clonic movements, seizures, nerve injury near the injection site, restlessness, anxiety, and emergence delirium.

Metabolism: Methohexital is extensively metabolized by the liver.

Elimination: Eliminated via the kidneys

Overdose: In the event of an overdose, maintenance of a patent airway and respiratory and cardiovascular support are required.

Dosage: Individualization and titration of dosage are required. Decreased dose in elderly and debilitated patients. Should not be administered intravenously in a concentration form greater than 1% (10 mg/ml).

For conscious sedation procedures: 10 mg increments have been used to augment the effects of benzodiazepines and opioids. To avoid deep sedation states or general anesthesia, extreme caution must be used when administering supplemental methohexital. Incremental doses must be given slowly over several minutes, with adequate circulation time allowed to assess the pharmacologic effect.

Supplied: In powder form for injection: 500 mg, 2.5 and 5.0 g, with diluent.

Midazolam
(Versed)

Classification: Benzodiazepine agonist

Schedule: Midazolam is subject to Schedule IV control under the Controlled Substances Act of 1970. FDA approved 1986.

Clinical Pharmacology: Midazolam is a water-soluble benzodiazepine. It is classified as a short-acting benzodiazepine CNS depressant with potent amnestic activity. The pharmacologic effect of benzodiazepines is primarily exerted via facilitated action of the inhibitory neurotransmitter gamma-aminobutyric acid (GABA). This GABA interaction enhances the inhibitory effects of various neurotransmitters. Benzodiazepines affect the limbic system, thalamus, and hypothalamus, producing a calm, sedate state. The effects of midazolam on the central nervous system are based on

- Dose administered
- Route of administration
- Presence of other premedicants
- Concurrent medications administered (opioids)

Specific advantages of midazolam use include a short half-life, superior sedation, amnesia, and anxiolysis when compared with other benzodiazepines. Midazolam has three to four times the sedative potency of diazepam. Midazolam is a water-soluble benzodiazepine. Diazepam and lorazepam use a propylene glycol suspension, which causes pain on injection, venous irritation, and phlebitis.

Onset: *IV:* 1 to 5 minutes; *IM:* 5 to 15 minutes; *intranasal:* < 5 minutes; *oral:* 30 minutes

Peak Effect: *IV:* immediate; *IM:* 15 to 60 minutes; *intranasal:* 10 minutes; *oral:* 2 to 6 hours

Duration: 2 to 6 hours

Indications: Preoperative medication, conscious sedation, and intravenous induction agent for general anesthesia

Contraindications: Known hypersensitivity to midazolam. Dosage reduction in debilitated patients, shock, coma, or acute alcohol intoxication

Protein Binding: 97%

Half-Life: 1 to 4 hours

Considerations: Individualized dosage. Reduce dose in elderly patients. Titrate medication to effect. Midazolam must never be used without individualization of dose. Bolus administration is not recommended for conscious sedation procedures.

Drug Interactions: Drug effect is accentuated (synergism) by concomitant use of sedatives, hypnotics, or narcotic analgesics. Drug dosage should be decreased according to the type, amount, and time of administration of adjunct medications. Patients receiving erythromycin and cimetidine may have a decrease in the plasma clearance of midazolam.

Respiratory Effects: Potent respiratory depressant. Decrease in respiratory rate and tidal volume. Apnea, respiratory depression, and cardiac arrest. Patients with chronic obstructive pulmonary disease are extremely sensitive to the respiratory depressant effects associated with midazolam.

CV Effects: Hypotension and bradycardia occur more frequently in patients premedicated with a narcotic. Patients with congestive heart failure eliminate midazolam more slowly.

CNS Effects: Agitation, involuntary movement, hyperactivity, and combativeness. These reactions may be due to

- Excessive dosing
- Inadequate dosing
- Hypoxia

Use of other CNS-depressant medications accentuates the respiratory depressant effects of midazolam.

Metabolism: Midazolam undergoes hepatic microsomal metabolism. Hepatic clearance may be decreased with use of enzyme-inhibiting drugs.

Elimination: Metabolites are excreted in the urine.

Overdose: In the event of an overdose (respiratory depression, apnea, cardiovascular collapse), maintenance of a patent airway and respiratory and cardiovascular support are required. Reversal with flumazenil, which is a specific benzodiazepine antagonist, generally restores the patient to a clear-headed state. Patients must be continuously monitored after the procedure to assess for

- Resedation
- Respiratory depression
- Residual depressant effects of benzodiazepines

A complete pharmacologic profile of flumazenil and dosage guidelines are listed in this appendix.

Dosage: *Conscious sedation:* Individualized and titrated for effect. Do not administer by rapid or single bolus injection. Titration to effect includes administration of drug until somnolence, nystagmus, or slurring of speech occurs.

Healthy patients: Prior to the procedure, small increments (0.5 mg) of midazolam are administered over a 2-minute period. Initial intravenous dose should not exceed 2.5 mg. Some patients may respond to as little as 0.5 to 1 mg.

Adults 60 years of age or older: Elderly, debilitated, chronically ill patients, or patients with decreased pulmonary reserve require small incremental (0.25 to 0.5 mg) doses administered over a 2-minute period. Initial intravenous dose should not exceed 1.5 mg. If additional sedation is required, it is imperative to wait several minutes to evaluate the pharmacologic effect before administering additional sedation.

Supplied: 1 mg/ml (in vials of 2, 5, and 10 ml), 5 mg/ml (in vials of 1, 2, 5, and 10 ml)

Manufacturer Recommendation: Intravenous Versed has been associated with respiratory depression and respiratory arrest, especially when used for conscious sedation. In some cases, where this was not recognized promptly and treated effectively, death or hypoxic encephalopathy has resulted. Intravenous Versed should be used only in hospital or ambulatory care settings, including physicians' offices, that provide for continuous monitoring of respiratory and cardiac function. Immediate availability of resuscitative drugs and equipment and personnel trained in their use should be assured.

The initial intravenous dose for conscious sedation may be as little as 1 mg but should not exceed 2.5 mg in a normal healthy adult. Lower doses are necessary for older (over 60) or debilitated patients and for patients receiving concomitant narcotics or other CNS depressants. The initial dose and all subsequent doses should never be given as a bolus; administer over at least 2 minutes and allow an additional 2 or more minutes to fully evaluate the sedative effect. The use of the 1 mg/ml formulation or dilution of the 1 mg/ml or 5 mg/ml formulation is recommended to facilitate slower injection.

Morphine Sulfate

Classification: Opioid agonist
Schedule: Morphine sulfate is subject to Schedule II control under the Controlled Substances Act of 1970.
Clinical Pharmacology: Morphine is an alkaloid of opium, which produces analgesia, sedation, euphoria, and dose-related respiratory depression. Hypotension and decreased systemic vascular resistance are related to the degree of histamine release. Nausea and vomiting associated with morphine sulfate administration are associated with stimulation of the chemoreceptor trigger zone.

Onset: *Oral:* within 1 hour; *IM:* 10 to 30 minutes; *IV:* < 5 minutes
Peak Effect: *Oral:* 1 to 2 hours; *IM:* 30 to 60 minutes; *IV:* 20 minutes

Duration: *Oral:* 4 to 12 hours; *IM:* 4 to 5 hours; *IV:* 4 to 5 hours

Indications: Morphine is a systemic narcotic analgesic that may be administered through a variety of routes, which include oral, intramuscular, and intravenous. Morphine may be used as a narcotic analgesic for the relief of moderate to severe pain.

Contraindications: Known hypersensitivity to morphine or natural opioids, **bronchial asthma,** decreased respiratory reserve, and increased intracranial pressure.

Protein Binding: 33%

Half-Life: 2 to 4 hours

Considerations: As with all narcotic adjuncts, individualized dosing is required with titration to patient effect.

Drug Interactions: Histamine release (urticaria, skin wheals, local tissue irritation), constipation, headache, anxiety, depression, convulsions, bradycardia, dysphoria, pruritus, nausea, vomiting, urinary retention, and biliary colic, as well as interference with thermal regulation

Respiratory Effects: Caution must be used in patients with decreased respiratory reserve and increased intracranial pressure. Acute respiratory failure and bronchospasm may occur in patients with COPD, acute asthma, or signs of respiratory embarrassment. The degree of bronchostriction is dependent on the magnitude of histamine release associated with the administration of morphine sulfate. Facilities must be fully equipped to monitor and treat respiratory depression.

CV Effects: Hypotension, bradycardia, and chest wall rigidity. Extreme caution must be exercised in patients with decreased circulating blood volume or impaired myocardial function. Hypotension may occur after IV injection secondary to histamine-mediated vasodilatation.

CNS Effects: Euphoria, somnolence. The use of CNS-depressant drugs, sedatives, and hypnotics potentiates morphine sulfate's CNS-depressant effects.

Metabolism: The principal site of metabolism is the liver.

Elimination: 90% of urinary excretion occurs within 24 hours; 7% to 10% of morphine is excreted in the feces.

Overdose: Signs and symptoms of narcotic overdose include decreased respiratory rate and volume, extreme somnolence, cold clammy skin, bradycardia, and hypotension. In the event of an overdose, maintenance of a patent airway, coupled with cardiac and respiratory support, is required. Ventilation and oxygenation must be maintained until the respiratory depressant effects have dissipated.

Reversal: Naloxone (Narcan) is a narcotic antagonist that will reverse the respiratory and cardiovascular depressant effects associated with morphine overdose. Naloxone may also reverse side effects associated with narcotic administration. These side effects include urinary retention, pruritus, respiratory depression, nausea, and vomiting. Careful titration is required to avoid full reversal of analgesia.

Patients treated with naloxone must remain adequately monitored and reassessed after the procedure to avoid the development of renarcotization and respiratory depression.

Dosage: *Analgesia:* IV 2 to 15 mg (0.05 to 0.2 mg/kg)

Should be individualized and reduced in the elderly, debilitated, patients with renal/hepatic disease, or patients with hypothyroidism. Titration to individual patient response is required. If used for conscious sedation, slow IV injection is required.

Supplied: *Oral tablets:* 15 to 30 mg; *soluble tablets:* 10, 15, and 30 mg; *injection:* 0.5, 1, 3, 5, 8, and 10 mg/ml

Naloxone Hydrochloride
(Narcan)

Classification: Opiate receptor antagonist

Clinical Pharmacology: Naloxone hydrochloride is a pure narcotic antagonist with no agonist activity. Through competitive inhibition at the opiate receptors, respiratory depression, hypotension, hypercapnia, sedation, and euphoria associated with the administration of narcotics are reversed. Naloxone has not been shown to produce tolerance or physical or psychologic dependence. In the presence of physical dependence, naloxone will produce withdrawal symptoms.

Onset: IV: 2 minutes

Peak Effect: 5 to 15 minutes

Duration: 1 to 4 hours

Indications: Complete or partial reversal of narcotic depression (respiratory depression, sedation, and hypotension) induced by the administration of opioids. Additional indications include diagnosis of suspected acute opioid overdosage.

Contraindications: Known hypersensitivity to naloxone. Caution must be used when administering to patients with pre-existing cardiac disease or patients with known or suspected physical dependence on opioids.

Half-Life: 0.5 to 1.5 hours

Considerations: Titrate slowly to the desired effect. Excessive reversal with naloxone may result in total reversal of analgesia with additional side effects (hypertension, excitation, etc.). The duration of action of some narcotics may exceed that of naloxone; therefore patients must be carefully monitored after the procedure. Repeated doses of naloxone may be administered as required.

Respiratory Effects: Reversal of respiratory depression. Rapid intravenous administration may induce pulmonary edema.

CV Effects: Hypotension, hypertension, ventricular tachycardia/fibrillation

CNS Effects: Excitement, tremors, seizures

Metabolism: Hepatic conjugation

Elimination: Renal

Overdose: Larger than necessary doses of naloxone may result in significant reversal of analgesic effects (hypertension, tachycardia, etc.).

Dosage: 0.1 to 0.2 mg titrated to patient response. May repeat every 2 to 3 minutes to a total dose of 10 mg. Additional doses of Narcan may be required, depending on total dose, type, and time interval since the last administration of narcotic. Low doses (1 to 4 µg/kg) have been used to reverse the respiratory depression associated with general anesthesia and MAC sedation.

Neonates and children: 10 to 100 µg/kg; *infusion:* 5 to 15 µg/kg/hr

Supplied: 0.4 mg/ml in 10 ml vials; 0.4 mg/ml in 1, 2, and 5 ml ampules; 1 mg/ml in 10 ml vial; 0.02 mg/2 ml ampule and 2 ml vial

Propofol
(Diprivan)

Classification: Sedative hypnotic

Schedule: Not a controlled substance

Clinical Pharmacology: Propofol is a sedative hypnotic for intravenous use. Produces rapid hypnosis with minimal excitation. It produces nonspecific cortical depression and produces a more complete and rapid awakening than Pentothal or Brevital. It has intrinsic antiemetic effects and has no analgesic properties.

Onset: 40 seconds

Peak Effect: 1 minute

Duration: 5 to 10 minutes

Indications: For the induction and maintenance of general anesthesia and as an adjunct to IV conscious sedation

Contraindications: Known hypersensitivity to propofol

Protein Binding: 97% to 99%

Considerations: Individualized dose and titration to effect. Reduce dose in elderly, hypovolemic, and high-risk patients. Potentiation occurs when combined with narcotic analgesics and CNS depressants. Pain on injection is decreased with the addition of IV lidocaine, 0.1 mg/kg, added to the propofol emulsion.

Special Handling Procedures: Propofol is available as an oil-in-water emulsion (intralipid), which contains soybean oil, glycerol, and egg lecithin. A history of egg allergy is not a definitive contraindication to its use. Patients with egg allergies generally have a reaction to egg whites (albumin), whereas egg lecithin is extracted from egg yolk. When originally released from production, propofol contained no antimicrobial preservatives. The CDC has reported sepsis and death related to contaminated propofol solution. Propofol now contains 0.005% disodium edetate. Disodium edetate retards the rate of growth of microorganisms in the event of contamination. Strict aseptic technique must be maintained in its handling.

Manufacturer Handling Instructions: Diprivan injection should be prepared just prior to the initiation of each procedure.

The ampule neck surface or vial stopper should be disinfected with 70% isopropyl alcohol, and Diprivan injection should be drawn into sterile syringes immediately after ampules or vials are opened.

When withdrawing Diprivan injection from vials, a sterile vent spike should be used.

The syringe(s) should be labeled with appropriate information, including the date and time the ampule or vial was opened.

Administration should commence promptly and must be completed within 6 hours after the ampules or vials have been opened.

Diprivan injection should be prepared for single patient use only.

Any unused portions of Diprivan Injection, reservoirs, dedicated administration tubing, or solution containing Diprivan injection must be discarded at the end of the procedure or at 6 hours, whichever occurs sooner.

The IV line should be flushed every 6 hours and at the end of the procedure to remove residual Diprivan Injection.

Respiratory Effects: Dose-dependent respiratory depression, apnea, hiccoughs, laryngospasm, bronchospasm, wheezing, and coughing

CV Effects: Hypotension associated with a decrease in cardiac output, cardiac contractility and preload, arrhythmias, tachycardia, bradycardia, decreased cardiac output

CNS Effects: Headache, dizziness, confusion, euphoria, myoclonic/clonic movement, seizures, sexual illusions, and possible additive effect with other CNS drugs, sedatives, and opioids

Metabolism: Hepatic conjugation to inactive metabolites

Elimination: Inactive metabolites are eliminated via urine.

Overdose: In the event of an overdose, maintenance of a patent airway and respiratory and cardiovascular support are required.

Dosage: *For conscious sedation procedures:* 10 mg increments have been used to augment the effects of benzodiazepines and opioids. To avoid deep sedation states or general anesthesia, extreme caution must be used in the administration of supplemental propofol. Incremental doses must be given slowly over several minutes and adequate circulation time allowed to assess full pharmacologic effect.

Supplied: 10 mg/ml (20 ml ampule, 50 ml vial, 100 ml infusion vial), 10 mg/ml (prefilled syringe)

Remifentanil Hydrochloride
(Ultiva)

Classification: Opioid agonist
Schedule: Remifentanil is subject to Schedule II control under the Controlled Substances Act of 1970.
Clinical Pharmacology: Remifentanil is an opioid agonist with a rapid onset of action, peak effect, and short duration of action. Unique pharmacokinetic properties include nonspecific esterase metabolism, rapid clearance independent of renal and hepatic function, and lack of accumulation regardless of total dose or duration of infusion. Rapid clearance and lack of accumulation result in rapid offset of analgesic effects (5 to 10 minutes) after discontinuation of the drug. Postoperative pain must be treated effectively with adequate postoperative analgesia.
Onset: *IV:* 1 to 2 minutes
Peak Effect: 5 to 10 minutes
Duration: Dose dependent (single dose or infusion technique). Rapid recovery 5 to 10 minutes after discontinuation of drug.
Indications: Analgesic action of short duration, as an analgesic agent for induction and maintenance of general anesthesia, as an analgesic component of IV conscious sedation
Contraindications: Patients with known hypersensitivity to fentanyl analogs
Protein Binding: 92%
Half-Life: 1.5 to 2 hours
Considerations: Titration to effect is required. Dosage reduction and caution must be used when administered to elderly, debilitated patients and patients susceptible to respiratory depression. Chest wall rigidity is related to total dose administered and speed of injection. The pharmacokinetics of remifentanil have not been studied in patients under 2 years of age.
Drug Interactions: Circulatory and respiratory depression may occur in the presence of concomitant administration of sedatives and CNS-depressant medications.

Respiratory Effects: Dose-dependent ventilatory depression. Extreme caution must be exercised when administered to patients with COPD, decreased pulmonary reserve, and compromised respiratory status. Facilities must be fully equipped to monitor and treat respiratory depression.
CV Effects: Dose-dependent hypotension and bradycardia, which are effectively treated with vagolytic doses of atropine or glycopyrrolate.
CNS Effects: Euphoria, dysphoria, sedation. Extreme caution should be exercised in patients with increased intracranial pressure. Addition of CNS-depressant drugs produces a synergistic effect and potentiates the effects of remifentanil.
Metabolism: Esterase metabolism. Hydrolysis by nonspecific esterases in the blood and tissues yields inactive carboxylic acid metabolites.
Elimination: Inactive metabolites are excreted in the urine.
Overdose: Signs and symptoms of narcotic overdose include decreased respiratory rate and volume, extreme somnolence, cold clammy skin, bradycardia, and hypotension. In the event of an overdose, maintenance of a patent airway, coupled with cardiac and respiratory support, is required. Ventilation and oxygenation must be maintained until the respiratory depressant effects have dissipated.
Reversal: Naloxone (Narcan) is a narcotic antagonist that will reverse the respiratory and cardiovascular depressant effects associated with remifentanil overdose. Naloxone may also reverse side effects associated with narcotic administration. These side effects include urinary retention, pruritus, respiratory depression, nausea, and vomiting. Careful titration is required to avoid full reversal of analgesia.

Patients treated with naloxone must remain adequately monitored and reassessed after the procedure to avoid the development of renarcotization and respiratory depression.

Dosage: *Remifentanil alone:* 1 μg/kg administered over 30 to 60 seconds approximately 90 seconds prior to the procedure.

Remifentanil in conjunction with 2 mg of midazolam: 0.5 μg/kg administered over 30 to 60 seconds approximately 90 seconds prior to the procedure.

Should be individualized and reduced in the elderly and debilitated and in patients with hypothyroidism. Titration to individual patient response is required.

Supplied: 1 mg of remifentanil base lyophilized powder, 3 ml vial; 2 mg of remifentanil base lyophilized powder, 5 ml vial; 5 mg of remifentanil base lyophilized powder, 10 ml vial

Thiopental Sodium
(Pentothal)

Classification: Barbiturate

Schedule: Thiopental is subject to Schedule III control under the Controlled Substances Act of 1970.

Clinical Pharmacology: Thiopental is an ultra-short-acting barbiturate, which causes CNS depression, a hypnotic state, and anesthesia. Its primary mechanism of action is via its effect on the reticular activating center and interaction with the gamma-aminobutyric acid receptor complex. It is not an analgesic agent. Repeated doses lead to accumulation of the drug secondary to its increased lipid solubility and prolonged elimination phase.

Onset: *IV:* 10 to 20 seconds; *rectal administration:* 8 to 10 minutes

Peak Effect: *IV:* 30 to 40 seconds

Duration: *IV:* 5 to 15 minutes

Indications: For the induction of general anesthesia, as an adjunct for supplementary regional anesthesia and monitored anesthesia care procedures. Use as an anticonvulsant and induction agent for barbiturate coma (to decrease cerebral metabolic rate and intracranial pressure).

Contraindications: Porphyria, known hypersensitivity to barbiturates, status asthmaticus, shock, severe heart disease

Protein Binding: 80%

Half-Life: 3 to 8 hours

Considerations: Thiopental should be administered only by qualified, trained personnel. Because of its high pH (10 to

12), signs and symptoms of extravascular injection (necrosis, pain) or intra-arterial injection (gangrene, spasm, or thrombosis of vessel) require immediate intervention. Treatment includes infiltration of the area with 5 to 10 mg of phentolamine diluted in 10 ml of normal saline solution.

Intra-arterial injection of papaverine (40 to 80 mg) may decrease the incidence of smooth muscle spasm.

Respiratory Effects: Decreased tidal volume and rate secondary to depression of the medullary breathing centers; apnea, laryngospasm, histamine release, bronchospasm, sneezing, and coughing

CV Effects: Venous dilation, decreased cardiac output, hypotension, decreased systemic vascular resistance and coronary perfusion pressure

CNS Effects: Potentiates CNS, sedative, narcotic, and hypnotic medications; headache, prolonged recovery, somnolence, emergence delirium. Thiopental decreases cerebral blood flow, intracranial pressure, and cerebral metabolic rate. Depresses EEG and evoked potentials.

Metabolism: Primary mechanism of metabolism is the liver.

Elimination: Inactive metabolites are excreted via the kidneys.

Overdose: In the event of overdose, maintenance of a patent airway and respiratory and cardiovascular support are required.

Dosage: *For conscious sedation procedures:* 10 to 20 mg increments have been used to augment the effects of benzodiazepines and opioids. To avoid deep sedation states or general anesthesia, extreme caution must be used when administering supplemental doses of Pentothal. Incremental doses must be given slowly, with adequate circulation time allowed to assess the pharmacologic effect.
Supplied: *Injection (syringes):* 250, 400, and 500 mg; *vials with diluent:* 500 and 1000 mg; *kits:* 1, 2.5, and 5 g

SCHEDULE OF CONTROLLED SUBSTANCES

Drugs that come under the jurisdiction of the Controlled Substances Act are divided into five schedules. Adherence to Federal and State guidelines regarding administration, dispensing, distribution, and accountability is imperative. Copies of the Controlled Substances Act may be obtained from the Superintendent of Documents, U.S. Government Printing Office, Washington, D.C. 20402.

Schedule I

The substances in this schedule are those that have no accepted medical use in the United States but have a high abuse potential. Some examples are heroin, LSD, peyote, and methaqualone.

Schedule II

The substances in this schedule have a high abuse potential with severe psychic or physical dependence. Schedule II substances consist of specific narcotics, stimulants, and depressant medications. Examples of Schedule II controlled substances are opium, morphine, codeine, fentanyl, sufentanil, hydromorphone, meperidine, oxycodone. Additional Schedule II medications are amphetamines, methylphenidate (Ritalin), pentobarbital, and secobarbital.

Schedule III

Schedule III substances have an abuse potential less than those in Schedules I and II and include compounds containing limited quantities of certain narcotic and nonnarcotic medications. Examples of Schedule III drugs include derivatives of barbituric acid (except those identified in earlier schedules), phentermine, paregoric, and any compound, mixture, preparation, or suppository dosage form containing amobarbital, secobarbital, or pentobarbital.

Schedule IV

The substances in this schedule have an abuse potential less than those listed in Schedules I, II, and III. Examples of Schedule IV medications include chloral hydrate, meprobamate, paraldehyde, methohexital, diazepam, midazolam, lorazepam, and pentazocine.

Schedule V

The substances in this schedule have an abuse potential less than those listed in Schedules I, II, III, and IV. These substances consist primarily of medications containing limited quantities of narcotics and stimulant drugs used for their antitussive, antidiarrheal, and analgesic effects. Examples include buprenorphine and propylhexedrine.

BIBLIOGRAPHY

Barash P. *Clinical Anesthesia.* 2nd ed. Philadelphia: Lippincott; 1992.

Cummins R. *Textbook of Advanced Cardiac Life Support.* Dallas, Tex: American Heart Association; 1994.

Davidson J, Eckhardt W, Perese D. *Clinical Anesthesia Procedures of the Massachusetts General Hospital.* 4th ed. Boston: Little, Brown; 1993.

Duke J, Rosenberg S. *Anesthesia Secrets.* St. Louis: Mosby; 1996.

Estafanous F. *Opioids in Anesthesia.* 2nd ed. Boston, Mass: Butterworth-Heinemann, 1991.

Furniss S, Munger M. Understanding ACLS pharmacotherapy. *Anesthesia Today.* 1996;7:1.

Jacobs E. *Saunders Review for NCLEX-RN.* 2nd ed. Philadelphia: WB Saunders; 1994.

Kanarek B. *Glaxo Wellcome Announces New ULTIVA: Remifentanil HCl for Injection.* Research Triangle Park, NC: Glaxo Wellcome Co.; 1996.

Katz J. *Anesthesiology: A Comprehensive Study Guide.* New York: McGraw-Hill; 1997.

Miller R. *Anesthesia.* 4th ed. New York: Churchill Livingstone; 1994.

Moragan E, Mikhail M. *Clinical Anesthesiology.* 2nd ed. Stamford, Conn: Appleton & Lange; 1996.

Omoigui S. *The Anesthesia Drugs Handbook.* 2nd ed. St. Louis: Mosby; 1995.

Rice T. *The Physician's Desk Reference.* 50th ed. Montvale, NJ: Medical Economics Company; 1996.

Roizen M, Fleisher L. *The Essence of Anesthesia Practice.* Philadelphia: WB Saunders; 1997.

Advanced Cardiac Life Support Algorithms

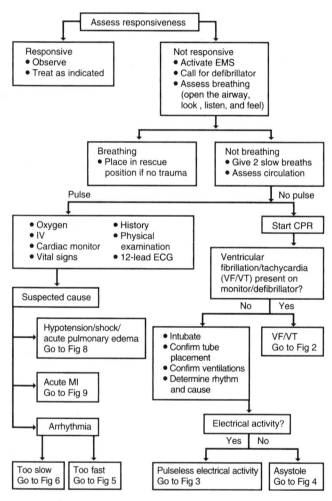

FIGURE 1. Universal algorithm for adult emergency cardiac care (ECC). (From *JAMA* 268:2216, Oct 28, 1992. Copyright 1992, American Medical Association.)

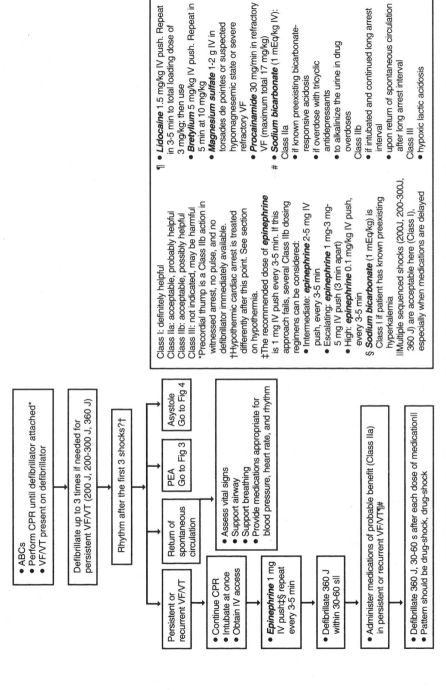

FIGURE 2. Algorithm for ventricular fibrillation and pulseless ventricular tachycardia (VF/VT). (From *JAMA* 268:2217, Oct 28, 1992. Copyright 1992, American Medical Association.)

PEA includes
- Electromechanical dissociation (EMD)
- Pseudo-EMD
- Idioventricular rhythms
- Ventricular escape rhythms
- Bradyasystolic rhythms
- Postdefibrillation idioventricular rhythms

• Continue CPR • Intubate at once	• Obtain IV access • Assess blood flow using Doppler ultrasound

↓

Consider possible causes
(Parentheses=possible therapies and treatments)
- Hypovolemia (volume infusion)
- Hypoxia (ventilation)
- Cardiac tamponade (pericardiocentesis)
- Tension pneumothorax (needle decompression)
- Hypothermia (see hypothermia algorithm, Section IV)
- Massive pulmonary embolism (surgery, ***thrombolytics***)
- Drug overdoses such as tricyclics, digitalis, β-blockers, calcium channel blockers
- Hyperkalemia*
- Acidosis†
- Massive acute myocardial infarction (go to Fig 9)

↓

- ***Epinephrine*** 1 mg IV push, *‡ repeat every 3-5 min

↓

- If absolute bradycardia (<60 beats/min) or relative bradycardia, give ***atropine*** 1 mg IV
- Repeat every 3-5 min up to a total of 0.04 mg/kg§

Class I: definitely helpful
Class IIa: acceptable, probably helpful
Class IIb: acceptable, possibly helpful
Class III: not indicated, may be harmful
Sodium bicarbonate 1 mEq/kg is Class I if patient has known preexisting hyperkalemia.
†***Sodium bicarbonate*** 1 mEq/kg:
  Class IIa
  - if known preexisting bicarbonate-responsive acidosis
  - if overdose with tricyclic antidepressants
  - to alkalinize the urine in drug overdoses
  Class IIb
  - if intubated and long arrest interval
  - upon return of spontaneous circulation after long arrest interval
  Class III
  - hypoxic lactic acidosis
‡The recommended dose of ***epinephrine*** is 1 mg IV push every 3-5 min.
If this approach fails, several Class IIb dosing regimens can be considered.
  - Intermediate: ***epinephrine*** 2-5 mg IV push, every 3-5 min
  - Escalating: ***epinephrine*** 1 mg-3 mg-5 mg IV push (3 min apart)
  - High: ***epinephrine*** 0.1 mg/kg IV push, every 3-5 min
§ Shorter ***atropine*** dosing intervals are possibly helpful in cardiac arrest (Class IIb).

FIGURE 3.   Algorithm for pulseless electrical activity (PEA) (electromechanical dissociation [EMD]). (From *JAMA* 268:2219, Oct 28, 1992. Copyright 1992, American Medical Association.)

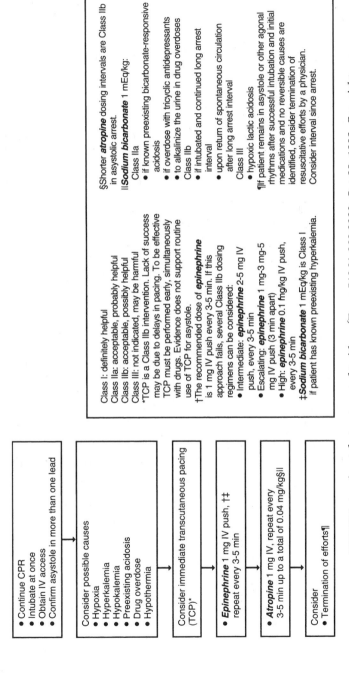

FIGURE 4. Asystole treatment algorithm. (From *JAMA* 268:2220, Oct 28, 1992. Copyright 1992, American Medical Association.)

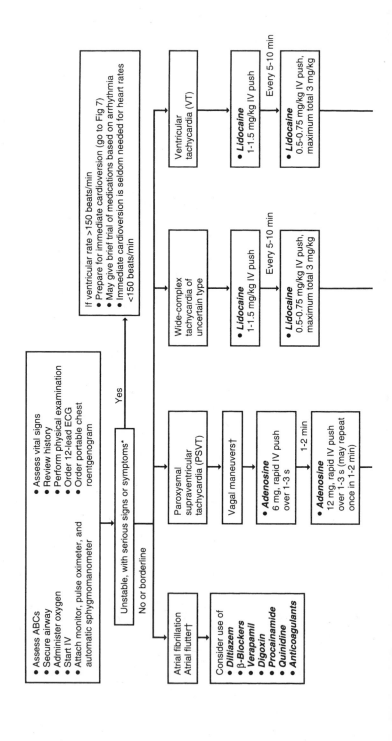

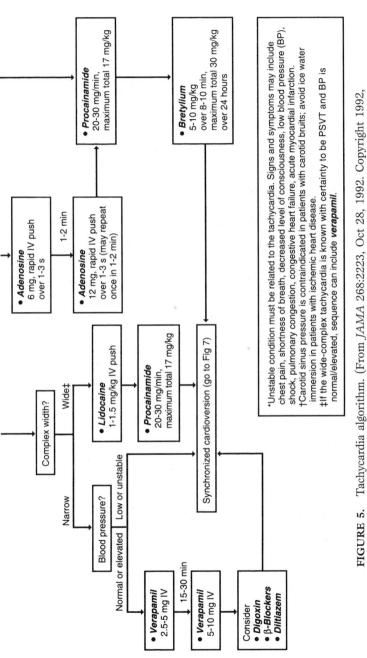

FIGURE 5. Tachycardia algorithm. (From *JAMA* 268:2223, Oct 28, 1992. Copyright 1992, American Medical Association.)

Complex width?

Narrow

Wide‡

Blood pressure?

• **Lidocaine**
1-1.5 mg/kg IV push

• *Adenosine*
6 mg, rapid IV push
over 1-3 s

1-2 min

• *Adenosine*
12 mg, rapid IV push
over 1-3 s (may repeat
once in 1-2 min)

• *Procainamide*
20-30 mg/min,
maximum total 17 mg/kg

• *Bretylium*
5-10 mg/kg
over 8-10 min,
maximum total 30 mg/kg
over 24 hours

Normal or elevated

Low or unstable

• *Procainamide*
20-30 mg/min,
maximum total 17 mg/kg

Synchronized cardioversion (go to Fig 7)

• *Verapamil*
2.5-5 mg IV

15-30 min

• *Verapamil*
5-10 mg IV

Consider
• *Digoxin*
• *β-Blockers*
• *Diltiazem*

*Unstable condition must be related to the tachycardia. Signs and symptoms may include chest pain, shortness of breath, decreased level of consciousness, low blood pressure (BP), shock, pulmonary congestion, congestive heart failure, acute myocardial infarction.
†Carotid sinus pressure is contraindicated in patients with carotid bruits; avoid ice water immersion in patients with ischemic heart disease.
‡If the wide-complex tachycardia is known with certainty to be PSVT and BP is normal/elevated, sequence can include *verapamil*.

293

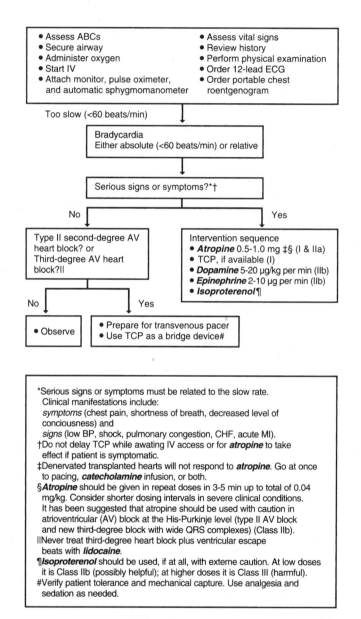

FIGURE 6. Bradycardia algorithm (with the patient not in cardiac arrest). (From *JAMA* 268:2221, Oct 28, 1992. Copyright 1992, American Medical Association.)

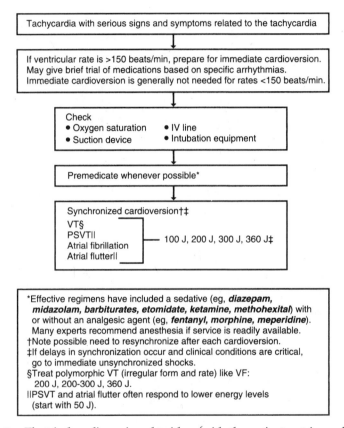

FIGURE 7.   Electrical cardioversion algorithm (with the patient not in cardiac arrest). (From *JAMA* 268:2224, Oct 28, 1992. Copyright 1992, American Medical Association.)

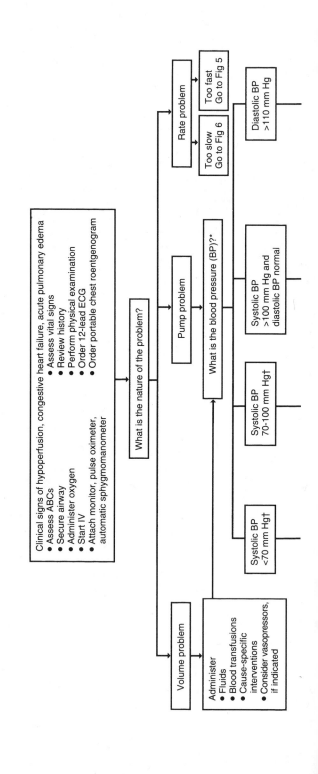

Clinical signs of hypoperfusion, congestive heart failure, acute pulmonary edema
- Assess ABCs
- Secure airway
- Administer oxygen
- Start IV
- Attach monitor, pulse oximeter, automatic sphygmomanometer
- Assess vital signs
- Review history
- Perform physical examination
- Order 12-lead ECG
- Order portable chest roentgenogram

What is the nature of the problem?

Volume problem

Administer
- Fluids
- Blood transfusions
- Cause-specific interventions
- Consider vasopressors, if indicated

Pump problem

What is the blood pressure (BP)?*

Systolic BP <70 mm Hgt

Systolic BP 70-100 mm Hgt

Systolic BP >100 mm Hg and diastolic BP normal

Rate problem

Too slow
Go to Fig 6

Too fast
Go to Fig 5

Diastolic BP >110 mm Hg

296

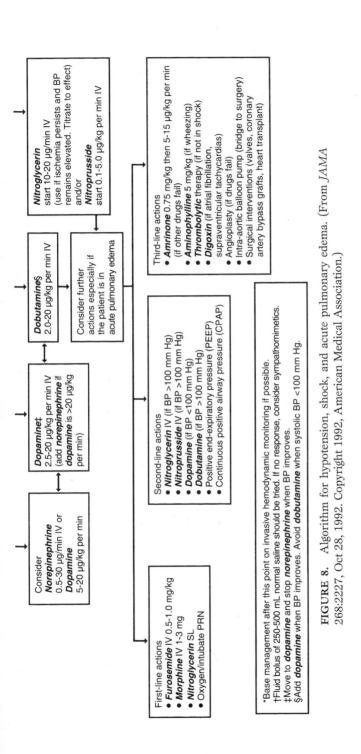

FIGURE 8. Algorithm for hypotension, shock, and acute pulmonary edema. (From *JAMA* 268:2227, Oct 28, 1992. Copyright 1992, American Medical Association.)

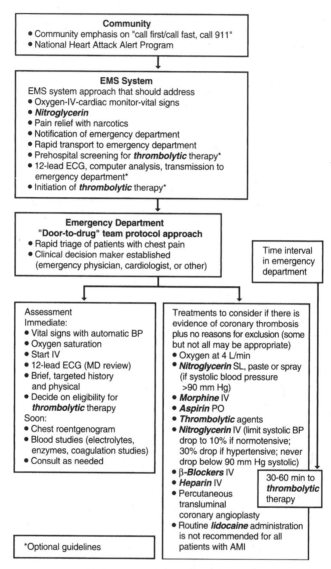

Community
- Community emphasis on "call first/call fast, call 911"
- National Heart Attack Alert Program

EMS System
EMS system approach that should address
- Oxygen-IV-cardiac monitor-vital signs
- *Nitroglycerin*
- Pain relief with narcotics
- Notification of emergency department
- Rapid transport to emergency department
- Prehospital screening for *thrombolytic* therapy*
- 12-lead ECG, computer analysis, transmission to emergency department*
- Initiation of *thrombolytic* therapy*

Emergency Department
"Door-to-drug" team protocol approach
- Rapid triage of patients with chest pain
- Clinical decision maker established (emergency physician, cardiologist, or other)

Time interval in emergency department

Assessment
Immediate:
- Vital signs with automatic BP
- Oxygen saturation
- Start IV
- 12-lead ECG (MD review)
- Brief, targeted history and physical
- Decide on eligibility for *thrombolytic* therapy
Soon:
- Chest roentgenogram
- Blood studies (electrolytes, enzymes, coagulation studies)
- Consult as needed

Treatments to consider if there is evidence of coronary thrombosis plus no reasons for exclusion (some but not all may be appropriate)
- Oxygen at 4 L/min
- *Nitroglycerin* SL, paste or spray (if systolic blood pressure >90 mm Hg)
- *Morphine* IV
- *Aspirin* PO
- *Thrombolytic* agents
- *Nitroglycerin* IV (limit systolic BP drop to 10% if normotensive; 30% drop if hypertensive; never drop below 90 mm Hg systolic)
- β-*Blockers* IV
- *Heparin* IV
- Percutaneous transluminal coronary angioplasty
- Routine *lidocaine* administration is not recommended for all patients with AMI

30-60 min to *thrombolytic* therapy

*Optional guidelines

FIGURE 9. Acute myocardial infarction (AMI) algorithm. Recommendations for early treatment of patients with chest pain and possible AMI. (From *JAMA* 268:2230, Oct 28, 1992. Copyright 1992, American Medical Association.)

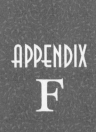

American Academy of Pediatrics Committee on Drugs

APPENDIX F

GUIDELINES FOR MONITORING AND MANAGEMENT OF PEDIATRIC PATIENTS DURING AND AFTER SEDATION FOR DIAGNOSTIC AND THERAPEUTIC PROCEDURES

GENERAL GUIDELINES

CANDIDATES

Patients who are ASA class I and II are frequently considered appropriate candidates for conscious or deep sedation (Appendix 2). Patients in ASA class III or IV present special problems that require additional and individual consideration.

RESPONSIBLE PERSON

The pediatric patient shall be accompanied to and from the treatment facility by a parent, legal guardian, or other responsible person.

FACILITIES

The practitioner who uses sedation must have immediately available the facilities, personnel, and equipment to manage emergency situations. Possible complications include, but are not limited to, vomiting, seizures, anaphylaxis or anaphylactoid reactions, and cardiorespiratory impairment, which may lead to a cardiopulmonary arrest.

BACK-UP EMERGENCY SERVICES

A protocol for access to back-up emergency services shall be clearly identified, with an outline of the procedures necessary for immediate use. For nonhospital

---

Used with permission of the American Academy of Pediatrics from Kaurman RE, Banner W, Berlein C, et al. Guidelines for monitoring and management of pediatric patients during and after sedation for diagnostic and therapeutic procedures. *Pediatrics.* 1993;89: 1110–1115.

facilities, an emergency assist system should be established, and ready access to ambulance service must be assured.

On-Site Equipment

Equipment must be suitable for children of all ages and sizes being treated. A positive-pressure oxygen delivery system, capable of administering greater than 90% oxygen for at least 60 minutes, and a functional suction apparatus with appropriate suction catheters must be immediately available. Note that if a self-inflating type bag is used, 15 L/min flow is required.[1-4] Equipment for noninvasive measurement of blood pressure (sphygmomanometer and blood pressure cuffs) and oxygen saturation monitoring (pulse oximetry) must be available. Airway management and breathing equipment must be checked for appropriate function before each sedation.

An emergency cart or kit must be immediately accessible. This cart or kit must contain equipment to provide the necessary age-appropriate drugs and equipment to resuscitate a nonbreathing and unconscious patient. The contents of the kit must allow for the provision of continuous life support while the patient is being transported to a medical facility or to another area within a medical facility. All equipment and drugs must be checked and maintained on a scheduled basis. (See Appendix 3 for suggested drugs and Appendix 4 for emergency life support equipment.)

Inhalation sedation equipment must (1) have the capacity of delivering 100% and never less than 25% oxygen concentration at a flow rate appropriate to the size of the patient, and (2) be used in conjunction with a calibrated and functional oxygen analyzer.

Consideration should be given to the National Institute of Occupational Safety and Health Standards for the scavenging of waste gases.[5]

Documentation

Documentation shall include, but not be limited to, the guidelines that follow.

Before Sedation

1. *Informed consent.* The patient record shall document that appropriate informed consent was obtained according to local, state, and institutional requirements.
2. *Instructions and information provided to the responsible person.* The practitioner shall provide verbal and/or written instructions to the responsible person. Information shall include objectives of the sedation and anticipated changes in behavior during and after sedation. A 24-hour telephone number for the practitioner or his/her associates should be provided to all patients and their families. Instructions shall include limitations of activities and appropriate dietary precautions.

Dietary Precautions

The use of sedation must be preceded by an evaluation of food and fluid intake (see Appendix 5).

Documentation at the Time of Sedation

1. *Health evaluation.* Before conscious or deep sedation, a health evaluation shall be performed by an appropriately licensed practitioner and reviewed at the time of treatment. This health evaluation should include:

   - Age and weight;
   - Health history, including (1) allergies and previous allergic or adverse drug reactions; (2) drug use including dosage, time, route, and site of administration for prescription, over-the-counter, or illicit drugs; (3) relevant diseases, physical abnormalities, and pregnancy status; (4) a summary of previous relevant hospitalizations; (5) history of sedation or general anesthesia, and any complications; and (6) relevant family history;
   - Review of systems;
   - Vital signs, including heart rate, blood pressure, respiratory rate, and temperature;
   - Physical examination, including an evaluation of the airway;
   - Physical status evaluation (ASA classification, see Appendix 2);
   - Name, address, and telephone number of the child's or family's physician.

   For hospitalized patients, the current hospital record may suffice for adequate documentation of presedation health; however, a brief note shall be written documenting that the chart was reviewed, positive findings were noted, and a management plan was formulated. If the clinical or emergency condition of the patient precludes acquiring complete information before sedation, this health evaluation should be obtained as soon as feasible.

2. *Prescriptions.* When prescriptions are used, a copy of the prescription or a note describing the content of the prescription should be in the patient's chart along with a description of the instructions that were given to the responsible person.

Documentation during Treatment

The patient's chart shall contain documentation at the time of treatment that the patient's level of consciousness and responsiveness, heart rate, blood pressure, respiratory rate, and oxygen saturation were monitored until the patient satisfied predetermined discharge criteria (see Appendix 1). The patient's chart shall also contain a time-based record that includes the name, route, site, time, dosage, and patient effect of administered drugs. During administration, the inspired concentrations of oxygen and inhalation sedation agents and the duration of their administration shall be documented. Adverse events shall be documented. Special attention must be paid to calculation of dosage, ie, mg/kg or mg/lb.

Documentation after Treatment

The time and condition of the child at discharge from the treatment area or facility shall be documented; this should include documentation that the child's level of consciousness has returned to a state that is safe for discharge by recognized criteria (see Appendix 1).

SPECIFIC GUIDELINES FOR LEVEL OF SEDATION

CONSCIOUS SEDATION

Conscious sedation is a medically controlled state of depressed consciousness that (1) allows protective reflexes to be maintained; (2) retains the patient's ability to maintain a patent airway independently and continuously; and (3) permits appropriate response by the patient to physical stimulation and/or verbal command, eg, "open your eyes." A minimally depressed level of consciousness should be used for the very young or handicapped child incapable of the usually expected verbal responses.

The caveat that loss of consciousness should be unlikely is a particularly important aspect of the definition of conscious sedation, and the drugs and techniques used should carry a margin of safety wide enough to render unintended loss of consciousness highly unlikely. Since the patient who receives conscious sedation may progress into a state of deep sedation and obtundation, the practitioner should be prepared to increase the level of vigilance corresponding to that necessary for deep sedation. Sedatives should only be administered at the health care facility where appropriate monitoring can be instituted.

Personnel

THE PRACTITIONER. The practitioner responsible for the treatment of the patient and/or the administration of drugs for sedation must be competent to use such techniques, to provide the level of monitoring provided in these guidelines, and to manage complications of these techniques. The practitioner must be trained in, and capable of providing, at the minimum, pediatric basic life support; training in pediatric advanced life support is strongly encouraged.

SUPPORT PERSONNEL. The use of conscious sedation shall include provision of a person, in addition to the practitioner, whose responsibility is to monitor appropriate physiologic parameters and to assist in any supportive or resuscitation measures, as required. It is strongly encouraged that this individual be trained in pediatric basic life support. The support person shall have specific assignments in the event of an emergency and, thus, current knowledge of the emergency cart inventory.

The practitioner and all ancillary personnel should participate in periodic reviews of the facility's emergency protocol, to ensure proper function of the equipment and staff interaction.

Monitoring and Documentation

BASELINE. Before administration of sedative medications, a baseline determination of vital signs shall be documented.

DURING THE PROCEDURE. The practitioner shall document the name, route, site, time of administration, and dosage of all drugs administered. There shall be continuous quantitative monitoring of oxygen saturation (eg, pulse oximetry) and heart rate, and intermittent recording of respiratory rate and blood pressure; these should be monitored and recorded in a time-based record. Restraining devices should be checked to prevent airway obstruction or chest restriction. The child's head position should be checked frequently to ensure airway patency. If a restraint device is used, a hand or foot should be kept exposed. A functioning suction apparatus must be present.

AFTER THE PROCEDURE. The child who has received conscious sedation must be observed in a suitably equipped facility; ie, the facility must have functioning suction apparatus, as well as the capacity to deliver more than 90% oxygen and positive-pressure ventilation, eg, bag and mask. The patient's vital signs should be recorded at specific intervals. If the patient is not fully alert, oxygen saturation (pulse oximetry) and heart rate monitoring shall be used continuously until appropriate discharge criteria are met (see Appendix 1).

The Use of Nitrous Oxide for Conscious Sedation

The use of nitrous oxide for conscious sedation is defined as the administration of nitrous oxide—50% or less, with the balance as oxygen, without any other sedative, narcotic, or other depressant drug before or concurrent with the nitrous oxide—to an otherwise healthy ASA class I or II patient. The patient is able to maintain verbal communication throughout. A second individual whose responsibility is to monitor the patient may also assist with the procedure. While pulse oximetry is not required under this specific method of sedation, it is strongly encouraged.

DEEP SEDATION

Deep sedation is a medically controlled state of depressed consciousness or unconsciousness from which the patient is not easily aroused. Deep sedation may be accompanied by a partial or complete loss of protective reflexes, including the inability to maintain a patent airway independently and to respond purposefully to physical stimulation or to verbal command. The state and risks of deep sedation may be indistinguishable from those of general anesthesia.

Personnel

The state of deep sedation, regardless of how it is achieved, requires that there must be one person available whose only responsibility is to constantly observe the patient's vital signs, airway patency, and adequacy of ventilation, and to either administer drugs or direct their administration. At least one individual must be present who is trained in, and capable of, providing pediatric basic life support, and who is skilled in airway management and cardiopulmonary resuscitation; training in pediatric advanced life support is strongly encouraged.

Equipment

In addition to the equipment previously cited for conscious sedation, an electrocardiograph monitor and a defibrillator for use in pediatric patients should be readily available.

Vascular Access

Patients receiving deep sedation should have an intravenous line in place or have immediately available a person skilled in establishing vascular access in pediatric patients.

Monitoring

The patient shall be observed continuously by a competent individual, and monitoring shall include all parameters described for conscious sedation. Vital signs, including oxygen saturation and heart rate, must be documented at least every 5 minutes in a time-based record. The use of a precordial stethoscope or capnograph to aid in monitoring adequacy of ventilation is encouraged. The practitioner shall document the name, route, site, time of administration, and dosage of all drugs administered. The inspired concentrations of inhalation sedation agents and oxygen and the duration of administration shall be documented.

Postsedation Care

The facility and procedures followed for postsedation care shall conform to those described under "Conscious Sedation."

SPECIAL CONSIDERATIONS

LOCAL ANESTHETIC AGENTS. All local anesthetic agents are cardiac depressants and may cause central nervous system excitation or depression. Particular attention should be paid to dosage in small children. To ensure that the patient will not receive an excessive dose, the maximum allowable safe dosage (eg, mg/kg or mg/lb) should be calculated prior to administration. There may be enhanced sedative effects when local anesthetic drugs are used with other sedatives or narcotics.[6-10]

INHALATION SEDATION. The use of nitrous oxide poses special risks. Except under the direction of an anesthesiologist or anesthetist, nitrous oxide should not be used in patients of ASA physical status 3 and 4, in patients with an altered level of consciousness, or in patients for whom sequential assessment of level of consciousness is critical. Using inhalation sedation with nitrous oxide in conjunction with sedatives, narcotics, or other depressant medications may rapidly produce a state of deep sedation or general anesthesia and requires the level of monitoring described under "Deep Sedation."

SPECIAL CONSIDERATIONS FOR MONITORING DURING MAGNETIC RESONANCE IMAGING

The special technologic problems associated with monitoring patients in a magnetic resonance imaging scanner—specifically, the powerful magnetic field and the generation of radiofrequency—necessitate the use of special equipment to provide continuous patient monitoring throughout the scanning procedure. Pulse oximeters capable of continuous function even during scanning are now available and should be used in any sedated or restrained pediatric patient. Thermal injuries can result if appropriate precautions are not taken; avoid coiling the oximeter wire and place the probe as far from the magnetic coil as possible to diminish the possibility of injury. Electrocardiogram monitoring during magnetic resonance imaging has been associated with thermal injury, and it should be used with caution in this setting.[11-14]

ACKNOWLEDGMENTS

The committee on Drugs wishes to thank the Committee on Standards, American Society of Anesthesiologists, Burton Epstein, MD, Chairman; the Committee on Pediatric Anesthesia, American Society of Anesthesiologists, Stephen Hall, MD, Chairman; and the Society for Pediatric Anesthesia, Theodore Striker, MD, Liaison, for their extensive review and helpful suggestions.

COMMITTEE ON DRUGS, 1991 TO 1992
Ralph E. Kauffman, MD, Chairman
William Banner, Jr, MD, PhD
Cheston M. Berlin, MD
Jeffrey L. Blumer, MD, PhD
Richard L. Gorman, MD
George H. Lambert, MD
Geraldine S. Wilson, MD

Liaison Representatives
Donald R. Bennett, MD, PhD, American Medical Association
José F. Cordero, MD, MPH, Centers for Disease Control
Charles J. Coté, MD, Chairman, Section on Anesthesiology, American Academy of Pediatrics
Paul Tomich, MD, American College of Obstetricians and Gynecologists
Sam A. Licata, MD, Bureau of Drugs, Health Protection Branch, Canada
Paul Kauffman, MD, Pharmaceutical Manufacturers Association
Gloria Troendle, MD, Food and Drug Administration
Sumner J. Yaffe, MD, National Institute of Child Health and Human Development

Consultants
Mary Ellen Mortensen, MD
Wayne R. Snodgrass, MD, PhD
Anthony R. Temple, MD

APPENDIX 1. RECOMMENDED DISCHARGE CRITERIA

1. Cardiovascular function and airway patency are satisfactory and stable.
2. The patient is easily arousable, and protective reflexes are intact.
3. The patient can talk (if age-appropriate).
4. The patient can sit up unaided (if age-appropriate).
5. For a very young or handicapped child, incapable of the usually expected responses, the presedation level of responsiveness or a level as close as possible to the normal level for that child should be achieved.
6. The state of hydration is adequate.

APPENDIX 2. ASA PHYSICAL STATUS CLASSIFICATION

Class I   A normally healthy patient.
Class II   A patient with mild systemic disease.
Class III A patient with severe systemic disease.
Class IV   A patient with severe systemic disease that is a constant threat to life.
Class V   A moribund patient who is not expected to survive without the operation.

APPENDIX 3. SUGGESTED EMERGENCY DRUGS[15]

Oxygen
Glucose (50%)
Atropine
Epinephrine (1:1000; 1:10,000)
Phenylephrine
Dopamine
Diazepam
Isoproterenol
Calcium chloride or calcium gluconate
Sodium bicarbonate

Lidocaine (cardiac lidocaine, local infiltration)
Naloxone hydrochloride
Diphenhydramine hydrochloride
Hydrocortisone
Methylprednisolone
Succinylcholine
Aminophylline
Racemic epinephrine
Albuterol by inhalation
Ammonia spirits

NOTE: The choice of emergency drugs may vary according to individual need.

APPENDIX 4. SUGGESTED EMERGENCY EQUIPMENT

Intravenous Equipment
Intravenous catheters
    24-, 22-, 20-, 18-, and 16-gauge
Tourniquets
Alcohol wipes
Adhesive tape
Assorted syringes
    1 mL, 3 mL, 6 mL, and 12 mL
Intravenous tubing
    Pediatric drip (60 drops/mL)
    Pediatric burette type
    Adult drip (10 drops/mL)
    Extension tubing
Intravenous fluid
    Lactated Ringer's solution
    Normal saline
Three-way stopcocks
Pediatric intravenous (IV) boards

Assorted IV needles
 22-, 20-, and 18-gauge
Intraosseous bone marrow needle
Sterile gauze pads

Airway Management Equipment
Face masks
 Infant, child, small adult, medium adult, large adult
Breathing bag and valve set
Oral airways
 Infant, child, small adult, medium adult, large adult
Nasal airways
 Small, medium, large
Laryngoscope handles
Laryngoscope blades
 Straight (Miller) No. 1, 2, 3
 Curved (Macintosh) No. 2, 3
Endotracheal tubes
 2.5, 3.0, 3.5, 4.0, 4.5, 5.0, 5.5, 6.0 uncuffed
 6.0, 7.0, 8.0 cuffed
Stylettes (appropriate sizes for endotracheal tubes)
Surgical lubricant
Suction catheters (appropriate sizes for endotracheal tubes)
Nasogastric tubes
 Yankauer-type suction
Nebulizer with medication kits
Gloves

APPENDIX 5. RECOMMENDED DIETARY PRECAUTIONS

1. Before elective sedation. The use of sedation must be preceded by an evaluation of food and fluid intake. Intake of food and liquids should be as follows: (1) infants 0 to 5 months, no milk or solids for 4 hours before scheduled procedure; (2) infants 6 to 36 months, no milk or solids for 6 hours before scheduled procedure; and (3) children older than 36 months, no milk or solids for 8 hours before scheduled procedure. Oral intake of clear liquids may continue, but in no instance should oral intake occur less than 2 hours before sedation. Patients known to be at risk for pulmonary aspiration of gastric contents (eg, those with a history of gastroesophageal reflux, extreme obesity, pregnancy, a history of previous esophageal dysfunction) may benefit from appropriate pharmacologic treatment to reduce gastric volume and increase gastric pH.

2. For the emergency patient. The use of sedation must be preceded by an evaluation of food and fluid intake. When protective airway reflexes are lost, gastric contents may be regurgitated into the airway. Therefore, patients with a history of recent oral intake or with other known risk factors, such as trauma, decreased level of consciousness, extreme obesity, pregnancy, or bowel motility dysfunction, require careful evaluation before administration of sedatives. If possible, such patients may benefit from delaying the procedure and administering appropriate pharmacologic treatment to reduce gastric volume and increase gastric pH. When proper fasting has not been assured, the increased risks of sedation must be carefully weighed against its benefits, and the lightest effective sedation should be used. An emergency patient may require protection of the airway before sedation.

REFERENCES

1. Finer NN, Barrington KJ, Al-Fadley F, Peters KL. Limitations of self-inflating resuscitators. *Pediatrics.* 1986;77:417–420.
2. Boidin MP, Mooi B, Erdmann W. Controlled administration of oxygen with self-inflating resuscitation bags. *Acta Anaesthesiol Belg.* 1980;31:157–165.
3. Carden E, Hughes T. Evaluation of manually operated self-inflating resuscitation bags. *Anesth Analg.* 1975;54:133–138.
4. Kanter RK. Evaluation of mask-bag ventilation in resuscitation of infants. *AJDC.* 1987;141:761–763.
5. National Institute for Occupational Safety and Health (NIOSH). *Criteria for a Recommended Standard. Occupational Exposure to Waste Anesthetic Gases and Vapors.* Cleveland, OH: US Department of Health, Education, and Welfare; 1977. NIOSH publication 77-140.
6. Goodson JM, Moore PA. Life-threatening reactions after pedodontic sedation: an assessment of narcotic, local anesthetic, and antiemetic drug interaction. *J Am Dent Assoc.* 1983;107:239–245.
7. Aubuchon RW. Sedation liabilities in pedodontics. *Pediatr Dent.* 1982;4:171–180.
8. Fitzmaurice LS, Wasserman GS, Knapp JF, et al. TAC use and absorption of cocaine in a pediatric emergency department. *Ann Emerg Med.* 1990;19:515–518.
9. Tipton GA, DeWitt GW, Eisenstein SJ. Topical TAC (tetracaine, adrenaline, cocaine) solution for local anesthesia in children: prescribing inconsistency and acute toxicity. *South Med J.* 1989;82:1344–1346..
10. Bonadio WA, Wagner V. Half-strength TAC topical anesthetic, for selected dermal lacerations. *Clin Pediatr.* 1988;27:495–498.
11. Shellock FG, Crues JV. MRI: Safety considerations in magnetic resonance imaging. *Magn Reson Imaging Decisions.* 1988;2:25–30.
12. Kanal E, Shellock FG, Talagala L. Safety considerations in MR imaging. *Radiology.* 1990;176:593–606.
13. Shellock FG, Slimp GL. Severe burn of the finger caused by using a pulse oximeter during MR imaging. *Am J Roentgenol.* 1989;153:1105.
14. Wendt RE III, Rokey R, Vick GW III, Johnston DL. Electrocardiographic gating and monitoring in NMR imaging. *Magn Reson Imaging.* 1988;6:89–95.
15. American Academy of Pediatrics, Committee on Drugs. Emergency drug doses for infants and children. *Pediatrics.* 1988;81:462–465.

Clinical Competencies for Conscious Sedation

CLINICAL COMPETENCY PROFILE		
GOALS, OBJECTIVES, LEGAL SCOPE OF PRACTICE **Chapter One**		
Intravenous Conscious Sedation Nursing Competencies	**Comments/Goals**	**Competency Met Date and Initial**
1. Identify AORN Recommended Practice I, intent and rationale.		Date: Initials:
2. Discuss the rationale for the increased use of intravenous conscious sedation.		Date: Initials
3. Define Conscious Sedation.		Date: Initials
4. Delineate the components of conscious sedation vs. deep sedation.		Date: Initials
5. Discuss the objectives of conscious sedation.		Date: Initials:
6. List the clinical endpoints of conscious sedation.		Date: Initials:
7. Identify the regulatory bodies which impact on the administration of intravenous conscious sedation in your practice setting.		Date: Initials:
8. Delineate components of the State of _____ Nurse Practice Act or position statement related to the administration of intravenous conscious sedation.		Date: Initials:
9. Identify JCAHO standards related to the administration of intravenous conscious sedation in your practice setting.		Date: Initials:
10. List regulatory, statutory and recommended practice patterns associated with the administration of conscious sedation.		Date: Initials

CLINICAL COMPETENCY PROFILE		
PREPROCEDURE ASSESSMENT AND PATIENT SELECTION Chapter Two		
Intravenous Conscious Sedation Nursing Competencies	**Comments/Goals**	**Competency Met Date and Initial**
1. List the goals of preprocedure patient assessment.		Date: Initials:
2. Describe mechanisms to enhance preprocedure patient rapport.		Date: Initials
3. Define hyper/hypotension.		Date: Initials
4. Describe the preprocedure care of the hypertensive patient presenting for intravenous conscious sedation.		Date: Initial:
5. Identify components of preprocedure assessment for patients with a history of coronary artery disease.		Date: Initial:
6. Describe preprocedure pulmonary evaluation of patient's presenting for the administration of intravenous conscious sedation.		Date: Initial:
7. Delineate recommended treatment protocol for the asthmatic patient prior to the administration of conscious sedation.		Date: Initial:
8. Identify the significance of past medical history in the evaluation of the patient for intravenous conscious sedation.		Date: Initial:
9. Describe the purpose of eliciting past surgical history and anesthesia history.		Date: Initial:
10. List the components of the preprocedure medication evaluation.		Date: Initial:

PREPROCEDURE ASSESSMENT AND PATIENT SELECTION—Continued
Chapter Two

Intravenous Conscious Sedation Nursing Competencies	Comments/Goals	Competency Met Date and Initial
11. List 3 clinical manifestations associated with a true allergic reaction.		Date: Initial:
12. Identify the clinical management of patients presenting for intravenous conscious sedation with a history of latex allergy.		Date: Initial:
13. Delineate pertinent criteria in the selection of preprocedure laboratory data prior to the administration of intravenous conscious sedation.		Date: Initial:
14. Identify the rational and components of a complete preprocedure informed consent.		Date: Initial:
15. Describe mechanisms to decrease preprocedure patient anxiety.		Date: Initial:
16. Identify current NPO (nothing by mouth) guidelines for patients scheduled to receive intravenous conscious sedation.		Date: Initial:

CLINICAL COMPETENCY PROFILE		
INTRODUCTION TO PHARMACOLOGIC CONCEPTS Chapter Three		
Intravenous Conscious Sedation Nursing Competencies	**Comments/Goals**	**Competency Met Date and Initial**
1. Define pharmacokinetics.		Date: Initials:
2. List three mechanisms utilized to achieve the transfer of pharmacologic agents across cell membranes.		Date: Initials:
3. Identify the effect of protein binding on the pharmacologic action of intravenous medications.		Date: Initials:
4. State two advantages/disadvantages associated with oral, sublingual, intramuscular and intravenous routes of medication administration.		Date: Initials:
5. Describe pharmacologic drug distribution as proposed by the two compartmental model.		Date: Initials:
6. Identify four major sites of drug metabolism.		Date: Initials:
7. Define pharmacodynamics and the clinical implications associated with the administration of intravenous conscious sedation medications.		Date: Initials:
8. Differentiate the role of pharmacologic agonist vs. antagonist.		Date: Initials:
9. Delineate the role of the kidneys in the excretion of pharmacologic compounds.		Date: Initials:

CLINICAL COMPETENCY PROFILE		
MANAGEMENT OF RESPIRATORY COMPLICATIONS Chapter Four		
Intravenous Conscious Sedation Nursing Competencies	Comments/Goals	Competency Met Date and Initial
1. Identify nursing responsibilities in the recognition of respiratory insufficiency.		Date: Initials:
2. List four factors which contribute to the development of respiratory insufficiency.		Date: Initials:
3. State the importance of maintaining the gag reflex during the administration of intravenous conscious sedation.		Date: Initials:
4. Describe four components of a comprehensive airway evaluation.		Date: Initials:
5. Identify signs and symptoms associated with airway obstruction.		Date: Initials:
6. Demonstrate the proper technique of the following airway maneuvers: ~Head Tilt ~Chin Lift ~Jaw Thrust ~Insertion of a nasal/oral airway		Date: Initials:
7. List variables which impact on mask fit when positive pressure ventilation is required.		Date: Initials:
8. State common size endotracheal tubes required for emergency resuscitation in your practice setting.		Date: Initials:
9. Describe the function of the laryngo-scope blade and handle as part of emergency resuscitative equipment.		Date: Initials:
10. Identify the advantages and disadvantages associated with utilization of: ~Nasal Cannula ~O2 Face Mask ~Non Rebreathing Masks ~Bag Valve Devices		Date: Initials:

CLINICAL COMPETENCY PROFILE

CONSCIOUS SEDATION MEDICATIONS, TECHNIQUES OF ADMINISTRATION Chapter Five		
Intravenous Conscious Sedation Nursing Competencies	**Comments/Goals**	**Competency Met Date and Initial**
1. List the ideal characteristics of injected pharmacologic agents utilized to produce sedation.		Date: Initials:
2. Identify the advantages, disadvantages and limitations associated with the following agents: ~Benzodiazepines ~Opioids ~Barbiturates ~Ketamine ~Local anesthetics		Date: Initials:
3. Describe the cardiovascular, respiratory and central nervous system effects associated with the administration of: ~Benzodiazepines ~Opioids ~Barbiturates ~Ketamine ~Local anesthetics		Date: Initials:
4. Describe the clinical use of single dose injection technique to achieve the sedative state.		Date: Initials:
5. Identify the advantage of pharmacologic combination (synergism) in the administration of intravenous sedatives.		Date: Initials:
6. Discuss the administration of intravenous sedative medications via the bolus technique.		Date: Initials:

CLINICAL COMPETENCY PROFILE		
MONITORING MODALITIES Chapter Six		
Intravenous Conscious Sedation Nursing Competencies	Comments/Goals	Competency Met Date and Initial
1. Identify appropriate ECG lead placement for identification of myocardial ischemia vs. dysrhythmia detection.		Date: Initials:
2. Describe the 5 waves of the cardiac cycle.		Date: Initials:
3. Discuss signs and symptoms associated with the following cardiac rhythms: ~Sinus bradycardia ~Atrial fibrillation ~Premature ventricular contractions ~Ventricular tachycardia ~Ventricular fibrillation		Date: Initials:
4. Define hypo/hypertension.		Date: Initials:
5. List 3 factors which contribute to the development of hypotension.		Date: Initials:
6. Outline recommended treatment protocol for hypotension.		Date: Initials:
7. Identify recommended treatment protocol for hypertension.		Date: Initials:
8. Describe factors which impact on pulse oximeter sensor selection.		Date: Initials:
9. Discuss recommended monitoring practices as prescribed by regulatory state statutes, and professional organizations related to the administration of conscious sedation.		Date: Initials:
10. Identify nursing implications related to the use of automated blood pressure cuffs.		Date: Initials:

CLINICAL COMPETENCY PROFILE		
SPECIFIC PATIENT POPULATIONS **Chapter Seven**		
Intravenous Conscious **Sedation Nursing Competencies**	**Comments/Goals**	**Competency Met** **Date and Initial**
1. List components of the physiologic aging process.		Date: Initials
2. Identify preprocedure considerations of the geriatric patient that may require additional evaluation or consultation.		Date: Initials:
3. Describe pharmacologic considerations which render the geriatric patient more sensitive to sedative medications.		Date: Initials:
4. Delineate the core components of an airway evaluation in the geriatric patient.		Date: Initials:
5. Describe the anatomic and physiologic differences which impact on the administration of sedatives in the pediatric patient population.		Date: Initials:
6. State recommended NPO guidelines for the pediatric patient presenting for the administration of sedation.		Date: Initials:
7. List the anatomic and physiologic variations which may lead to the rapid development of hypoxemia in the pediatric patient.		Date: Initials:
8. List methods to decrease shivering in the pediatric patient.		Date: Initials:

CLINICAL COMPETENCY PROFILE		
PRINCIPLES OF INTRAVENOUS THERAPY **Chapter Eight**		
Intravenous Conscious **Sedation Nursing Competencies**	**Comments/Goals**	**Competency Met** **Date and Initial**
1. Identify complications associated with intravenous access in patients with previous mastectomy, lymph node dissection or renal access grafts.		Date: Initials:
2. Describe local and systemic complications associated with intravenous catheter placement.		Date: Initials:
3. List common intravenous solutions used during the administration of conscious sedation.		Date: Initials:

CLINICAL COMPETENCY PROFILE		
CONSCIOUS SEDATION LOCATIONS AND SPECIFIC PROCEDURES Chapter Nine		
Intravenous Conscious Sedation Nursing Competencies	Comments/Goals	Competency Met Date and Initial
1. Identify 4 environmental challenges associated with the delivery of intravenous conscious sedation.		Date: Initials:
2. List 3 procedures performed in radiology suites which may require the administration of intravenous conscious sedation.		Date: Initials:
3. State the percent of the patient population which experience a reaction to the injection of contrast media.		Date: Initials:
4. List 5 manifestations of a contrast media allergic reaction.		Date: Initials:
5. Discuss treatment protocol for patients experiencing a reaction to contrast media. (Mild and severe reactions)		Date: Initials:
6. Identify 4 procedures which may be performed in the cardiology suite and patient considerations associated with each procedure.		Date: Initials:
7. Identify 3 requirements of office based conscious sedation practice.		Date: Initials:
8. List the contents of a full E cylinder of oxygen.		Date: Initials:
9. Discuss the practitioners role in the safe handling and transport of medical gas cylinders.		Date: Initials:
10. Identify patients who require monitoring during MRI procedures.		Date: Initials:

Continued on following page

CONSCIOUS SEDATION LOCATIONS AND SPECIFIC PROCEDURES—Continued
Chapter Nine

Intravenous Conscious Sedation Nursing Competencies	Comments/Goals	Competency Met Date and Initial
11. List 4 methods to prevent the development of burns in patients during MRI procedures.		Date: Initials:
12. Delineate the documentation of the return of a gag reflex in a post-procedure upper endoscopy patient.		Date: Initials:
13. Identify the signs and symptoms of respiratory embarrassment associated with the insertion of a peritoneal dialysis catheter and the infusion of the dialysate.		Date: Initials:
14. Describe the phenomena known as Compartment Syndrome.		Date: Initials:
15. List 3 absolute contraindications for utilization of lithotrpsy.		Date: Initials:
16. Describe the treatment and etiology of apnea following insertion of a retrobulbar block.		Date: Initials:
17. Describe the postprocedure care of a patient status post oral surgery.		Date: Initials:
18. Identify localization methods to anesthetize the oropharynx in patients scheduled for bronchoscopy, upper endoscopy or TEE.		Date: Initials:
19. Delineate the role of the magnet with regard to the MRI and its impact on accurate patient monitoring.		Date: Initials:

CLINICAL COMPETENCY PROFILE		
POSTPROCEDURE MONITORING AND DISCHARGE CRITERIA Chapter Ten		
Intravenous Conscious Sedation Nursing Competencies	Comments/Goals	Competency Met Date and Initial
1. Identify the purpose of postprocedure monitoring in patients receiving conscious sedation.		Date: Initials:
2. Delineate the requirements for postprocedure documentation.		Date: Initials:
3. List the core components of postprocedure documentation		Date: Initials:
4. State the 5 objective criteria developed by Aldrete to assess postprocedure recovery.		Date: Initials:
5. Discuss the purpose of "criteria" based postprocedure parameters.		Date: Initials:
6. Discuss the advancement of post-procedure activity level.		Date: Initials:
7. Describe nursing responsibilities related to the postprocedure teaching process.		Date: Initials:
8. Indicate the purpose of specific conscious sedation discharge instructions and their purpose.		Date: Initials:
9. Identify characteristics unique to perianesthesia nursing practice: Phase I vs. Phase II recovery.		Date: Initials:
10. List 5 components of a postprocedure report.		Date: Initials:
11. Delineate postprocedure treatment options for the following complications: ~Pain ~Airway obstruction ~Hypertension/hypotension		Date: Initials:

CLINICAL COMPETENCY PROFILE

EFFECTIVE RISK MANAGEMENT STRATEGIES AND IMPLEMENTATION OF A CONSCIOUS SEDATION EDUCATIONAL PROGRAM
Chapter Eleven

Intravenous Conscious Sedation Nursing Competencies	Comments/Goals	Competency Met Date and Initial
1. Identify 4 individual injury prevention strategies the registered nurse may utilize to improve quality patient care.		Date: Initials:
2. List core components of a conscious sedation data base program.		Date: Initials:
3. Describe state nurse practice requirements related to the administration of intravenous conscious sedation within your Commonwealth.		Date: Initials:
4. State the contents of the practitioner portfolio.		Date: Initials:
5. Identify the requirement of biomedical certification for medical equipment.		Date: Initials:
6. Delineate mechanisms of information dissemination within a department or clinical area.		Date: Initials:
7. Describe the continuous quality improvement process.		Date: Initials:
8. State mechanisms utilized in the successful implementation of a conscious sedation educational program.		Date: Initials:

Index

Note: Page numbers in *italics* refer to illustrations; page numbers followed by t refer to tables.

A

You've read the book, now get the credit—

Interested in obtaining continuing education credit for *Manual of Conscious Sedation*? **Nursing Spectrum** will mail you a free multiple-choice test packet. You choose whether to take a test for an individual chapter, multiple chapters, or the entire book. For a nominal price, you can earn contact hours at home. Discounts are available for multiple chapters or the entire book.

Call our corporate continuing education office at 800-866-0919 and request the conscious sedation test today!

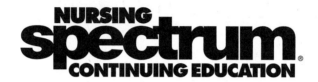

Nursing Spectrum is accredited as a provider of continuing education in nursing through the American Nurses Credentialing Center's Commission on Accreditation, by the State of Florida, Board of Nursing (provider no. 2711768), and by the American Association of Critical-Care Nurses (96 01 07). **This is a Category A offering.**

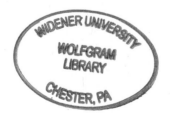